Crimmigration in the Age of COVID-19

Crimmigration in the Age of COVID-19

Editor

Robert Koulish

MDPI • Basel • Beijing • Wuhan • Barcelona • Belgrade • Manchester • Tokyo • Cluj • Tianjin

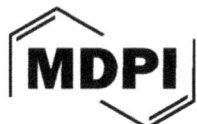

Editor
Robert Koulish
College of Behavioral and Social Sciences,
University of Maryland,
College Park, MD, USA

Editorial Office
MDPI
St. Alban-Anlage 66
4052 Basel, Switzerland

This is a reprint of articles from the Special Issue published online in the open access journal *Social Sciences* (ISSN 2076-0760) (available at: https://www.mdpi.com/journal/socsci/special_issues/Crimmigration_in_the_Age_of_COVID-19).

For citation purposes, cite each article independently as indicated on the article page online and as indicated below:

LastName, A.A.; LastName, B.B.; LastName, C.C. Article Title. *Journal Name* **Year**, *Volume Number*, Page Range.

ISBN 978-3-0365-6424-1 (Hbk)
ISBN 978-3-0365-6425-8 (PDF)

© 2023 by the authors. Articles in this book are Open Access and distributed under the Creative Commons Attribution (CC BY) license, which allows users to download, copy and build upon published articles, as long as the author and publisher are properly credited, which ensures maximum dissemination and a wider impact of our publications.

The book as a whole is distributed by MDPI under the terms and conditions of the Creative Commons license CC BY-NC-ND.

Contents

About the Editor vii

Preface to "Crimmigration in the Age of COVID-19" ix

Robert Koulish
COVID-19 and the Creeping Necropolitics of Crimmigration Control
Reprinted from: *Soc. Sci.* **2021**, *10*, 467, doi:10.3390/socsci10120467 1

Witold Klaus
The Porous Border Woven with Prejudices and Economic Interests. Polish Border Admission Practices in the Time of COVID-19
Reprinted from: *Soc. Sci.* **2021**, *10*, 435, doi:10.3390/socsci10110435 7

José A. Brandariz and Cristina Fernández-Bessa
Coronavirus and Immigration Detention in Europe: The Short Summer of Abolitionism?
Reprinted from: *Soc. Sci.* **2021**, *10*, 226, doi:10.3390/socsci10060226 21

Maartje Van Der Woude and Nanou Van Iersel
Governing Migration through COVID-19? Dutch Political and Media Discourse in Times of a Pandemic
Reprinted from: *Soc. Sci.* **2021**, *10*, 379, doi:10.3390/socsci10100379 39

Regina C. Serpa
The Exceptional Becomes Everyday: Border Control, Attrition and Exclusion from Within
Reprinted from: *Soc. Sci.* **2021**, *10*, 329, doi:10.3390/socsci10090329 59

Henrietta McNeill
Dealing with the 'Crimmigrant Other' in the Face of a Global Public Health Threat: A Snapshot of Deportation during COVID-19 in Australia and New Zealand
Reprinted from: *Soc. Sci.* **2021**, *10*, 278, doi:10.3390/socsci10080278 71

Joanna Tsiganou, Anastasia Chalkia and Martha Lempesi
COVID-19 Crisis as the New-State-of-the-Art in the Crimmigration Milieu
Reprinted from: *Soc. Sci.* **2021**, *10*, 457, doi:10.3390/socsci10120457 85

Dora Schriro
On the Other Side of the Looking Glass: COVID-19 Care in Immigration Detention
Reprinted from: *Soc. Sci.* **2021**, *10*, 353, doi:10.3390/socsci10100353 103

Justine N. Stefanelli
Detained during a Pandemic: Human Rights behind Locked Doors
Reprinted from: *Soc. Sci.* **2021**, *10*, 276, doi:10.3390/socsci10070276 125

Wenjie Liao, Kim Ebert, Joshua R. Hummel and Emily P. Estrada
The House Is on Fire but We Kept the Burglars Out: Racial Apathy and White Ignorance in Pandemic-Era Immigration Detention
Reprinted from: *Soc. Sci.* **2021**, *10*, 358, doi:10.3390/socsci10100358 141

About the Editor

Robert Koulish

Robert Koulish, Professor. Robert Koulish, Ph.D., is a Research Professor and Director of MLaw Programs, administered through the College of Behavioral and Social Sciences (BSOS) at the University of Maryland. Koulish is also a Lecturer of Law at the UMD Carey School of Law in Baltimore, where he teaches a seminar in immigration law and policy. Dr. Koulish is a co-author of the forthcoming book, Detaining Immigrants, Scoring Criminals, and has several books, including Crimmigrant Nations: Resurgent Nationalism and the Closing of Borders (Fordham University Press, 2020), with Maartje van der Woude, and he authored Immigration and American Democracy, Subverting the Rule of Law (Routledge Press, 2010). He was co-editor, with Maria Joao Guia, and Valsamis Mitsilegas for Immigration Detention, Risk and Human Rights: Studies on Immigration and Crime, by Springer, in 2016. He has authored numerous peer-reviewed academic articles, law review articles, book chapters, and op-ed columns, and is a founding member of CINETS (Crimmigration Control International Net of Studies; http://www.crimmigrationcontrol.com), a growing network of critical immigration law scholars, which hosts bi-annual international conferences, book volumes, and research collaborations.

Preface to "Crimmigration in the Age of COVID-19"

In 2020–2022, much of the world was at risk for catching COVID-19. This book, "Crimmigration in the Age of COVID-19," contributes to understanding immigration during the pandemic. It engages a cross-national and interdisciplinary case-study approach to show how countries carved out exceptions to public health protocols for migrants. In the immigration context a variety of governments weaponized public health protocols to criminalize and exclude migrants.

The Trump Administration sadistically misplayed the pandemic at almost every turn. Trump came to power on the backs of migrants, referring to them as murderers and rapists. The intersection of Trump's COVID-19 and migration policies carved out space for the exceptional dehumanization of migrants in 2020–2021.

This book documents the weaponization of public through crimmigration. Crimmigration is the criminalization of migration and migrants via state-of-the-art surveillance and militarized technologies. During the worst of COVID-19, crimmigration strategies–mandatory detention and harsh exclusions—exacerbated the risk of transmission among migrants. Policies not migrants were to blame here. The ostensibly public health related Title42 actually pushed migrants, already at great risk, into unregulated shantytowns controlled by Mexican drug cartels. Additionally, migrants contended with detention facilities, medium security prisons, that functioned as Petrie dishes for the disease.

We hope this book contributes to understanding the intersection of public health and crimmigration, and border penologies during these exceptional times.

Robert Koulish
Editor

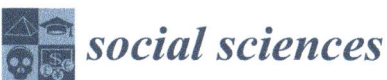

Editorial

COVID-19 and the Creeping Necropolitics of Crimmigration Control

Robert Koulish [1,2]

[1] MLAW Programs, University of Maryland, College Park, MD 20742, USA; rkoulish@umd.edu
[2] Department of Government and Politics, University of Maryland, College Park, MD 20742, USA

Citation: Koulish, Robert. 2021. COVID-19 and the Creeping Necropolitics of Crimmigration Control. *Social Sciences* 10: 467. https://doi.org/10.3390/socsci10120467

Received: 1 December 2021
Accepted: 1 December 2021
Published: 6 December 2021

Publisher's Note: MDPI stays neutral with regard to jurisdictional claims in published maps and institutional affiliations.

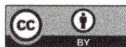

Copyright: © 2021 by the author. Licensee MDPI, Basel, Switzerland. This article is an open access article distributed under the terms and conditions of the Creative Commons Attribution (CC BY) license (https://creativecommons.org/licenses/by/4.0/).

The COVID-19 pandemic has had a drastic impact on migration and migrants and immigration policies worldwide. Considering that over 250 million people have contracted the disease globally, including in that figure 5.1 million deaths, there is hardly any part of the globe which has escaped government attempts to control migration in order to stop the spread of disease. Migrants, particularly those in detention, have been the most susceptible to COVID-19, and the most vulnerable to punitive COVID-19 politics, as the pandemic has had a disproportionate impact on institutionalized populations (Turcotte 2021).

Governments have responded to COVID-19 with border closures, travel bans, and other disruptions to migrant flows world-wide. At first, these initial immigration responses were generally accepted as reasonable attempts to mitigate the spread of disease (Banulescu-Bogdan et al. 2020; O'Brien 2021). However, the obvious fact is that viruses are not easily deterred by border walls or gated ports of entry. Short of stopping the return of nationals or at least quarantining them upon arrival to their home country, deploying public health protocols for contact-tracing, social distancing, and supplying masks, immigration authorities can achieve little to mitigate the spread of the infectious disease.

This Special Issue was inspired by the observation that migration controls flourished despite their inability to mitigate the spread of the Coronavirus. More than 750,000 people in the U.S. died after former President Trump first imposed COVID-19 inspired travel restrictions in March 2020. Many countries including the U.S. have since deployed migration penologies as a pretext to deter and punish new arrivals. Migrant penologies include anti-immigrant narratives intended to distract public opinion from the governments' own inabilities to remain ahead of the virus and redirect growing public anxiety towards immigrants as a convenient and regrettably hate-filled scapegoat.

The Special Issue contends with this pretext, in particular the pattern of *how*, why and when (and also, who) migration-centered COVID-19 policies ended up punishing rather than protecting immigrants through this public health nightmare. The Issue follows a recent book Maartje van der Woude and I co-edited called *Crimmigrant Nations: Resurgent Nationalism and the Closing of Borders* (Koulish and van der Woude 2020). The book was published about a week before the virus hit and governments shut down borders around much of the world in spring 2020. The articles in this Special Issue grapple with regulating crimmigration in relation to COVID-19, following along similar lines as to those in our book. That is to say, the articles in this Special Issue draw direct and indirect reference to three overlapping theories of migration control catalogued by Weber and McCulloch (2018). The theories are (1) crimmigration, (2) new penology, and (3) enemy penology. These theories help understand efforts to criminalize, securitize, and even terrorize immigrants in the name of protecting public safety and national security. As much as these theories interrogate the harsh regulation of migrant life through controls, COVID-19 directs attention to the necropolitics of migration control.

Crimmigration highlights the *how* of migration and border control, with a focus on legal form and process (Weber and McCulloch 2018; Stumpf 2006). Crimmigration drew its name from immigration policies enacted during the 1990s that perversely blurred the distinctions between crime control and immigration law. This occurred within an immigration law framework that dilutes due process and other procedural safeguards for immigrants while importing a robust carceral regime to immigration driven by the private prison complex.

Second, new penology responds to the *why* of migration and border control, to bring immense and sophisticated technologies to bear on migration and migrant communities. Technologies are purposed to control mobility and migrants through surveillance, detention, and removal (Weber and McCulloch 2018). A deeper dive connects mobility and migration control to larger shifts in political economy and the preservation of white elite hegemony (Miller 2019; Mercille 2011; Xenakis and Cheliotis 2020; Koulish and van der Woude 2020). New penology scholars, including van der Woude and Van Lersel, have in this Issue applied Jonathan Simon's *Governing Through Crime* thesis to migration control (Bosworth and Guild 2008). Governing through migration rather than governing migration shifts from regulating borders through entry and exit requirements, to regulating migrants through punitive bordering, detention, and harsh expulsions (Koulish and van der Woude 2020).

Third, enemy penology describes the *who and when* of migration and border control (Krasmann 2007; Weber and McCulloch 2018). It starts with a triggering event (*the when*) by a perceived enemy (*the who*). The event could be real (the 9/11 catastrophe or COVID-19) or manufactured (migrant caravans heading to the U.S. border in 2018; border closures to asylum seekers in Poland during COVID-19). Similarly, *the who* can be real or imagined. The triggering event rationalizes the deployment of august state power: border closures, travel bans, and state of emergency declarations, followed by military deployment. Migrant control mechanisms also include surveillance, detention, and removal. What turns executive power into august power is the combination of vast resource allocation with the lack of accountability and oversight from the courts or legislature. Almost always, the who is constituted by people of color: Muslims after 9/11 and AAPI during COVID-19.

Anti-immigrant narratives inform public opinion against immigrants and increase their vulnerability to attack from governments and right-wing vigilantes. Throughout immigration history, pandemics have been associated with exclusionary narratives against foreigners. Nation-states have sought to blame racial and ethnic minorities as responsible for human suffering internally for the purpose of diverting attention from the governments' own failure to protect its people. Scapegoating the ethnic and racial 'other' during pandemics provides a through line for anti-immigration discourses generally. The anti-Asian message in Trump's "china-virus" tweets for example can be traced back to Justice Fields' opinion referring to *unassimilable alien hordes* in the *Chae Chan Ping* case in 1889. Chinese were similarly blamed for spreading smallpox at the end of the 19th century, and more recently for SARs, just as Muslims were put on alert by the moral panic generated after September 11.

This Special Issue features a critical examination of administering migration penologies and crimmigration during Covid in a variety of countries in Europe, Australia, and the United States. The reader will notice that the countries' immigration responses to COVID-19 can be pinpointed along a loosely defined spectrum of punitiveness from abolition to necropolitics. Where they fall on the spectrum is due to a variety of factors beyond the scope of this Special Issue, but include the following: governing type (democratic versus authoritarian) and currents of liberal rights versus ethnonationalism. A country's willingness to engage punitive migrant penologies presumably indicates the salience of ethnonationalism and authoritarianism within a country's politics. Were there a law and policy that foreshadows a country's embrace of authoritarian ethnonationalism, it is immigration law and policy. The through-line is to structural racism, overwhelming executive power, and a pre-Warren Court era application of due process and other procedural rights.

My reading of the authors shows government responses were the most punitive in the United States, U.K., Greece, and Poland, showing, for example, the rising tide of ethnonationalism in the U.S. The Dutch response was more temperate, hence coinciding with its social democratic institutions. The article on Spain highlights temporary abolition.

The U.S. case under former President Trump, written by three authors, highlights the former President's infatuation with authoritarian and ethnonationalist power grabs at immigrants' expense, garnering a spot at the punitive side of this sliding scale. Poland's right leaning regime (Bartyzel 2021) similarly steers a punitive turn, and the U.K.'s Brexit policies and fancy with Trumpism helps explain its punitive governing of crimmigration under COVID-19.

The contributions in this Special Issue should be read through the three theoretical frames: The *how* of crimmigration, which focuses on law and policies that are intendedly punitive or punitive in their effects. Migrant penologies focus on the administration of the technologies of power regulating the life of migrant populations. The *why* is to render migrant populations productive or docile. The *who and when* that enemy penologies responds to occupy a similar terrain but on securitization rather than criminalization grounds. Enemy penologies helps authorities to distinguish Syrians and Belarusians at the Polish border (the former as enemy), for example, and ban Muslims from U.S. airports (Klaus 2020; Koulish and van der Woude 2020).

Additionally is the necropolitics of crimmigration informed by COVID-19. As much as the three theories contend with the harsh regulation of migrant life, necropolitics addresses the regulation of migrant death. The concept borrows from Giorgio Agamben's *Homo Sacer* (Agamben 1998) and was coined by Achille Mbebe (2019). Mbebe describes necropolitics as "the power to manufacture an entire crowd of people who specifically live at the edge of life, or even on its outer edge—people for whom living means continually standing up to death ... (where) Nobody even bears the slightest feelings of responsibility or justice ... " (Mbebe 2019, pp. 37–38).

The concept helps to understand how in the thick of the pandemic governments refused to release immigrants from detention facilities, creating as an outcome the utterly avoidable risk of exposing large numbers of densely populated immigrants to COVID 19. Additionally, it describes the dehumanizing efforts to stigmatize, injure, and humiliate "those not considered to be one of us" (Mbebe 2019, p. 58). The necropolitics of crimmigration in the U.S. is associated with two Trumpian COVID-19 era enforcement practices: Migrant Protection Protocols (MPP), forcing asylum seekers back into Mexico, and Title 42, expelling undocumented immigrants on public health grounds. MPP and Title 42 highlight the government's indifference to "small doses" of death at the border. As Human Rights First recently reported, "When the U.S. government delivers people seeking safety to danger in Mexico, through Title 42, or MPP, they face unimaginable violence and persecution" (21 October 2021). In sum, the concept of necropolitics sheds light on efforts to govern migrants through COVID-19.

In the following, I briefly introduce the authors' arguments in order from the least punitive to most punitive country case studies, from abolition to cruelty for its own sake.

In the first article, *Coronavirus and Immigration Detention in Europe: The Short Summer of Abolition?* Jose Angel Brandariz and Fernandez-Bessa provide a case study of Spain drawing on "the multi-scalar nature of mobility governance" in the EU. The case study of the national policy agenda in Spain demonstrates it as an outlier in the E.U. crimmigration-verse. Whereas most countries used COVID-19 to combat immigrants, Spain introduced an abolitionist detention stance during the summer of 2020. Spain closed detention centers and released immigrants as Spanish courts interpreted international law. Additionally, the authors contend with the harsh realities in other detention centers in the Canary Islands and elsewhere under Spanish control to show Spain's position is far from ideal. Still, the authors take a lessons-learned approach to consider a future in Europe that minimizes detention.

Maartje van der Woude and Van Lersel in *Governing Migration through Covid-19? Dutch Political and Media Discourse in Times of a Pandemic*, borrow Jonathan Simon's (Simon 2007) new penology framework to frame empirical research into the Dutch response to COVID-19 using crimmigration. Following Simon, the authors analyze the governing through migration thesis using key factors from Simon's original theory, the proximity and proportionality of government response to the (COVID-19) problem. They find the

Netherland's anti-immigration response is more temperate than some but more punitive than many EU countries.

In *The Exceptional Becomes Everyday: Border Control, Attrition and Exclusion from Within*, Regina Serpa compares crimmigration in the U.K. and the Netherlands. Of the two, the UK has the more coercive crimmigration environment, compared to the Netherland's spiriting a more temperate approach to immigrants in the time of COVID-19. The gist of Serpa's analysis focuses on 'welfare penalism', in which local U.K. housing authorities played 'soft cop' during COVID-19 by reporting homeless migrants to immigration authorities for removal.

In *Dealing with the 'Crimmigrant Other' in the face of a Global Public Health Threat: A Snapshot of Deportation during Covid-19 in Australia and New Zealand*, Henrietta McNeill addresses the tension between using crimmigration to fight COVID-19 and using COVID-19 to exacerbate crimmigration. She focuses on the challenge of detaining and deporting immigrants in the face of the pandemic to discover in both Australia and New Zealand that governments prioritized the constructed securitized threat over the real threat posed by COVID-19.

Byron Villagomez Moncayo's article, The Stigma of Being Venezuelan in Ecuador in the Pandemic Context, frames the crimmigration analysis through the tension between the Constitutional provision opening the door to immigrants and national security restrictions influenced by the United States. The arrival of Venezuelan refugees pushed Ecuador into the punitive camp of harsh xenophobic exclusions.

In *Covid-19 as the New State-Of-The-Art in Crimmigration Milieu*, Joanna Tsiganou, Anastasia Chalkia, and Martha Lempesi focus on Greece's crimmigration in the age of COVID-19. The authors' analysis shows similarities to the Polish situation but highlighting techniques of control over asylum seekers unprotected from COVID-19. Here the Greek state failed to provide for the public health of asylum seekers, specifically concrete screening. By caging asylum seekers in dystopian camps where social distancing is impossible, and excluding them from vaccines and COVID-19 tests, the authors identify new crimmigrant identities under the rubric of public health discrimination.

Witold Klaus in *The Porous Border Woven with Prejudices and Economic Interests: Polish Border Admission Practices in the Time of Covid-19,* shows how COVID-19 accentuates the harsh realities of crimmigration on migrants. As Klaus reports, Poland's COVID-19 response is "more of the same, only worse." Poland opened and closed the border in pursuit of economic and political interests rather than in response to the public health crisis. Borders were closed to asylum seekers following dictates of xenophobia to prevent entrance to Muslim asylum seekers, but were issuing protocols to accommodate Belarusian refugees, while also opening the border to migrant workers despite the pandemic. Klaus shows that the Polish asylum policy preferred to be governed by old demons rather than public health concerns and followed demands of the Polish labor market for migrant workers over concerns for the pandemic. At the same time, and Belarus refugees were still denied access to protocols protecting them from COVID-19.

Of all the countries' responses to COVID-19 using crimmigration, U.S. policy under Trump was extreme. The border wall could not prevent 750,000 deaths. Although detention decreased from approximately 50,000 per day in 2019, to 19,000 per day in 2020, detainees were excluded from anti-COVID-19 protocols, and, as a result, about 10% of detainees tested positive, with nine reported deaths. Although detention decreased from approximately 50,000 per day in 2019, to 19,000 per day in 2020 due to a federal court order, detainees were excluded from anti-COVID-19 protocols, and as a result about 10% of detainees tested positive, and there were nine reported deaths.

In *On the Other Side of the Looking Glass: Covid-19 Care in Immigration Detention*, Dora Schriro (Schriro 2009) provides an inside perspective on the U.S. detention system. Schriro is a former upper-level policy official inside DHS and the author of the "Schriro Report," a 2009 report that recommended decriminalizing detention through alternatives to detention and risk assessment. Unfortunately, ICE systematically undermined many of the report's recommendations, positioning Schriro to take a more critical stance towards U.S. detention policy.

In *Detained During a Pandemic: Human Rights Behind Locked Doors*, Justine Stephanelli's take is similarly critical of U.S. detention during COVID-19. Stephanelli frames detention using human rights to show how far U.S. detention has strayed from human rights norms, and even fails much lower domestic standards still designed to mitigate substandard conditions and outright abuse. Stephanelli examines access to health care and counsel, two important tools to advance overriding public health concerns during the pandemic.

In *The House is on Fire but We Kept the Burglars Out: Racial Apathy and White Ignorance in Pandemic-Era Immigration Detention*, Wenjie Liao, Kim Ebert, Joshua Hummel, and Emily Estrada make use of content analysis to discover how activists and direct stakeholders responded to the COVID-19 crisis. Activists and stakeholders were represented by the ACLU, ICE, and the private prison industry (CoreCivic and GEO group). The article is framed by the recognition that crises have the potential and carry opportunities for radical change. They query the responses of stakeholders in the business of detaining immigrants for signs of new approaches to detention. To follow the thread of the Special Issue, the authors show that the health of detainees are not much of a concern for ICE during COVID-19. Additionally, ICE manufactured an alternative storyline featuring "COVID fraud" which adds to the growing list of enemy penologies.

The articles in this Special Issue show how the pandemic exacerbated the perversions of crimmigration to the immigrants' harm. Perversions that flipped a civil process into a largely privatized criminal juggernaut and that endeavors to fill detention beds and contain migrants by the thousands in closely confined spaces.

The authors share the intent to unpack the criminalization of migration. Their contributions help to understand how different countries governed migrants through COVID-19. This introduction is in part intended to guide the comparison along a heuristic scale of punitiveness from abolition to regulating death.

It is my hope that this issue contributes to a growing movement of activist scholarship pointing away from the punitive narratives and techniques that deny justice under immigration law, and towards a process that is fair and respects human dignity. As much as COVID-19 shows governments manipulating crisis as a tool to exacerbate migrant controls, it also reveals a yearning for an alternative paradigm that applies due process and fair procedures to immigrants and provides them with safe routes to membership status in their new destination.

Funding: This research received no external funding.

Conflicts of Interest: The author declares no conflict of interest.

References

Agamben, Giorgio. 1998. *Homo Sacer: Sovereign Power and Bare Life*. Stanford: Stanford University Press.

Banulescu-Bogdan, Natalia, Meghan Benton, and Susan Fratzke. 2020. *Coronavirus is Spreading across Borders, But It Is Not a Migration Problem*. Washington: Migration Policy Institute.

Bartyzel, Dorota. 2021. Anti-Migrant Stance helps Boost Polish Ruling Party's Popularity. Available online: https://www.bloomberg.com/news/articles/2021-09-14/anti-migrant-stance-helps-boost-polish-ruling-party-s-popularity (accessed on 23 November 2021).

Bosworth, Mary, and Mhairi Guild. 2008. Governing Through Migration Control: Security and Citizenship in Britain. *British Journal of Criminology* 48: 703–19. [CrossRef]

Klaus, Witold. 2020. How Does Criminalization Unfold in Poland? Between Securitization Introduced to Polish Migrants by its Europeanization and Polish Xenophobia. In *Koulish and van der Woude, Crimigrant Nations: Resurgent Nationalism and the Closing of Borders*. New York: Fordham University Press.

Koulish, Robert, and Maartje van der Woude. 2020. *Crimmigrant Nations: Resurgent Nationalism and the Closing of Borders*. New York: Fordham Press.

Krasmann, Susanne. 2007. The Enemy on the Border: Critique of a Programme in Favor of the Preemptive State. *Punishment & Society* 9: 301–18.

Mbebe, Achille. 2019. *Necropolitics*. Durham: Duke University Press.

Mercille, Julien. 2011. Violent Narco-Cartels or U.S. Hegemony? The Political Economy of the 'war on drugs' in Mexico. *Third World Quarterly* 32: 1637–53. [CrossRef]

Miller, Todd. 2019. *Empire of Borders: The Expansion of the US Border Around the World*. Brooklyn: Verso.

O'Brien, Michelle. 2021. Suppression, Spikes, and Stigma: How Covid-19 will Shape International Migration and Hostilities towards It. *International Migration Review* 55: 640–59. [CrossRef]

Schriro, Dora. 2009. *Immigration Detention Overview and Recommendations*. Washington: DHS.

Simon, Jonathan. 2007. *Governing Through Crime: How the War on crime Transformed American Democracy and Created a Culture of Fear*. Oxford: Oxford University Press.

Stumpf, Juliet. 2006. The Crimmigration Crisis: Immigrants, Crime, and Sovereign Power. *International Organizations Law Review* 56: 356–420.

Turcotte, Maura. 2021. Virus Cases are Surging at crowded Immigration Detention Centers in the U.S. *NYT*. September 6. Available online: https://www.nytimes.com/2021/07/06/us/covid-immigration-detention.html (accessed on 21 November 2021).

Weber, Leanne, and Jude McCulloch. 2018. Penal Power and Border Control: Which Thesis? Sovereignty, Governmentality, or the Pre-emptive State. *Punishment & Society* 21: 496–514.

Xenakis, Sappho, and Leonidas K. Cheliotis. 2020. The Trumping of Neoliberal Penality? Trump's Presidency and the Rise of Nationalist Authoritarianism in the United States. In *Koulish and van der Woude, Crimigrant Nations: Resurgent Nationalism and the Closing of Borders*. New York: Fordham University Press.

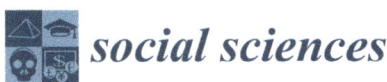

Article

The Porous Border Woven with Prejudices and Economic Interests. Polish Border Admission Practices in the Time of COVID-19

Witold Klaus

Institute of Law Studies, Polish Academy of Sciences, Nowy Swiat 72, 00-33 Warsaw, Poland; witold.klaus@gmail.com

Abstract: The COVID-19 pandemic has severely restricted global movement, thus affecting migration processes and immigrants themselves. The paper focuses on the evaluation of bordering procedures and practices introduced by the Polish government in the time of the pandemic. The aim is to highlight the duality in the admission processes at Polish borders between labour and forced migrants, which have been driven, as I argue, by economic interests and the xenophobic attitudes of the government. The paper is based on interviews with experts assisting migrants during the pandemic in Poland, whose direct contact with thousands of clients has allowed them to acquire broad knowledge of how the new legal provisions have affected different groups of immigrants. The data confirms that the Polish border is very porous. It has been almost completely closed to asylum seekers, especially those fleeing from Muslim countries, for whom the only option is to cross the border illegally. Only one exception was made for Belarusians, who were cordially welcomed at the border while escaping persecution in their home country in the wake of their protests against Lukashenko's regime. Economic migrants, on the other hand, exist on the other side of the spectrum. For immigrant workers, borders have remained open throughout the whole pandemic. Moreover, some further measures facilitating their arrival were introduced, such as de facto lifting of quarantine for seasonal farm workers.

Keywords: border practices; asylum seekers; economic migrants; Poland; pushbacks at the border; COVID-19 pandemic; governmental xenophobia

Citation: Klaus, Witold. 2021. The Porous Border Woven with Prejudices and Economic Interests. Polish Border Admission Practices in the Time of COVID-19. *Social Sciences* 10: 435. https://doi.org/10.3390/socsci10110435

Academic Editor: Robert Koulish

Received: 31 July 2021
Accepted: 9 November 2021
Published: 13 November 2021

Publisher's Note: MDPI stays neutral with regard to jurisdictional claims in published maps and institutional affiliations.

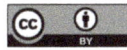

Copyright: © 2021 by the author. Licensee MDPI, Basel, Switzerland. This article is an open access article distributed under the terms and conditions of the Creative Commons Attribution (CC BY) license (https://creativecommons.org/licenses/by/4.0/).

1. Introduction

The COVID-19 pandemic has caused an unprecedented process of immobility for billions of people globally. Not only was traffic across borders stopped, but any mobility within countries as well. However, at the same time, many people were forced to leave their country of residence, while others were unable to return home, although they wanted to (Chamie 2020). As Thomas Nail aptly noted, 'The COVID world is just like it was before, only more so. (...) Things were awful before COVID, now they are worse' (Nail 2020, pp. 889, 891). This observation very accurately reflects the deepening segregation of immigrants on Polish borders after March 2020.

There is an extensive body of literature about the ambivalent attitude of Polish authorities towards immigration: the far-right government of 'Law and Justice' party, which has been ruling since the end of 2015, came to power using anti-immigrant and xenophobic slogans in the election campaign. They stoked fear of 'others' caused by the so-called refugee crisis of 2015–2016 (Koulish and van der Woude 2020), resulting in a drastic deterioration of the public's attitude towards refugees in Poland (Pędziwiatr and Legut 2016; Jaskułowski 2019). This fear was artificially orchestrated by politicians, because no people from the Mediterranean region, Africa or Central Asia had come to Poland seeking international protection—whether in an illegal manner (the Balkan route bypassed Poland), nor legally, i.e., through resettlement or relocations in which Poland refused to participate

(CJEU 2020). Despite this, the government successively developed laws and policies based on xenophobia, the aim of which was to prevent refugees from entering Poland (Klaus 2017; 2020b). Quite quickly, however, the practices of the Polish authorities became steeped in ambivalence. A huge antipathy to refugees and the intention to drive them away from Polish borders was accompanied by relatively high receptiveness to economic migrants—although mainly those from neighbouring countries, i.e., primarily from Ukraine (Klaus 2020a). The trend could be attributed to the demands of employers who faced significant shortages of workers. As a result of this process (which the government neither supported nor opposed), from 2018 onwards, Poland began to gradually emerge as a country of immigration. In recent years, it has, in fact, been leading the list of EU countries with the highest number of newly admitted immigrants (Solga and Tereszkiewicz 2020). In this respect, with the reluctance of the government and society's restraint towards migration and the simultaneous blending of many migrants into the local labour markets, Poland is not unlike, say, Italy from the first decade of the 21st century (Ambrosini 2013).

In this paper, I would like to present how the above processes were affected by the COVID-19 pandemic. I will focus on the possibilities of entering and staying in Poland for different groups of immigrants. I will demonstrate how many facilitating measures have been introduced for economic migrants, especially for Ukrainians (yet not necessarily so for people from more distant and other ethnically different countries) when it comes to their arrival and work. At the same time, the border for asylum seekers was tightly closed, but only in one direction—the government did not allow them to enter Poland. Meanwhile, return procedures were ongoing and people were held in detention awaiting them. An interesting breakthrough in this policy came in the autumn of 2020, when the government decided to introduce far-reaching facilitating measures exclusively for asylum seekers fleeing Belarus.

2. Two-Folding '3D'—Unwanted and 'Essentially' Wanted Immigrants Vis-à-Vis Governmental Xenophobia

The problem of segregating migrants into wanted and unwanted, better and worse, has long featured in the literature (Aas 2011; Kmak 2015). The extremely unwanted group is represented by asylum seekers. It is against them that governments try to apply deterrence processes (Hamlin 2012; Gilbert 2009) using practices referred to as '3D': desertion, detention, and deportation (Kalir 2020), i.e., implementing the policy of deportability and detainability (De Genova 2019). All these activities constitute what could be described as governmental xenophobia (Valluy 2011, pp. 116–17), because they are based on the prejudices and resentment of people in power towards 'Others' (an approach of this manner bears all the hallmarks of pure racism, even though Valluy himself does not use this term), and their goal is stigmatisation and labelling of migrants—both as a whole and those belonging to specific groups (such as asylum seekers)—as problematic and threatening. As a result, governments introduce public policies and regulations whose task is to not allow migrants in, to expel them or make their stay unpleasant by creating a hostile environment for them (Kalir 2019).

During the pandemic it transpired, however, that some migrants are indispensable to the countries of the Global North, hence the borders for them must remain open. Much was said then about essential workers—in the case of migrants, they were people who primarily looked after dependent people, especially the elderly (Nowicka et al. 2021), or agricultural workers—because someone had to plant and then harvest the crops. This is the second group of '3D' migrants, i.e., those who performed dirty, dangerous, and demanding work (Ambrosini 2013, p. 184). Not only were borders opened for these workers, but some countries even organised transports to bring them over (Bejan 2020; Parmet 2020). Most often, however, they were not provided with appropriate COVID-secure conditions and treated differently in relation to the citizens of the host country.

What is happening is the separation of two types of subjects: those who deserve protection and those who do not. The deserving are the German subjects, whose lives and health are valued and should be protected from the foreign, potentially infected intruders; the undeserving are the Romanian seasonal workers, the disposable subjects, those whose work matters more than their health, and whose health becomes vital only in relation to the domestic population, that is, only in terms of not contaminating them. (Bejan 2020, p. 2)

In addition, the arrival of this group of migrants was treated as temporary in nature and for work purposes only, so their rights were additionally limited, e.g., by preventing the arrival of migrants' family members or by introducing restrictions on access to healthcare, including also assistance in the case of COVID-19 infection or vaccination against it (Parmet 2020, p. 242).

In the case of both types of migrants described above, one can speak of the xenophobia of the people governing the country. It is blatantly obvious with regards to asylum seekers: the xenophobia is expressed directly in the statements of the governing bodies and their actions. However, even when it comes to migrant workers, we see the process of their differentiation from citizens, resulting from the perception that whites are superior to non-whites, and proving that some postcolonial white supremacy still exists (Kalir 2019). In the case of people from different parts of Europe (the richer West and the poorer East) we can talk about different shades of whiteness, where two identities overlap—nationality and ethnicity, i.e., being an immigrant and a stranger (Fox et al. 2012), and class, i.e., being poor (Webster 2008). In the case of Germany, it will be a distinction between Germans and Romanians or Poles; in Poland—between Poles and Ukrainians.

Polish xenophobia has its roots in centuries-old antisemitism (Bilewicz et al. 2012) and the legacy of the communist regime. Not only did communism render Poland a nationally and ethnically homogeneous state, but it also combined it with a homogenic and nationalist ideology, which strengthened the society's suspicion of others, including foreigners, and even made some groups national enemies (Libman and Obydenkova 2020; Burjanek 2001; Zarycki 2008). All this is combined with the process of Poles abandoning European values, set in motion in 2015, known as de-Europeanisation, which includes departure from tolerance (Vermeersch 2019).

Moreover, it is important to consider the specific Polish attitude towards its eastern neighbours—Ukraine and Belarus, which can easily be called postcolonial. Centuries ago, these societies formed one state organism. In it, Poles played a dominant role—the role of 'civilisers', who looked down on the inhabitants of the areas in the east. To this day, many politicians believe them to be a Polish zone of political influence (Zarycki 2008), hence the great involvement of Polish politicians of all parties in the democratic transformations taking place in Ukraine (including Maidan in 2014) or in supporting Belarusians protesting against the regime of Lukashenko in 2020. Still, the air of superiority towards eastern neighbours and their inhabitants is never absent, driven by matters of culture and identity. This deeply rooted perception of neighbours located further to the East as more backward is common to many societies of central and eastern Europe, and its aim is to present oneself (also to oneself) as better and Europe-worthy. To belong to the 'West' is to belong to civilisation (Melegh 2006, pp. 115–16). At the same time, this 'superiority' has an economic and class background, resulting from the stereotypical perception of Ukrainians mainly through the prism of their economic migration, poverty, backwardness, or poor economic development of the country, etc. Belarusians are probably perceived in a similar way, but there is no detailed research here (and besides, Poles tend to treat all eastern neighbours as one, and do not distinguish Belarusians from Ukrainians and Russians) (Koval et al. 2021). On the other hand, migrants from these countries are generally accepted by the Polish society as similar and familiar. The authorities perceive them in a similar way—as people from a similar culture and therefore more wanted (if migrants must come to Poland at all) than those from more distant countries and a different ethnic or religious background (Klaus 2020a).

3. Methodology of the Research

The aim of the research was to examine how the pandemic itself, as well as the regulations introduced by the government in the field of border management, influenced the lives of immigrants in Poland. Because it was impossible to reach a large and diverse group of immigrants who could assess these processes, in-depth interviews with experts working with migrants were conducted instead. The main goal was to reach people who have been providing advice and support to a large number of migrants for years. We assumed that these people would have a comprehensive picture of not only the practical functioning of the new regulations, but also the problems arising from the stay of migrants in Poland during the pandemic.

Between December 2020 and January 2021, fifteen in-depth expert interviews were carried out with 16 persons (9 women and 7 men). The group comprised six individuals offering legal advice and six assistants (who provide information and support but are not lawyers themselves). A total of nine respondents represented civil society organisations (CSOs) (of which three were grass-root immigrant organisations), three people worked for private law firms, two in public administration and a further two were experts—a researcher and a representative of an employers' organisation. The group of experts consisted of prominent representatives of organisations and institutions (especially on the national level) working in the area of migration for years. All interviewees shared the experience of working with diverse migrant groups—both forced and economic, as well as with people from different parts of the world. The main criterion used to invite experts to the study was a premise that the organisations or institutions they worked for should provide direct legal assistance to immigrants (in the form of legal advice or information). The group was also geographically diverse and included cities of various sizes located in different regions of Poland. Due to the composition of the researched group, the study has its limitations, as it focuses mostly on a general overview of the situation of immigrants during the pandemic (on the national level and in just several regions in Poland) and thus it could have overlooked some more nuanced and personal problems, especially in vulnerable groups, that people did not decide to share with the legal consultants in the first place and then the experts could not refer to during interviews.

The interviews were semi-structured, conducted on the basis of a common protocol (which was modified depending on the individual expertise of the interviewee), and the average duration was between 40 min and 1.5 h. The interviews were transcribed and then coded using the inductive approach and the MaxQDA software, although the basic categories were taken from the main categories of the interview protocol (Petintseva et al. 2020).

4. Better and Worse Asylum Seekers—I.e., Who May Enter the Country

Since 2015, Polish authorities have been gradually closing borders to asylum seekers. Refugees have been approaching the Polish border applying for international protection, but the border guards 'fail' to hear these requests and do not accept their applications, sending most of the asylum seekers back to Belarus. Over the years, the number of people who have managed to enter has gradually decreased—from over 12.6 thousand in 2015 to just over 4 thousand in 2019. Entry was refused mainly to Chechens and Tajiks; in other words, Muslims (Klaus 2020a; Szczepanik 2018). These practices have been recognised by the European Court of Human Rights as a violation of the non-refoulement principle and as an example of prohibited collective expulsions (ECtHR 2020; 2021). Those illegal expulsions and refusals to accept asylum claims took place mainly at one border guard post on the Polish–Belarusian border, in the city of Terespol. For many years, this railway border crossing has received the greatest number of asylum applications in Poland, as it is located on the Moscow–Berlin railway route. Hence, it was the most convenient place to cross the Polish border for refugees from the former USSR countries, i.e., the vast majority of people who applied for asylum in Poland.

The outbreak of the pandemic, which reached Poland in March 2020, resulted in the government closing the borders on 15 March 2020, which remained relatively impenetrable to migrants without Polish citizenship until 13 June 2020 (Nowicka et al. 2021, p. 5). The list of individuals who were allowed entry into Poland, although short at first, expanded over time. From the very beginning it included people who had the right to work in Poland (Princ 2020) and never included migrants seeking international protection. When asked about the absence (it could hardly be interpreted as an oversight) of this group, the Border Guard explained that such migrants could enter the country based on a provision, which allows people to be admitted 'in particularly justified cases' and after obtaining permission from the Commander-in-Chief of the Border Guard in this specific case[1]. In reality, however, the provision did not work in the case of refugees (except for Belarusians, as discussed below).

The railway crossing in Terespol was closed on 15 March and the train service to Belarus was suspended. This resulted in the discontinuation of asylum applications in Terespol; from 15 March until the end of 2020, only 32 applications in total were accepted in this facility (compared to 540 in 2019). Throughout 2020, only 1535 applications (which covered 2656 asylum seekers) were accepted in the whole country (KGSG 2021).

In 2021, the closure of the border continued, so the desperate refugees from other countries waiting in Belarus began to cross the Polish border illegally. According to the information published on the website of the Border Guard, 45 Chechens, 4 Tajiks and 93 Afghans who crossed the Polish–Belarusian border illegally have been apprehended since the beginning of 2021. All these people were placed in detention and most of them then submitted applications for international protection. Some of them had earlier tried to submit asylum applications on the Polish border, to no avail. The conduct of the Polish authorities not only forced them to pay the smugglers to arrange an illegal border crossing for them, but they were additionally punished for entering Poland—both by deprivation of liberty in detention centres, as well as by having proceedings initiated against them for illegal border crossing, along with a criminal conviction in a simplified procedure and without their presence in court—a standard practice in such cases (Kaciupska 2021). This practice is highly questionable, not least because it contravenes the provision of Article 31, paragraph 2 of the Geneva Convention that prohibits the punishment of refugees for illegal border crossing. What is also particularly relevant in this case is that those asylum seekers were not coming from a safe country. Belarus is no longer one, as declared by the ECtHR (ECtHR 2020, para. 177–78).

The situation at the border changed in August 2020 when, following Alexander Lukashenko's regime's brutal suppression of protests against the rigging of the presidential election, many protesters had to flee Belarus. It was at that time that Polish authorities began to introduce numerous measures to facilitate their entry, such as humanitarian visas (which had practically never been issued before), as well as other types of visas:

> consulates were issuing [. . .] repatriate visas to hide those people [from Belarusian authorities]. It mostly concerned the families of members of the Coordination Council against whom criminal proceedings were initiated in Belarus. There was a big problem whether such people would be allowed to leave or banned from leaving Belarus. Polish consulates here were trying to save such people. *Activist for a Belarusian organisation in Poland* (W6)

Belarusians were admitted to Poland on the basis of any visa (even one not explicitly mentioned in the COVID-19 regulations as granting entitlement to entry), or even without any visa at all—in which case, border guards themselves tried to obtain permission to enter from the Commander-in-Chief of the Border Guard. On 22 September, after Sviatlana Tsikhanouskaya's visit to Poland, the Polish government put Belarusians on the list of foreigners who, as the only nationality, could cross the Polish border regardless of the purpose of entry and the entry document. This is how this phenomenon was recounted by the participants of the research:

It really is a cosmic exception of some sort. I won't criticise Polish authorities for allowing Belarusians to enter but it is a textbook example of unfair treatment and you'd be hard pressed to find a better illustration of it. We've got better and worse refugees. It isn't bad to assume in advance that some groups […] deserve protection so we're letting them in. However, you mustn't assume [...] the opposite with regard to any other group, which is exactly what is happening to Chechens, Tajiks [they are thought not to deserve protection]. *Activist from an organisation helping refugees* (W3)

Indeed, Belarusians get preferential treatment when it comes to entering the country at the moment. We've seen how the situation in Terespol looked before—other foreigners were never let in like that […]. If anything, I reckon it's a political gesture of goodwill on the part of the Polish state, to allow Belarusians to enter Poland. *Activist for a Belarusian organisation* (W6)

The same respondent witnessed the extent of border guards' helpfulness:

a family of Belarusians wanted to cross the Polish border with their dog, which had no documents, and they went 'why won't you let us in with the dog—we're refugees and so is the dog'. Never before in my career had I seen border guards apologise and promise to do all they can to let the people in, including calling a vet and getting them to examine the dog and authorise its entry. I, for one, was very surprised.

Without doubt, the sense of cultural familiarity must have been playing a part in border guards' perception of Belarusians as people who are basically the same as us—a neighbour in need. The fundamental difference in the treatment of Belarusians can also be attributed to political will and a keen interest of Polish authorities in what is happening in a country considered to be a Polish political sphere of influence (Zarycki 2008). Furthermore, not without significance is the fact that officials are able to single out Belarusians amongst other refugees seeking protection in Poland, most of whom are Muslims. This element seems to have been of special importance when comparing the treatment of immigrants from the Middle East, Afghanistan and African countries who started to appear at the Polish border in the late spring of 2021. A ploy orchestrated by Lukashenko's regime in order to destabilise the situation on the eastern border saw the immigrants being brought by planes from the Middle East with Belarusian tourist visas with a view to crossing the border. Those illegal border crossings by thousands of people who were dispatched by the regime to Lithuanian, Latvian and Polish borders resulted in a fence being built along the stretch of the EU eastern borders, which provoked violent responses by both border guards of the targeted EU countries (with a significant number of push-backs to Belarus) as well as Belarusian authorities, and caused the deaths of several people in the Polish forests, mostly as a result of hypothermia (ECRE 2021; Parliamentary Assembly 2021).

5. One-Side Open Border—Deportability and Detainability in the Time of the Pandemic

Although the admission of migrants to Poland was very limited during the pandemic, the reverse practice was very much business as usual. Various types of expulsions from the territory of Poland continued throughout the entire period, also during the full closure of the borders. Between 15 March and 15 June 2020, a total of 799 people were expelled from Poland—the vast majority by land to neighbouring countries, mainly to Ukraine (KGSG 2021). While some countries, such as the Netherlands, suspended deportations in the first phase of the pandemic, i.e., spring 2020 (Kalir 2020), Poland did not follow this path. This was probably due to the exact fact that many people could be expelled by land to one of the neighbouring countries.

One of the forms of bordering practices is placing migrants in detention centres. This measure is not only intended to deter illegal border crossings (Bosworth et al. 2018), but also to facilitate the expulsion process (De Genova 2019). Worldwide, the facilities introduced a range of practices in response to the COVID-19 pandemic. Spain followed the path of full abolition, and all detained immigrants were released (Brandariz and Fernández-Bessa 2021). In the US, a lot depended on the courts, but overall, the number of migrants in the said facilities had decreased; the courts also ordered the release of all children who had been in detention for more than 20 days (Parmet 2020, p. 242). By contrast, Poland recorded no spike in the number of people released from detention due to the pandemic.

> When the first wave came in spring there were releases which were off the record, so to speak. What happened was they released a fair number of people, but it was all hush-hush, [...] and nobody would admit officially that it was because of the pandemic.
> *Lawyer for CSO* (W12)

The authorities officially confirmed this fact, stating that, in their judgment, there was no need to release detained individuals due to the pandemic[2]. The facilities introduced various COVID-secure precautions, effectively cutting the residents off from the rest of the world, as all visits were forbidden (RPO 2021a, pp. 205–10). Contact with the world was possible only online, as were meetings with lawyers, which in practice significantly limited detainees' access to legal aid. A lawyer shared her opinion about these visits:

> different rules apply [to online visits], depends on which centre we are talking about. [...] in one of the centres a 'virtual visit' can be scheduled with a specific person one wishes to talk to. [...] the lawyer must know in advance who they wish to speak with. Inevitably, if they don't know the name of the client, they will not be able to submit their name and the virtual visit will not be possible at all. (W12)

However, statistical data show that during the first wave of the virus, i.e., in the spring of 2020, the number of people in detention was reduced by informal means. In the period from March to May 2020, the number of people in the centres decreased from 241 in March to 150 in May, only to increase again as of June, reaching 387 people in December 2020. New people were also admitted to the centres all the time—it was only in the period between 13 March and 30 June 2020 that the number of new arrivals stood at 129. In total, 658 people were admitted from 15 March until the end of the year (KGSG 2021). The situation changed dramatically in 2021, due to a vast influx of people illegally crossing the eastern border. The number of places in detention increased (tripled) and new centres were opened. However, despite those changes, detention facilities remained overcrowded, and conditions were heavily criticised by the Polish ombudsman who visited them in October 2021 (RPO 2021b).

As for releases from detention, only a small number of those released received alternatives to detention. The pandemic had not changed much in this respect—from March to December 2020, these alternatives were only offered to 127 people (KGSG 2021). It is difficult to clearly determine how many people were released due to the impossibility of expulsion. In theory, the role of detention in return procedures is to facilitate the efficient expulsion of migrants. Hence, in a situation where there is no real possibility of carrying out deportation, detention should be considered illegal, as it does not fulfil the purpose for which it was used (Kalir 2020). However, experts remained divided on this point. Some confirmed that such releases did take place:

> I'm sure there was a certain number of people who were released at the very beginning, but I don't know if it had anything to do with the pandemic or a simple realisation that they could be expelled so there was no point in keeping them. *Activist for a CSO* (W3)

Others (members of CSOs as well), on the other hand, did not corroborate this account:

> I remember writing away all through March, April, and May—'hello, the borders are closed so there's no risk of an illegal crossing [of the border]'. [...] I had these guys you couldn't deport either, and they had partners in Poland. [...] [Regardless, they are all] still remained in detention. (W5)

they [border guards] only have one mode: that some expulsions will surely be possible any time soon. They schedule subsequent dates and go—well, next week for sure then. If it doesn't happen next week then they set another date for another week. They haven't got this mindset that allows them to take stock of the situation: ok, it's not going to be possible for the next two months. [...] They are stuck operating in the expulsion mode. (W12)

Perhaps such differences result from different practices followed in different detention centres (there are six in Poland) as well as informal actions undertaken by the authorities. It is noteworthy that, in fact, some expulsion did occur during the pandemic—only between 15 March and 30 April, in which as many as 88 people were deported directly from the centres (KGSG 2021). It would seem that the border was closed primarily to those who wanted to come to Poland, but it remained open when it was necessary to get rid of unwanted migrants.

6. 'It's the Economy, Stupid'

While the borders were closed to refugees, they remained very much open to people coming to work. However, in Poland's case, the caveat did not only concern essential workers, a term which basically covers people doing seasonal work in agriculture. The borders remained open to all migrants who could produce any document entitling them to work in Poland. In addition, further facilitating measures for migrant workers were introduced quite quickly: the validity of their visas, residence permits, and work permits were automatically extended (Princ 2020), so that they would not be required to apply for new ones issued during a pandemic or return to their country of origin to have them replaced.

These provisions, however, resulted not so much from the willingness to make things easier for migrant workers, but rather for those who employ them. They were prompted by the inefficiency of the Polish system of legalisation of work and stay, in which the procedures for obtaining documents can last for several months:

it takes around 6–7 months to have the work permit issued in normal circumstances, let alone during a pandemic. The same goes for changing the temporary residence and work permit when switching employers. The pandemic situation has made the wait even longer, causing more and more foreigners to take up work without a valid permit or to work illegally altogether. *Migration lawyer* (W8)

The government was well aware that the delays in completing formalities would only increase with offices working at reduced capacity due to the pandemic, which indeed happened (Cope et al. 2020, pp. 11–13). Hence, the introduction of the new regulations was intended to prevent the illegalisation of hundreds of thousands of migrant workers.

At face value these provisions appear to facilitate the functioning of migrants during the pandemic, and they really worked, at the start. However, these temporary regulations have now been in force for 1.5 years and it is not known when they will cease to apply (they are to be in force until the state of the epidemic emergency is cancelled by the government and for another 30 days after that date). Therefore, they create a sense of uncertainty and limbo with regards to what will happen later, when the new rules have been abandoned and new documents will not be issued by relevant offices on time.

The COVID-19 regulations also assumed the continuity of work with one employer, in a bid to eliminate the problem with extending employment. However, in the event of a change of employer (not least due to redundancies caused by the economic slowdown or the closure of certain sectors, such as gastronomy), the migrant is not able to quickly obtain new documents necessary to start work with another employer. However, they need a job to support themselves (because most often they are not eligible to receive social benefits). Hence, they often work illegally or in some sort of semi-legal arrangements (Kubal 2013), as indicated by the migration lawyer quoted above (W8).

Special regulations were introduced for seasonal workers in agriculture—their supposed quarantine at the contracted farm did not consist of complete self-isolation, as they could normally carry out all field work on the farm, which basically released them from having to quarantine at all. Another problem was that migrant workers were not adequately protected—they stayed in common rooms in larger groups and did not receive appropriate personal protective equipment (the fact that they often disregarded the epidemic threat themselves did not help either).

> In a nutshell the requirements stated that those who arrive during the pandemic must be accommodated in separate rooms. This never happened. I know, because I saw it with my own eyes: eight people would arrive to pick strawberries, each one on a different day. According to guidelines, they should each stay in their own room, and this never happened. They would be put together. [...] The face masks were just for show, in case of a spot check, but the workers themselves did not demand them—they felt that the fresh air made a difference. Mind you, when they were being transported [...] it did become problematic, because they were squeezed together in one delivery van. [...] they are squeezed together, there's no ventilation and all the facemasks are at the front, where the driver is, so that he can quickly throw them to people when he sees the police. You know, as in: put the masks on so that they can see everything's legit. A complete farce it was. *Seasonal work expert* (W1)

To summarize, the only ban enforced during this peculiar form of quarantine was the lack of contact with people outside the household, i.e., Poles. In fact, it was the safety of the latter that seemed to be a cause for concern for the authorities (as well as the state of the Polish economy, no doubt), rather than the well-being of migrant workers (cf. also Bejan 2020).

All the above regulations for migrant workers were 'tailored' primarily to Ukrainians and other workers from countries neighbouring Poland. Citizens from more distant (geographically but also ethnically) regions, i.e., people from Asian or African countries, were subject to obvious xenophobia, seeing as their arrival was obstructed in various ways—visas were not issued, those already issued were cancelled and consular posts were closed (cf. also Parmet 2020, p. 241).

The above regulations result from the Polish authorities' perception of migrant workers only in the context of immediate benefits for the economy, whereby disposable labourers come to work for a while when needed, and then leave. Such a setup relies on temporary and rather short-term migration, which is wholly untenable, as figures show different trends in this area. Still, hard facts will clearly not stand in the way of those who are in power and resent the presence of migrants in Poland for longer, let alone permanently.

7. Discussion and Conclusions

Most public policies introduced during a pandemic time are characterised by their uncertainty (Weible et al. 2020, p. 3), which stems from the unpredictability of what might happen and how the virus, as well as its mutations, will spread. The same uncertainty impacts on migration policies and then affects the lives of migrants. The second important effect of the pandemic is the deepening of existing inequalities (Weible et al. 2020, p. 5). Yet again, migrants pay the highest price for this state of affairs, especially those who are most vulnerable and in need of the greatest support, i.e., refugees. Meanwhile, on the EU level, not much is being enacted, be it on the level of individual states or in the EU as a whole (Dadusc and Mudu 2020), and the only evolution is visible in the language used with reference to migrants and refugees alike, which on a declarative level at least can be described as 'human and humane' (Panebianco 2021). This criticism applies to Poland as well, a country where the constitution guarantees the highest level of protection to refugees and where this very group of migrants has been overlooked the most during the pandemic, and experienced the greatest inconvenience as a result of the restrictions on movement (Princ 2020, p. 16).

On the whole, the pandemic has seen the return of governments shifting their attention to borders and societies closing in their national bubbles. Migration to many countries has been limited and migrants have often been accused of bringing along diseases (Ambrosini 2021, p. 389). In Poland, these processes have taken place to some extent only, emphasising the double standards that the government applies to different categories of migrants. Therefore, on the one hand, the borders have remained open throughout to migrant workers in response to economic demands and pressure from business owners which overrode the government's xenophobia. On the other hand, the borders have been almost entirely closed to refugees, who are perceived as undesirable and likely to generate additional costs (Barker 2018).

The pandemic has also exacerbated the division of migrants according to their ethnicity or religion. For many years now, various administrations in Poland have spoken about opening up, mainly to arrivals from culturally close societies, most notably citizens of neighbouring countries. Not only was this sentiment reflected in subsequent documents on migration policy but also while drafting custom-made regulations to cater to Ukrainians. The same happened during the pandemic, except this time the borders opened to a different single group of refugees—Belarusians. In a move without precedent (even when compared with the admission of Ukrainians after Russia's aggression against Ukraine in 2014), the government prepared regulations and protocols that opened the borders wide, offered significant help in crossing them as well as upon arrival. Belarusians were perceived not solely as people fleeing persecution but as individuals with agency, which was reflected in the launching of the 'Poland. Business Harbour' programme for entrepreneurs from Belarus (mainly from the IT sector) who wish to relocate to Poland.

Meanwhile, people from geographically, ethnically, and religiously distant countries (mainly Muslims), found themselves in an altogether different situation. Their arrival in Poland—whether as refugees or migrant workers—is rarely welcome and they themselves face many obstacles when trying to enter. To all intents and purposes, this level of government xenophobia bears all the marks of a phenomenon known as 'departheid' (Kalir 2019), which in Poland, due to the near absence of people from different ethnical or religious backgrounds, focuses on measures preventing their entry. Nonetheless, the main purpose of these practices is essentially the same—

> to protect the territory of White people, or what we can call 'White spaces,' from any 'invasion' by racialized Others. (. . .) [It's] an act of self-defense, protecting so-called Western civilization and Judeo-Christian values that are allegedly under attack from illegalized migrants. (Kalir 2019, pp. 28, 32)

Those 'values' are at the absolute forefront of the Polish government's policy at the moment. This fact became even more obvious in August 2021, when many immigrants found themselves stranded in the border zone, and the government contributed to the deaths of several people in the Polish forests by refusing to accept asylum claims from them while continuing to push them back to Belarus irrespective of their health condition.

Funding: The research presented in this article is part of the project 'Ensuring the safety and public order as a justification of criminalisation of migration' financed by the National Science Centre, Poland under the grant number 2017/25/B/HS5/02961.

Institutional Review Board Statement: The study was conducted according to the guidelines of the Declaration of Helsinki, and approved by the Ethical Committee of the Institute of Law Studies, Polish Academy of Sciences (decision 3/2018 of 29.03.2018).

Informed Consent Statement: Informed consent was obtained from all subjects involved in the study.

Data Availability Statement: Data available on request.

Acknowledgments: The author would like to thank Monika Szulecka for her cooperation in designing this research and for conducting several interviews within it.

Conflicts of Interest: The author declares no conflict of interest.

Notes

[1] Letter from the Border Guard Headquarters to the Commissioner for Human Rights, 21 May 2021, ref. KG-CU-ZSS.072.8.2020.
[2] Similar trends were also observed in Polish prisons. Again, the authorities (and the courts) decided against releasing imprisoned people due to the pandemic. A slight reduction in the prison population in 2020 resulted from a reduction in the number of new admissions to serve a sentence (Stańdo-Kawecka 2021).

References

Aas, Katja Franko. 2011. "Crimmigrant" Bodies and Bona Fide Travelers: Surveillance, Citizenship and Global Governance. *Theoretical Criminology* 15: 331–46. [CrossRef]

Ambrosini, Maurizio. 2013. Immigration in Italy: Between Economic Acceptance and Political Rejection. *Journal of International Migration and Integration* 14: 175–94. [CrossRef]

Ambrosini, Maurizio. 2021. The Battleground of Asylum and Immigration Policies: A Conceptual Inquiry. *Ethnic and Racial Studies* 44: 374–95. [CrossRef]

Barker, Vanessa. 2018. *Nordic Nationalism and Penal Order: Walling the Welfare State*. London and New York: Routledge.

Bejan, Raluca. 2020. COVID-19 and Disposable Migrant Workers. *Verfassungsblog: On Matters Constitutional (blog)*. April 16. Available online: https://intr2dok.vifa-recht.de/receive/mir_mods_00008555 (accessed on 8 November 2021).

Bilewicz, Michał, Mikołaj Winiewski, and Zuzanna Radzik. 2012. Antisemitism in Poland: Psychological, Religious, and Historical Aspects. *Journal for the Study of Antisemitism* 4: 423–42.

Bosworth, Mary, Katja Franko, and Sharon Pickering. 2018. Punishment, Globalization and Migration Control: "Get Them the Hell out of Here". *Punishment & Society* 20: 34–53. [CrossRef]

Brandariz, José A., and Cristina Fernández-Bessa. 2021. Coronavirus and Immigration Detention in Europe: The Short Summer of Abolitionism? *Social Sciences* 10: 226. [CrossRef]

Burjanek, Ales. 2001. Xenophobia among the Czech Population in the Context of Post-Communist Countries and Western Europe. *Sociologický Časopis/Czech Sociological Review* 9: 53–67. [CrossRef]

Chamie, Joseph. 2020. International Migration amid a World in Crisis. *Journal on Migration and Human Security* 8: 230–45. [CrossRef]

CJEU. 2020. *Commission v Poland, Hungary and the Czech Republic, Joined Cases C-715/17, C-718/17 and C-719/17*. Luxembourg: Court of Justice of the European Union. Available online: https://curia.europa.eu/juris/document/document.jsf;jsessionid=8B6C722352DED910A26DFC6A2360BC0F?text=&docid=224882&pageIndex=0&doclang=EN&mode=lst&dir=&occ=first&part=1&cid=40983794 (accessed on 8 November 2021).

Cope, Benjamin, Myroslava Keryk, and Ivanna Kyliushyk. 2020. *The Impact of COVID-19 on Ukrainian Women Migrants in Poland*. Warsaw: Foundation "Our Choice". Available online: https://pl.boell.org/sites/default/files/2021-03/NV_Boll_Raport_Covid_A4_EN.pdf (accessed on 8 November 2021).

Dadusc, Deanna, and Pierpaolo Mudu. 2020. Care without Control: The Humanitarian Industrial Complex and the Criminalisation of Solidarity. *Geopolitics*, 1–26. [CrossRef]

De Genova, Nicholas. 2019. Detention, Deportation, and Waiting: Toward a Theory of Migrant Detainability. *Gender a Výzkum/Gender and Research* 20: 92–104. [CrossRef]

ECRE. 2021. Poland: More Deaths at the Border, Poland Extends State of Emergency, Neither ECtHR Nor Commissioner Persuade Poland to End Pushbacks. European Council of Refugees and Exiles. Available online: https://ecre.org/poland-more-deaths-at-the-border-poland-seeks-to-extend-state-of-emergency-neither-ecthr-requests-nor-commissioner-visit-persuade-poland-to-end-pushbacks/ (accessed on 8 November 2021).

ECtHR. 2020. *M.K. and Others v. Poland*. Strasbourg: European Court of Human Rights. Available online: https://hudoc.echr.coe.int/eng#\{%22tabview%22:[%22document%22],%22itemid%22:[%22001-203840%22]\} (accessed on 8 November 2021).

ECtHR. 2021. *D.A. and Others v. Poland*. Strasbourg: European Court of Human Rights. Available online: https://hudoc.echr.coe.int/eng#\{%22fulltext%22:[%22D.A.%20and%20other%22],%22documentcollectionid2%22:[%22GRANDCHAMBER%22,%22CHAMBER%22],%22itemid%22:[%22001-210855%22]\} (accessed on 8 November 2021).

Fox, Jon E., Laura Moroşanu, and Eszter Szilassy. 2012. The Racialization of the New European Migration to the UK. *Sociology* 46: 680–95. [CrossRef]

Gilbert, Liette. 2009. Immigration as Local Politics: Re-Bordering Immigration and Multiculturalism through Deterrence and Incapacitation. *International Journal of Urban and Regional Research* 33: 26–42. [CrossRef]

Hamlin, Rebecca. 2012. Illegal Refugees: Competing Policy Ideas and the Rise of the Regime of Deterrence in American Asylum Politics. *Refugee Survey Quarterly* 31: 33–53. [CrossRef]

Jaskułowski, Krzysztof. 2019. *The Everyday Politics of Migration Crisis in Poland—Between Nationalism, Fear and Empathy*. Cham: Palgrave Macmillan.

Kaciupska, Zuzanna. 2021. Karanie uchodźców za nielegalne przekroczenie granicy. *Laboratorium Migracji (Blog)*, July 19. Available online: https://interwencjaprawna.pl/karanie-uchodzcow-za-nielegalne-przekroczenie-granicy/ (accessed on 8 November 2021).

Kalir, Barak. 2019. Departheid: The Draconian Governance of Illegalized Migrants in Western States. *Conflict and Society* 5: 19–40. [CrossRef]

Kalir, Barak. 2020. 3D Threats to Illegalised Migrants—Desertion, Detention, Deportation—During Pandemic. *Identities Journal Blog (Blog)*, April 27. Available online: http://www.identitiesjournal.com/4/post/2020/04/3d-threats-to-illegalised-migrants-desertion-detention-deportation-during-pandemic.html (accessed on 8 November 2021).

KGSG. 2021. *Statistical Data from Polish Border Guard*. Information of 01 February 2021, no KG-OI-VIII.0180.15.2021.JL. Warsaw: Polish Border Guard Headquarters.

Klaus, Witold. 2017. Closing Gates to Refugees: The Causes and Effects of the 2015 "Migration Crisis" on Border Management in Hungary and Poland. *Yearbook of the Institute of East-Central Europe* 15: 11–34.

Klaus, Witold. 2020a. Between Closing Borders to Refugees and Welcoming Ukrainian Workers: Polish Migration Law at the Crossroads. In *Europe and the Refugee Response: A Crisis of Values?* Edited by Elżbieta M. Goździak, Izabela Main and Brigitte Suter. London and New York: Routledge, pp. 74–90.

Klaus, Witold. 2020b. How Does Crimmigration Unfold in Poland? Between Securitisation Introduced to Polish Migration Policy by Its Europeanisation and Polish Xenophobia. In *Crimmigrant Nations: Resurgent Nationalism and the Closing of Borders*. Edited by Robert Koulish and Maartje var der Woude. New York: Fordham University Press, pp. 298–314.

Kmak, Magdalena. 2015. "The Ugly" of EU Migration Policy: The role of the Recast Reception Directive in Fragmentation of the Refugee Subject. In *Europe at the Edge of Pluralism*. Edited by Magdalena Kmak and Dorota A. Gozdecka. Cambridge, Antwerp and Portland: Intersentia Publishing, pp. 83–94.

Koulish, Robert, and Maartje van der Woude. 2020. Introduction. The "Problem" of Migration. In *Crimmigrant Nations: Resurgent Nationalism and the Closing of Borders*. Edited by Robert Koulish and Maartje van der Woude. New York: Fordham University Press, pp. 1–29.

Koval, Nadiia, Laurynas Vaičiūnas, and Iwona Reichardt. 2021. *Polacy i Ukraińcy w codziennych kontaktach*. Wrocław: Kolegium Europy Wschodniej im. Jana Nowaka-Jeziorańskiego we Wrocławiu. Available online: https://www.kew.org.pl/wp-content/uploads/2020/12/RAPORT-Polacy-i-Ukraincy-w-codziennych-kontaktach-05-07.pdf (accessed on 8 November 2021).

Kubal, Agnieszka. 2013. Conceptualizing Semi-Legality in Migration Research. *Law & Society Review* 47: 555–87. [CrossRef]

Libman, Alexander, and Anastassia V. Obydenkova. 2020. Proletarian Internationalism in Action? Communist Legacies and Attitudes Towards Migrants in Russia. *Problems of Post-Communism* 67: 402–16. [CrossRef]

Melegh, Attila. 2006. *On the East-West Slope: Globalization, Nationalism, Racism and Discourses on Central and Eastern Europe*. Budapest and New York: Central European University Press.

Nail, Thomas. 2020. Philosophy in the Time of COVID. *Philosophy Today* 64: 889–93. [CrossRef]

Nowicka, Magdalena, Susanne Bartig, Theresa Schwass, and Kamil Matuszczyk. 2021. COVID-19 Pandemic and Resilience of the Transnational Home-Based Elder Care System between Poland and Germany. *Journal of Aging & Social Policy* 33: 474–92. [CrossRef]

Panebianco, Stefania. 2021. Towards a Human and Humane Approach? The EU Discourse on Migration amidst the COVID-19 Crisis. *The International Spectator* 56: 19–37. [CrossRef]

Parliamentary Assembly. 2021. Instrumentalised migration pressure on the borders of Latvia, Lithuania and Poland with Belarus. Council of Europe. Resolution 2404. Available online: https://pace.coe.int/en/files/29537/html (accessed on 8 November 2021).

Parmet, Wendy E. 2020. Immigration Law's Adverse Impact on COVID-19. In *Assessing Legal Responses to COVID-19*. Edited by Scott Burris, Sarah de Guia, Lance Gable, Donna E. Levin, Wendy E. Parmet and Nicolas P. Terry. Boston: Public Health Law Watch, pp. 240–43.

Pędziwiatr, Konrad, and Agnieszka Legut. 2016. Polskie rządy wobec unijnej strategii na rzecz przeciwdziałania kryzysowi migracyjnemu. In *Uchodźcy w Europie—Uwarunkowania, istota, następstwa*. Edited by Konstanty A. Wojtaszczyk and Jolanta Szymańska. Warszawa: Wydawnictwa Uniwersytetu Warszawskiego, pp. 671–93.

Petintseva, Olga, Rita Faria, and Yarin Eski. 2020. *Interviewing Elites, Experts and the Powerful in Criminology*. Cham: Palgrave Macmillan. [CrossRef]

Princ, Marcin. 2020. Foreigners' Rights in The Age of Pandemics—Migration Aspects. *Wroclaw Review of Law, Administration & Economics* 10: 93–111. [CrossRef]

RPO. 2021a. *Raport RPO z działalności w Polsce Krajowego Mechanizmu Prewencji Tortur, nieludzkiego, poniżającego traktowania lub karania*; Biuletyn Rzecznika Praw Obywatelskich 2. Warszawa: Rzecznik Praw Obywatelskich. Available online: https://bip.brpo.gov.pl/sites/default/files/Raport_KMPT_2020_interaktywny.pdf (accessed on 8 November 2021).

RPO. 2021b. *Złe Warunki Mogą Pogłębiać Traumy. Wizytacje ad hoc w Ośrodkach dla Cudzoziemców*; Warszawa: Rzecznik Praw Obywatelskich. Available online: https://bip.brpo.gov.pl/pl/content/rpo-osrodki-cudzoziemcy-wizytacje-zle-warunki (accessed on 8 November 2021).

Solga, Brygida, and Filip Tereszkiewicz. 2020. Challenges of Poland's Migration Policy from the Perspective of the Experiences of Selected European Union Countries. *European Research Studies Journal* XXIII: 434–50. [CrossRef]

Stańdo-Kawecka, Barbara. 2021. Populacja Więzienna w Polsce w Pierwszym Roku Pandemii COVID-19. *Archiwum Kryminologii* 43: 1–23, online first. [CrossRef]

Szczepanik, Marta. 2018. Border Politics and Practices of Resistance on the Eastern Side of "Fortress Europe": The Case of Chechen Asylum Seekers at the Belarusian–Polish Border. *Central and Eastern European Migration Review* 7: 69–89. [CrossRef]

Valluy, Jérôme. 2011. The Metamorphosis of Asylum in Europe: From the Origins of "Fake Refugees" to Their Internment. In *Racial Criminalization of Migrants in the 21st Century*. Edited by Salvatore Palidda. Farnham, Burlington: Ashgate, pp. 107–18.

Vermeersch, Peter. 2019. Victimhood as Victory: The Role of Memory Politics in the Process of de-Europeanisation in East-Central Europe. *Global Discourse: An Interdisciplinary Journal of Current Affairs* 9: 113–30. [CrossRef]
Webster, Colin. 2008. Marginalized White Ethnicity, Race and Crime. *Theoretical Criminology* 12: 293–312. [CrossRef]
Weible, Christopher M., Daniel Nohrstedt, Paul Cairney, David P. Carter, Deserai A. Crow, Anna P. Durnová, Tanya Heikkila, Karin Ingold, Allan McConnell, and Diane Stone. 2020. COVID-19 and the Policy Sciences: Initial Reactions and Perspectives. *Policy Sciences* 53: 225–41. [CrossRef] [PubMed]
Zarycki, Tomasz. 2008. Polska i jej regiony a debata postkolonialna. In *Oblicze polityczne regionów Polski*. Edited by Małgorzata Dajnowicz. Białystok: Wyższa Szkoła Finansów i Zarządzania, pp. 31–48.

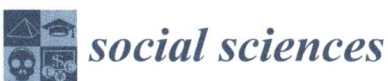

Article

Coronavirus and Immigration Detention in Europe: The Short Summer of Abolitionism?

José A. Brandariz * and Cristina Fernández-Bessa

ECRIM, Law School, University of A Coruña, Campus de Elviña, s/n, 15071 A Coruña, Spain; c.fernandezb@udc.es
* Correspondence: jose.angel.brandariz@udc.es

Abstract: In managing the coronavirus pandemic, national authorities worldwide have implemented significant re-bordering measures. This has even affected regions that had dismantled bordering practices decades ago, e.g., EU areas that lifted internal borders in 1993. In some national cases, these new arrangements had unexpected consequences in the field of immigration enforcement. A number of European jurisdictions released significant percentages of their immigration detention populations in spring 2020. The Spanish administration even decreed a moratorium on immigration detention and closed down all detention facilities from mid-spring to late summer 2020. The paper scrutinises these unprecedented changes by examining the variety of migration enforcement agendas adopted by European countries and the specific forces contributing to the prominent detention decline witnessed in the first months of the pandemic. Drawing on the Spanish case, the paper reflects on the potential impact of this promising precedent on the gradual consolidation of social and racial justice-based migration policies.

Keywords: coronavirus; immigration detention; migration enforcement; detention abolition

Citation: Brandariz, José A., and Cristina Fernández-Bessa. 2021. Coronavirus and Immigration Detention in Europe: The Short Summer of Abolitionism? *Social Sciences* 10: 226. https://doi.org/10.3390/socsci10060226

Academic Editors: Robert Koulish and Nigel Parton

Received: 15 May 2021
Accepted: 10 June 2021
Published: 12 June 2021

Publisher's Note: MDPI stays neutral with regard to jurisdictional claims in published maps and institutional affiliations.

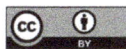

Copyright: © 2021 by the authors. Licensee MDPI, Basel, Switzerland. This article is an open access article distributed under the terms and conditions of the Creative Commons Attribution (CC BY) license (https://creativecommons.org/licenses/by/4.0/).

1. Introduction

The coronavirus pandemic, which started in early 2020, has deeply shaken the foundations of our social life, turning upside down every dimension of our world. Specifically, the COVID-19 pandemic has had a seismic impact on human mobility, since international—and, in many cases, even local—travel was immediately singled out as a critical risk factor of coronavirus infection. Consequently, public health policies aimed at curbing the pandemic have fuelled a wide variety of re-bordering processes (Genschel and Jachtenfuchs 2021; Wille and Kanesu 2020). In fact, more than 140 countries had imposed border crossing restrictions in April 2020, in the framework of the first phase of the public health crisis (Connor 2020).[1] In various regions, these were unprecedented measures. Schengen member states reintroduced border control at internal borders 122 times from 2006 to 2019, whilst these controls were reinstated 170 times from just March 2020 to April 2021, in all but seven cases for coronavirus-related reasons (source: European Commission 2021). Re-bordering processes, though, have gone far beyond measures aimed at re-erecting physical barriers. In many aspects, anti-coronavirus strategies have boosted chauvinist agendas, hampering previous international cooperation efforts. This shortcoming was especially evident in the case of the European Union (EU), for EU institutions largely failed to provide the much-needed leadership in the continental management of the crisis (Hall et al. 2020; Kluth 2021).

Given the far-reaching impact of anti-covid policies on human mobility, it is unsurprising that they have profoundly affected migration management practices. Travel bans and public health measures have significantly shifted a variety of border arrangements, including visa and legal residence policies, asylum practices and deportation procedures. Immigration detention has ranked high in this regard. As confinement institutions were reasonably tagged as critical hot spots for coronavirus infection since the onset of the crisis, they made up a major concern for national and international public health authorities (WHO 2020). This concern was focused on prisons but also on other facilities characterised by freedom of movement restrictions in which physical distancing measures are not feasible, such as asylum reception centres and migration detention facilities.

The COVID-19 crisis has resulted in various changes in the field of immigration detention. It has altered detention conditions in a variety of ways, from curtailing detention places and implementing distancing protocols to further isolating detainees by suspending visitation procedures (European Commission 2020a). In addition, the pandemic has called into question the role and goals and migration detention policies, in a period in which deportation efforts have been significantly eroded by the coronavirus turmoil. In this scenario, public health concerns have taken the lead over other public policy priorities, resulting in significant contingents of immigration detainees being released in many jurisdictions.

This paper explores the impact of the coronavirus pandemic on immigration detention by essentially spotlighting these exceptional release practices. A good reason to embrace this viewpoint is that those practices—at least during a "short summer"—might operate as a window of opportunity to reflect on detention abolition, that is, as a rare opportunity to envision new migration enforcement arrangements giving preference to alternatives to detention over confinement measures (Roman 2020; Weber 2020; see also Majkowska-Tomkin 2020). Having said that, neither immigration detention practices have a global reach (Brandariz 2021) nor recent release policies were implemented globally (Chew et al. 2020; Dehm 2020). Consequently, European countries make up a suitable (continental) case to examine how and to what extent the sanitary crisis has contributed to change immigration detention. More precisely, Spain was the only global north country that closed down all immigration detention facilities for some time in mid-2020. Therefore, Spain may be an appropriate point of reference to reflect on immigration enforcement goals and alternatives to detention in a post-pandemic world.

No wide-encompassing, comparative and detailed database on immigration detention changes implemented in the framework of the coronavirus has been released yet. Consequently, this paper largely draws on the information supplied by a wide number of reports published by NGOs and watchdog institutions,[2] as well as on media articles and some official law enforcement statistics. Building on these unsystematic data, the paper proceeds as follows. Initially, it presents the immigration detention changes implemented across Europe, and specifically in Spain to prevent coronavirus infections. Subsequently, the paper explores the forces and conditions contributing to the detention population decline witnessed in many European jurisdictions in mid-2020, as well as the strengths and weaknesses of those unprecedented policies for a detention abolition agenda. Drawing on this reflection, the paper outlines some conclusions on what can be learned from an exceptional time that we metaphorically call the "brief summer of abolitionism" in the field of immigration detention.

2. Public Health Policies and the Immigration Detention Decline

Immediately after the World Health Organization (WHO) qualified the coronavirus crisis as a global pandemic and national governments began to implement lockdown and quarantine measures globally in March 2020, public health authorities stressed that confinement institutions pose a critical challenge for anti-coronavirus policies. Prison facilities and other types of custodial sites were rapidly singled out as potential hotbeds for infection (Hawks et al. 2020; Hooks and Libel 2020; Hooks and Sawyer 2020). In fact, international organisations published guidelines providing advice to competent authorities on how to prevent the pandemic in these closed environments (WHO Europe 2020a).

In dealing with this concerning scenario, national administrations adopted a variety of policy agendas. Many countries imposed stringent quarantine restrictions, heightening the usual isolation of confinement facilities from the outside world. Therefore, both prisoners and immigration detainees were temporarily banned from receiving visits in many jurisdictions, sometimes with specific exceptions targeting lawyers and watchdog staff (see, e.g., Contrôleur Général des Lieux de Privation de Liberté CGLPL; Esposito et al. 2020; Home Office 2021). The Global Detention Project (GDP) COVID-19 Platform allows one to deduce that these quarantine measures gained particular traction in the course of the second and subsequent waves of the pandemic, when the "coronavirus fatigue" (WHO Europe 2020b) was beginning to affect national officials and infections behind bars were on the rise in various countries (Bulman 2021; Stuber and Zeier 2021; Vargas 2021).

In certain cases, these quarantine policies adopted xeno-racist and apartheid-like tones. In fact, anti-immigration agendas transpired in political decisions aimed at, e.g., completely closing off detention facilities and reception centres and extending quarantine measures targeting those facilities beyond national lockdown deadlines (International Commission of Jurists ICJ). Those practices frequently targeted overcrowded sites hosting particularly vulnerable asylum-seeking populations (Refugee Rights Europe 2020). These measures laid bare the "less eligibility" rationale (De Giorgi 2010) and the deterrence aims characterising immigration detention in many jurisdictions (Bosworth 2019; Campesi 2015; Leerkes and Broeders 2010), European and non-European alike.

These apartheid-like policies seem to have garnered particular traction in certain Mediterranean countries that have long disregarded human rights standards in enforcing their border policies such as Cyprus (Andreou 2021; European Council on Refugees and Exiles ECRE; Knews 2020a), Greece (Cossé 2020; International Commission of Jurists ICJ), and Malta (European Committee for the Prevention of Torture ECPT).[3] However, this has not been the case everywhere. On the contrary, in other jurisdictions, anti-coronavirus strategies pointed to a different, almost opposite direction. In stark contrast to those thanatopolitical agendas (Vaughan-Williams 2015), various European jurisdictions chose to follow international organisations' recommendations (see, e.g., Commissioner for Human Rights 2020) by reducing the capacity of custodial facilities, thereby curtailing occupancy rates. This did not lead national authorities to open up new detention facilities, but to halve their total detention capacity almost overnight, a measure taken in countries such as Belgium (Carretero 2020; Global Detention Project GDP), Finland (European Migration Network EMN), France (La Cimade 2020), and Sweden (European Council on Refugees and Exiles ECRE; Lindberg et al. 2020).

Release strategies, in turn, were unequivocally advocated by the medical community (see Lopez et al. 2021; Macmadu et al. 2020), which gave preference to healthcare concerns over law enforcement considerations. However, this agenda was also championed by various other critical actors, claiming that an exceptional scenario like the global pandemic justified relegating border control interests (United Nations Working Group on Alternatives to Immigration Detention UNWGATD). In several European jurisdictions such as France, Italy, Portugal, Sweden, Switzerland, and the UK this demand was heralded by numerous ombuds officials (ANSA 2020), politicians and lawmakers (Cassidy 2020), NGOs and migrant rights organisations (Expresso 2020; FARR 2020; Inquest 2020; Lasciateentrare 2020; Solidarité Sans Frontières SSF; Taylor 2020a), and evidently detained noncitizens themselves (Knews 2021; Loran 2020; Shenker 2021).

This public health agenda was partly successful. At least in the first stages of the pandemic, many European nations witnessed a significant decline in the number of prisoners (DLA Piper 2021). Aebi and Tiago (2020) show that prison population rates dwindled by more than 5 percent in fourteen EU and European Free Trade Association (EFTA) countries from January to September 2020, and especially in Bulgaria, France, Italy, Lithuania, and Portugal. The causes of this decline were varied. Lockdown measures hampering regular judicial activities reduced prison admissions. In addition, European jurisdictions released significant contingents of prisoners for coronavirus prevention motives. Indeed, Cyprus, France, Norway, Portugal, Slovenia, and Spain freed more than 10 percent of their incarcerated populations for COVID-19 reasons over the first nine months of 2020 (Aebi and Tiago 2020). Beyond wide-ranging release programmes implemented in countries such as Iran (Hafezi 2020) and Turkey (Kucukgocmen 2020), also in the US anti-coronavirus measures resulted in a prison population drop. It has been estimated that state prison populations plummeted by 17 percent from January 2020 to January 2021, although it is not clear the extent to which this drop was due to pandemic-driven measures (Sharma et al. 2020; Widra 2021).

As is illustrated by Table 1, release policies gained also significant momentum in the immigration detention field. Certainly, not all EU and EFTA countries adopted this detention downsizing approach to prevent coronavirus infections. Available data (sources: GDP COVID-19 Platform; European Council on Refugees and Exiles ECRE; Fundamental Rights Agency FRA) show that many European countries (e.g., Austria, Bulgaria, the Czech Republic, Denmark, Greece, and Romania, amongst others) were reluctant to reduce the occupancy rate of detention facilities by freeing detained noncitizens. By contrast, the onset of the pandemic led detention populations to quickly drop in other European jurisdictions. In fact, in these immigration enforcement systems, far-reaching release policies led the number of detainees to drastically diminish in the course of a few weeks. The result of this sudden change was that the number of detainees was counted to be a couple of hundreds in spring 2020 in various European countries such as Belgium (Coppens 2020; European Migration Network EMN), Italy (Coalizione Italiana Libertà e Diritti Civili CILD; Esposito et al. 2020; Roman 2020), the Netherlands (NOS 2020), and Sweden (Lindberg et al. 2020), whilst in Germany (European Council on Refugees and Exiles ECRE), and Norway (European Migration Network EMN; Trandum Supervisory Board 2021), this number ultimately dropped to several dozens. France stood out in this regard as well, since the French administration closed down a dozen detention facilities in the first weeks of the pandemic (Contrôleur Général des Lieux de Privation de Liberté CGLPL; Conxicoeur 2020). In Switzerland, in turn, certain cantonal governments such as that of Geneva also closed down detention facilities, whereas others did not adopt wide-ranging release strategies (Tribune de Genève 2020). Additionally, UK authorities implemented far-reaching anti-coronavirus measures in the field of immigration detention. Widespread release procedures led the number of immigration detainees to decline by around 70 percent in just the two first months of the pandemic (Home Office 2020).

Table 1. European jurisdictions particularly affected by coronavirus-related immigration enforcement changes.

Significant Decline in the Detention Population	Detention Facilities Almost Emptied	Closure of all Detention Facilities	Deportations More than Halved in 2020
Belgium, France, Italy, the Netherlands, Sweden, Switzerland, UK	Germany, Norway	Spain	Bulgaria, France, Italy, Poland, Slovakia, Spain

Sources: Eurostat (ec.europa.eu/eurostat/web/asylum-and-managed-migration/data/database; accessed on 4 May 2021), and various official and NGO reports, precisely referenced throughout the paper.

In addition to release procedures, occupancy rates were kept low by raising the threshold to impose detention measures and by excluding certain national groups from detention in several jurisdictions such as Finland, Norway and the UK (source: GDP COVID-19 Platform). Moreover, the number of issued removal decisions significantly declined in the vast majority of European jurisdictions in spring 2020 (European Migration Network EMN). Judicial actors, in turn, played a relatively significant role by both issuing release decisions and preventing the enforcement of detention measures in a number of jurisdictions such as France (Contrôleur Général des Lieux de Privation de Liberté CGLPL; Mucchielli 2020), Italy (Caprioglio and Rigo 2020; Roman 2020), and the UK (Harger 2020; Taylor 2020b). Specifically, the Swiss Federal Court handed down several critical decisions in this regard in June and July 2020 (24 Heures 2020a, 2020b).

Despite the relevant impact of these anti-coronavirus efforts on the immigration enforcement landscape, initiatives aimed at liberating all detained noncitizens and temporarily shutting down all detention facilities failed in a number of EU countries. This was the case in France, where a demand championed by ombudspersons (Contrôleur Général des Lieux de Privation de Liberté CGLPL), NGOs and lawyers (Observatoire de l'enfermement des étrangers OEE) was rejected by the Council of State, which considered it legally unjustified, in late March 2020 (Lecadre 2020). Likewise, in Britain, a legal challenge filed by a pro-migrant rights group (Detention Action 2020) was not upheld by the UK High Court, arguing that the number of released noncitizens was enough to safeguard detainees' right to healthcare (Ironmonger 2020).

3. Coronavirus and the Temporary Moratorium on Immigration Detention

In spite of the aforementioned institutional efforts, in Europe—as well as in the US-[4] anti-coronavirus policies fell short of imposing a moratorium on immigration detention and temporarily shutting custodial facilities. This was also the official stance adopted by the European Commission, which recommended EU member states to issue release decisions on a case-by-case basis (European Commission 2020a). The only exception to this widespread trend was the Spanish case (Jesuit Refugee Service JRS), since the Spanish administration actually released all detained immigrants and shut down its seven detention facilities on 6 May 2020 (Fernández-Bessa 2021; Martín 2020).

Spain has a long consolidated and relatively sizeable immigration enforcement system, which detains and deports significant contingents of unwanted noncitizens. More precisely, 132,448 noncitizens were confined in Spanish detention facilities from 2008 to 2019 (Fernández-Bessa 2021), and 214,470 foreign nationals were removed from Spain over the same twelve-year period (source: Eurostat). However, both dimensions of the mobility control apparatus have been shrinking in the recent past. The annual number of immigration detainees dwindled by 73.9 percent and that of removals declined by 58.5 percent from 2008 and 2019 (sources: Fernández-Bessa 2021; Eurostat). In stark contrast to this decline, Spain has witnessed a noteworthy increase in irregular border-crossing activities, particularly fuelled by the surge in the number of sea arrivals (Barbero Forthcoming),[5] which have had a significant impact on the Canary Islands in 2020 and 2021.

In Spain, immediately after the declaration of the state of alarm in mid-March 2020, various actors put the spotlight on the health measures to be taken in the field of immigration detention. Both migrant rights groups (Cies No 2020) and the National Ombudsman (Sainz 2020) called for the swift release of all detainees (see also Lopez-Sala 2021). The Spanish Minister of the Interior did not show an outright opposition to this demand; however, he claimed that release measures should be individually considered, rejecting any all-encompassing decision (Europa Press 2020a). However, the immigration enforcement scenario changed more rapidly than expected. Judicial actors stepped in issuing release injunctions based on the unsuitable sanitary conditions of detention facilities (Vargas 2020). By early April 2020, only 34 noncitizens remained in custody; four out of seven Spanish detention settings, including those of Madrid and Barcelona, had already been closed (Europa Press 2020b). Finally, less than eight weeks since the onset of the state of alarm, the last detainees were released in early May 2020 from CIE Algeciras, the detention facility located at the southern border. Spanish confinement facilities remained closed over a 4-month summer, until 23 September 2020 (Fernández-Bessa 2021; Muñoz and Vargas 2020). One month thereafter, the Spanish detention facilities were confining 186 noncitizens, the majority of whom had been detected while irregularly crossing the southern border (Sánchez 2020a). Reopening policies were gradually implemented, leading some detention sites to be put into operation again only in early 2021 (Fernández 2021).

Widespread release practices, and particularly the closure of the Spanish immigration detention estate are unexpected events that raise a number of questions. First, the forces contributing to the implementation of until recently unthinkable policies—which were not extended to the prison field—should be further scrutinised. This exploration may gain further insight into the nature, characteristics and operation of immigration detention policies in Europe. Second, the potentially lasting legacy of these exceptional events should be examined. This point will be analysed in the last section, whilst the remaining part focuses on the previous dilemma.

Crimmigration and border criminology scholars have long called into question the administrative law nature of immigration detention (Barker 2017; Bosworth 2019; García Hernández 2014), which is regulated as a precautionary measure exclusively aimed at preparing the eventual enforcement of a deportation order in the European case (Aas 2014; Bosworth 2012; Campesi 2013). Paradoxically, this legal nature was the basis of the far-reaching release schemes enacted in various European jurisdictions. The onset of the pandemic led to the immediate closure of borders in many countries, including global south countries of origin of irregular flows. This sudden re-bordering agenda made deportations unfeasible for some months in mid-2020, especially return procedures carried out by air and sea (European Migration Network EMN; Majkowska-Tomkin 2020).[6] The legal consequence of this unseen scenario is unambiguously laid down by Article 15(4) of the Return Directive (Directive 2008/115/EC of the European Parliament and of the Council of 16 December 2008), i.e., detained noncitizens must be immediately released when " ... reasonable prospect of removal no longer exist ... " (see Mitsilegas 2015; see also International Commission of Jurists ICJ).

The purposes of immigration detention policies have long been debated by the extant literature, which has elaborated a variety of theses on this topic. Border criminology scholars have scrutinised various immigration detention functions, both instrumental and symbolic, such as the management of destitute populations, the policing of membership boundaries, and the strengthening of national sovereignty (Bosworth 2019; Leerkes and Broeders 2010). The crimmigration thesis, in turn, underlines that immigration detention is being increasingly used for crime prevention purposes, rather than for its traditional mission related to immigration law breaches (García Hernández 2014; Turnbull 2017; see also Zedner 2016). Other authors embrace what might be called a "general deterrence" viewpoint, in which detention practices are geared towards dissuading unwanted noncitizens from coming, settling and staying in a given (national) community (Bosworth 2019; Campesi 2015; Leerkes and Broeders 2010). In addition, another strand of literature brings to the fore "special deterrence" goals, by claiming that detention policies are aimed at coercively persuading targeted noncitizens "to leave", by either collaborating in preparing their forced removals or signing in for so-called "voluntary return" programmes (Hasselberg 2016; Leerkes and Kox 2017; Martínez et al. 2018).

However, the public health crisis led the legal nature of immigration detention as a pre-removal precautionary measure to take precedence over any other detention goal. In fact, the extra-legal notion according to which detention procedures are also used to confine and incapacitate high-risk noncitizens, e.g., former prisoners, was only exceptionally alleged by certain national authorities in countries such as Belgium (Coppens 2020), Finland, the Netherlands (source: GDP COVID-19 Platform), and the UK (Ironmonger 2020) to justify the issuance or extension of detention orders (see though Esposito et al. 2020).

This analysis of the factors conditioning the immigration detention decline should also scrutinise why Spain was the only global north country closing down its detention sites in the framework of the pandemic. Immediately after Italy, Spain was one of the first European countries to be hardest hit by the COVID-19 pandemic. The MIPEX index ranks Spain relatively high in terms of migrant integration policies. In addition, despite the recent electoral impetus of the anti-immigration sentiments of far-right political party Vox, they do not seem to be particularly widespread in the Spanish case, if compared with other global north countries (D'Ancona 2016; Wonders 2017). Beyond all these background conditions, two more specific issues are what determined the exceptional decisions made by the Spanish authorities in the spring–summer of 2020. Their approach to anti-coronavirus measures in the field of immigration detention was particularly conditioned by legal provisions on the maximum length of detention (Piser 2020; Roman 2020). In Europe, detention time may be currently unlimited only in Ireland and the UK. These exceptional cases aside, detention time limits vary greatly among EU and EFTA countries. In the framework of these variations, Portugal and Spain have the shortest time limit, i.e., two months of detention, followed by France, with a three-month limit (Majcher et al. 2020). Consequently, especially tight time constraints played a pivotal role in the detention decline witnessed in the Spanish case.

Additionally, the impact of public health policies on the deportation field was also critical in fostering a temporary moratorium on immigration detention. Evidently, border closures and international travel restrictions dramatically affected removal activities in many European jurisdictions. However, a wide number of European jurisdictions such as Belgium, Cyprus (Knews 2020b), Finland, France (Contrôleur Général des Lieux de Privation de Liberté CGLPL), Germany (InfoMigrants 2020), the Netherlands, Norway, Poland, Portugal, Switzerland, and the UK managed to avoid a complete halt of their deportation practices even in the worst phases of the coronavirus pandemic (sources: GDP COVID-19 Platform; European Council on Refugees and Exiles ECRE; European Migration Network EMN; Fundamental Rights Agency FRA). Bulgaria, Croatia, Estonia, Slovakia and other countries, in turn, continued carrying out removals by land to neighbouring countries in spring 2020 (sources: GDP COVID-19 Platform; European Migration Network EMN; Fundamental Rights Agency FRA). In some jurisdictions, so-called Dublin returns aimed at re-settling asylum seekers among EU countries were particularly affected but other types of removals were not wholly hampered by travel ban provisions. Eurostat data also confirm that at least Greece, Italy, Poland, Slovenia, Sweden and the UK carried out hundreds of removals in the second quarter of 2020.[7] All in all, this official database reports that in various jurisdictions such as Bulgaria, France, Italy, Poland, and Slovakia the number of deportations was more than halved from 2019 to 2020, whilst in many other countries (Austria, Belgium, Croatia, Germany, Greece, Ireland, Latvia, Lithuania, the Netherlands, Romania, among others) this decline was from 20 percent to 50 percent.[8]

In Spain, the number of deportations dwindled by 57.5 percent from 2019 to 2020 (source: Eurostat). However, the aforementioned data show that Spain was not the only European country forced to scale down its removal practices. Consequently, the specific configuration of deportation policies in the Spanish case is what actually contributed to the enactment of a migration detention moratorium. In a jurisdiction suffering a significant "deportation gap" (Gibney 2008; Rosenberger and Küffner 2016) such as Spain,[9] deportation procedures are particularly and increasingly targeted. Removal operations carried out by land to neighbouring countries are irrelevant in the Spanish case. By contrast, return procedures targeting Moroccan and Algerian nationals make up the lion's share of Spanish deportation policies (Fernández-Bessa 2021; Fernández Bessa and Brandariz 2018); these two national groups combined accounted for 62.8 percent of the removal orders enforced in Spain from 2015 to 2019.[10] Therefore, the measures rapidly adopted in these countries and other critical countries for Spanish deportation policies such as Colombia to close borders and suspend international travel undermined the legal grounds of detention practices (Orejudo 2020).

Having said that, an additional point should be taken into consideration to understand immigration enforcement changes in Spain. In a country lacking a consolidated, far-reaching network of reception facilities, Spanish law enforcement agencies have long channelled immigrant and asylum-seeking newcomers into detention sites (Fernández-Bessa 2021). Evidently, the pandemic led to a significant change in the field of migration policing, since detected undocumented noncitizens were not directed towards detention resources any longer.[11] By contrast, irregular border-crossers were hosted in makeshift reception facilities and largely confined in the Canary Islands.[12] Surely, this migration policing shift was partly fostered by more general policing changes implemented in the framework of the anti-covid policy agenda. In fact, the Spanish administration concentrated policing resources in deploying an arguably unprecedented operation aimed at monitoring and penalising quarantine and lockdown breaches in spring 2020 (López-Riba 2020).

In sum, national policy agendas resulted in marked variations in the ways in which European states tackled infection risks in the field of immigration detention. This is unsurprising, since the multi-scalar nature of mobility governance in Europe (Brandariz and Fernández-Bessa 2020; Moffette 2018; Wonders 2017) gives shape to a notably diverse migration enforcement scenario (Brandariz 2021). This diversity was surely compounded by the re-bordering processes fuelled by the coronavirus pandemic, which reinforced chauvinist perspectives and agendas in managing the public health emergency. In this variegated framework, the Spanish administration went as far as to empty all detention facilities for a 4-month-and-17-day period. After having explored the forces and conditions contributing to that exceptional decision, the last section reflects on whether the widespread release practices set in motion in mid-2020 may pave the way for an enduring immigration detention decline in Europe.

4. Concluding Remarks: The Short Summer of Abolitionism?

In 1972, the German writer Hans Magnus Enzensberger published his book *The Short Summer of Anarchy* (*Der Kurze Sommer der Anarchie*). In between fiction and document, Enzensberger's essay narrates the life and death of the Spanish anarchist leader Buenaventura Durruti, with a special focus on the exceptional events that occurred in the summer of 1936. Back then, against the backdrop of the initial stages of the Spanish Civil War (1936–1939), anarchist activists and organisations engaged in a widespread revolutionary effort that actually eroded the capitalist rule in several Eastern Spain regions. This revolutionary impetus, though, did not last much longer than a short summer, before being completely defeated in spring 1937.

In a loose analogy to Enzensberger's book, a question arises as to whether the groundbreaking detention policies enacted in 2020 may reverberate beyond the brief summer of its legal validity (see also Roman 2020; Weber 2020). Certain evidence may lead one to infer that what happened in the European immigration detention scenario in mid-2020 was actually unique and unrepeatable. Despite the long-lasting impact of the public health crisis, immigration enforcement practices seem to have been largely brought back on track throughout Europe (Fundamental Rights Agency FRA; European Migration Network EMN; Jesuit Refugee Service JRS). Even in Spain, deportation practices resumed in late 2020 (Sánchez 2020b). In addition, a close look at what has happened inside the Spanish reception facilities located in northern Africa prevents any naïve conclusion associating Spain's immigration detention policies with any new, human rights-based agenda in the field of border and mobility management policies. In stark contrast to its approach to immigration detention, the Spanish Ministry of the Interior left the reception centres located in the enclave towns of Ceuta and Melilla unattended,[13] although the noncitizens sheltered in place had to cope with quarantine measures in these overcrowded and degraded facilities (Amnesty International 2020; Council of Europe 2020). This concerning scenario resonates with what has been happening in the Canary Islands since autumn 2020. A surge in the number of arrivals in the archipelago has been met by the Spanish administration by providing substandard reception conditions and impeding newcomers from travelling to the mainland (see, e.g., MacGregor 2021; Martín 2021; Human Rights Watch HRW). At least in this regard, the Spanish case is no exception. On the contrary, the policies adopted by Spain to tackle mobility flows have been worryingly similar to those recently implemented in other Mediterranean countries such as Cyprus and Greece.

These unpromising signs apparently forecast a rapid return to a business-as-usual scenario in immigration enforcement policies. However, there are certain reasons to think that what happened in the immigration detention field may actually reverberate well beyond the brief summer of 2020, having lasting consequences. In political terms, the pandemic created suitable conditions to spotlight detention practices and to rally a broad variety of actors behind an agenda aimed at putting human rights before border control interests. In empirical terms, the events of 2020 have been incidentally hailed as a pathway to detention abolition (Fialho and Moreno 2020). This may be an overstatement, especially if detention abolition is seen in the framework of a more far-reaching effort to abolish the carceral state (on this notion of prison abolition see García Hernández 2017; Shah 2021; Ybarra 2021). However, those events may operate as a humble albeit promising precedent, since national and EU authorities have verified that a significant reduction in the immigration detention estate does not lead the immigration enforcement apparatus to collapse (Esposito et al. 2020; Harger 2020; Saiz 2020). Consequently, this precedent might work as a political and policy resource to be leveraged for abolition purposes; in other words, it should be used to advocate a sharp, gradual and incremental reduction in immigration detention. In legal terms, what happened in Spain and other Western and Northern European countries in mid-2020 gave a significant boost to some easily overlooked legal principles regulating immigration detention in Europe. First, detention measures can only be imposed to prepare an eventual removal (Art. 15(1) and 15(5) of the Return Directive). Consequently, these law enforcement measures cannot be legally used to pursue any other competing goal, not even public protection purposes. Second, detention measures are not legally justified when other less coercive measures may warrant the eventual enforcement of the corresponding removal order (Art. 15(1) of the Return Directive). Third, detainees have to be released as soon as " ... a reasonable prospect of removal no longer exists ... " (Art. 15(4) of the Return Directive; see also Article 5(1)(f) of the European Convention on Human Rights).

Were this handful of legal tenets to be seriously taken into consideration, as it happened in 2020, they might significantly and enduringly alter the immigration detention landscape in Europe. As has been officially recognised (European Commission 2017, 2020b), a number of European jurisdictions are notably inefficient in enforcing their crimmigration policies. Eurostat data show that Belgium, Bulgaria, the Czech Republic, France, Italy, and Portugal had an average enforcement rate lower than 30 percent from 2008 to 2019. Detention policies do not seem to be of much use in bridging that deportation gap. In fact, in various European countries, wide swathes of the detained populations are placed under custody for relatively long periods without reasonable prospects of eventual deportation. Therefore, detention policies have long proven to be relatively ineffective, for significant percentages of detainees end up being released—or bailed—instead of deported. In Britain, 48.4 percent of the noncitizens detained from 2010 to 2019 were not removed but released on bail or after having been granted a leave to remain (source: Home Office; www.gov.uk/government/statistics/immigration-statistics-year-ending-march-2020/how-many-people-are-detained-or-returned; accessed on 19 April 2021). What is more, the removal rate has been constantly declining since the early 2010s. In the Spanish case, it is estimated that 50.5 percent of the undocumented noncitizens detained from 2010 to 2019 were not subsequently deported (Fernández-Bessa 2021). Similarly, official data report that no more than 49.8 percent of the detainees placed under custody in Italy from 2017 to 2019 were eventually removed (source: Garante Nazionale dei diritti delle persona detenute; www.garantenazionaleprivatiliberta.it/gnpl/it/pub_rel_par.page; accessed on 19 April 2021). Detention policies are even slightly less effective in a country such as France, which combines a sizeable immigration detention estate and relatively low deportation enforcement rates. La Cimade reports (www.lacimade.org/publication/?type-publication=rapports-sur-la-retention-administrative; accessed on 19 April 2021) estimate that only 45.6 percent of the noncitizens confined in French detention facilities from 2010 to 2019 were ultimately removed.

Although national and EU authorities are long aware of these shortcomings, they do not seem to be particularly willing to bring detention policies in line with EU (and national) law provisions. However, current detention strategies are untenable in both managerial and legal terms. The partly useless nature of detention practices for deportation practices has long been addressed by stressing that immigration detention actually pursues a number of goals unrelated to removal procedures themselves (Fernández-Bessa 2021). However, coronavirus-era detention policies have eroded the standing of these extra-legal purposes. Consequently, what happened in 2020 should be leveraged to significantly reduce the immigration detention estate in Europe, which has proven to be—at least—partly dispensable to carry out mobility management tasks. Those coronavirus-related events showed that this aspiration may join a broad variety of actors in the political and public sphere. This political agenda may be buttressed by a very simple fact, i.e., in contrast to what may be thought, not all EU and EFTA countries have sizeable detention systems (Brandariz 2021). In fact, national detention apparatuses are relatively tiny and narrow-ranging not only in small countries such as Estonia and Latvia but also in the Czech Republic, Ireland, Romania, and—to a certain extent—Germany and Italy (source: GDP data; www.globaldetentionproject.org/regions-subregions/europe; accessed 15 April 2021). Eurostat data confirm that these parsimonious detention policies do not inevitably lead those countries to rank particularly low in terms of either deportation numbers or deportation enforcement rates.[14] These cases, therefore, illustrate that EU jurisdictions may dispense away with or at least significantly curtail their detention systems without seriously compromising their border control policies (see also Piser 2020).

In stark contrast to the re-bordering processes triggered by the pandemic, this paper aimed to show that we should adopt a cross-national perspective in rethinking detention policies. The supranational level may supply key political and legal tools to build an immigration enforcement system focusing on alternatives to detention rather than on detention practices. This effort might take stock of the migration detention arrangements tested in the framework of the pandemic. In so doing, the events of 2020 would work as a powerful precedent, not as a memento of an increasingly distant, short summer in which immigration detention seemed to be a vulnerable carceral institution.

Author Contributions: J.A.B. explored detention changes across Europe (Section 2), whilst C.F.-B. scrutinised the Spanish case (Section 3). Both authors co-authored the introduction (Section 1) and the conclusions (Section 4). Both authors have read and agreed to the published version of the manuscript.

Funding: This research received no external funding.

Institutional Review Board Statement: Not applicable.

Informed Consent Statement: Not applicable.

Data Availability Statement: Publicly available datasets were analyzed in this study. This data can be found here: Eurostat. Asylum and managed migration data, ec.europa.eu/eurostat/web/asylum-and-managed-migration/data/database; Garante Nazionale dei diritti delle persona detenute, www.garantenazionaleprivatiliberta.it/gnpl/it/pub_rel_par.page; Global Detention Project, www.globaldetentionproject.org/regions-subregions/europe; Home Office, www.gov.uk/government/statistics/immigration-statistics-year-ending-march-2020/how-many-people-are-detained-or-returned; La Cimade, www.lacimade.org/publication/?type-publication=rapports-sur-la-retention-administrative; Migration Integration Policy Index, www.mipex.eu; National Mechanism for the Prevention of Torture; www.defensordelpueblo.es/informe-mnp/mecanismo-nacional-prevencion-la-tortura-informe-anual-2019/; Spanish Ministry of the Interior, www.interior.gob.es/gl/prensa/balances-e-informes/2020; UNHCR, data2.unhcr.org/en/situations/mediterranean/location/5226. (Links are accessed on 19 April 2021).

Acknowledgments: We thank the two anonymous reviewers and the editor of this special issue, Robert Koulish (University of Maryland, US), for their support and recommendations in preparing this article.

Conflicts of Interest: The authors declare no conflict of interest.

Notes

[1] On cross-border mobility restrictions implemented since mid-2020 see the KPMG (assets.kpmg/content/dam/kpmg/xx/pdf/2020/05/Interactive-GMS-Covid-Tracker.pdf; accessed on 19 April 2021) and nccr—on the move (public.tableau.com/profile/nccr.on.the.move#!/vizhome/Covid-19outbreak_15843550159920/Lists; accessed on 19 April 2021) databases.

[2] Specifically, the Global Detention Project (GDP) Covid-19 Platform (www.globaldetentionproject.org/covid-19-immigration-detention-platform; accessed on 7 April 2021) was a critical source of information for this study. In a peculiar period in which scholars were largely unaware of what was happening beyond their national borders, this platform provided vital information to carry out comparative explorations.

[3] The Migration Integration Policy Index 2020 ranks these three Mediterranean countries very low in terms of integration policies, well below the vast majority of Western and Nordic European nations and many other non-European jurisdictions such as Canada, New Zealand, Australia, USA, Brazil, and Argentina (see www.mipex.eu/; accessed on 8 April 2021).

[4] Release policies apparently garnered less traction in the US than in various Western and Northern European countries. However, also in the US the combination of an ongoing deportation effort with the scaling down of migration policing arrests resulted

5   in a significant decline in the number of detained noncitizens in mid-2020 (European Migration Network EMN). In fact, it is estimated that the US detained population dwindled by 42.5 per cent from late March to late July 2020 (Kerwin 2020; see also Erfani et al. 2021; Tosh et al. 2021).

5   UNHCR data show that the number of irregular sea arrivals mounted from 8162 in 2016 to 40,326 in 2020, after having peaked at 58,569 in 2018 (see data2.unhcr.org/en/situations/mediterranean/location/5226; accessed on 28 May 2021). The clousure of the Eastern and central Mediterranean routes following the agreements between the EU and Turkey and between Italy and Lybia since 2017 has particularly contributed to this surge.

6   Deportation restrictions made a relevant difference between European cases and the US case. The US administration managed to keep its deportation routes with global south countries relatively open even in the framework of the especially severe border closures imposed in the first wave of the pandemic. In fact, it is estimated that around 40,000 noncitizens were deported from the US in spring 2020 (Kassie and Marcolini 2020; see also European Migration Network EMN; Kerwin 2020).

7   Poland, Slovenia and Sweden were also particularly active in this field in the summer of 2020 (source: Eurostat; see also Fundamental Rights Agency FRA). By contrast, the European Migration Network reports (European Migration Network EMN) that the number of deportations only returned to pre-pandemic levels in summer 2020 in Cyprus, the Czech Republic, Poland, and Switzerland.

8   Paradoxically, the number of enforced deportations rose from 2019 to 2020 in the Czech Republic, and especially in Cyprus and Hungary.

9   In Spain, only 32.5 per cent of the issued deportation orders were actually enforced from 2008 to 2019 (source: Eurostat. Asylum and managed migration data).

10   Moroccan and Algerian nationals combined accounted for 44.1 per cent of the undocumented noncitizens under custody in Spanish detention facilities from 2014 to 2018 (Fernández-Bessa 2021). In addition, these two national groups accounted for 75.2 per cent of the noncitizens deported from Spain in 2019 after having been confined in one of the seven pre-removal facilities (source: National Mechanism for the Prevention of Torture; www.defensordelpueblo.es/informe-mnp/mecanismo-nacional-prevencion-la-tortura-informe-anual-2019/; accessed on 16 April 2021).

11   The Spanish Ministry of the Interior data (see www.interior.gob.es/gl/prensa/balances-e-informes/2020; accessed on 14 April 2021) show that around 12,750 irregular border-crossers arrived to Spain from 1 May 2020 to 30 September 2020.

12   In 2020, more than 23,000 noncitizens arrived to the Canary Islands, a Spanish archipelago in the Atlantic Ocean which is relatively close to the Western Sahara's coastline. Since August 2020, these border-crossers were hosted in an emergency camp sited in the Arguineguín pier, Grand Canary, which was set up for medical screening—including COVID-19 testing, police identification and registration purposes. This substandard facility was bitterly criticised by the Spanish Ombudsman, HRW, and other NGOs, for both its overcrowding and unsanitary conditions and the violation of asylum and police custody provisions. Empty hotel rooms were also used as an emergency accommodation solution in summer 2020. Both hotel rooms and the precarious Arguineguín facility were replaced with a new custodial centre, the Barranco Seco CATE, and with the transformation of former factories and administrative buildings into reception facilities since November 2020 (see Human Rights Watch HRW; Gobierno de España 2020).

13   The Spanish enclaves of Ceuta and Melilla are located in northern Africa and sorrounded by razor-wired border walls. Both towns have reception facilities called CETI (for their initials in Spanish), which are aimed at hosting mainly asylum seeking border-crossers while they are awaiting either to receive an international protection decision or to be transferred to the Iberian peninsula.

14   As far as the number of enforced deportations is concerned, the majority of the mentioned jurisdictions does not play a leading role in the European deportation apparatus; Germany, though, is a top deporting country. In terms of enforcement rates, the Czech Republic, Italy, and also Ireland have relatively low rates, whereas Estonia, Germany, Latvia, and Romania are particularly efficient in enforcing their deportation orders.

References

24 Heures. 2020a. Le TF Critique la Détention en vue du Renvoi. *24 Heures*. Available online: www.24heures.ch/le-tf-critique-la-detention-en-vue-du-renvoi-352216366834 (accessed on 12 April 2021).

24 Heures. 2020b. Asile: Pas de Détention si le Renvoi est empêché par le Coronavirus. *24 Heures*. Available online: www.24heures.ch/asile-pas-de-detention-si-le-renvoi-est-empeche-par-le-coronavirus-783597632491 (accessed on 12 April 2021).

Aas, Katja Franko. 2014. Bordered Penality: Precarious Membership and Abnormal Justice. *Punishment & Society* 16: 520–41.

Aebi, Marcelo Fernando, and Mélanie Tiago. 2020. *Prisons and Prisoners in Europe in Pandemic Times: An Evaluation of the Medium-Term Impact of the COVID-19 on Prison Populations*. Strasbourg: Council of Europe, Available online: https://wp.unil.ch/space/files/2021/02/Prisons-and-the-COVID-19_2nd-Publication_201109.pdf (accessed on 8 April 2021).

Amnesty International. 2020. Es Urgente el Traslado y Realojo en Condiciones Dignas de las Personas Migrantes y Solicitantes de Asilo en Melilla. Available online: www.es.amnesty.org/en-que-estamos/noticias/noticia/articulo/es-urgente-el-traslado-y-realojo-en-condiciones-dignas-de-las-personas-migrantes-y-solicitantes-de-a/ (accessed on 15 April 2021).

Andreou, Evie. 2021. UN agency Calls for Decongestion of Migrant Camp after Brawl. *Cyprus Mail*. Available online: https://cyprus-mail.com/2021/01/13/eu-asylum-support-office-sending-more-personnel-to-cyprus/ (accessed on 9 April 2021).

ANSA. 2020. Coronavirus: Italian Detainee Rights Guarantor Concerned about Migrants in Repatriation Centers. *InfoMigrants*. Available online: www.infomigrants.net/en/post/23685/coronavirus-italian-detainee-rights-guarantor-concerned-about-migrants-in-repatriation-centers (accessed on 9 April 2021).

Barbero, Iker. Forthcoming. Los Centros de Atención Temporal de Extranjeros como nuevo modelo de gestión migratorio: Situación actual, (des)regulación jurídica y mecanismos de control de derechos y garantías. *Derechos y Libertades* 45.

Barker, Vanessa. 2017. Penal Power at the Border: Realigning State and Nation. *Theoretical Criminology* 21: 441–57. [CrossRef]

Bosworth, Mary. 2012. Subjectivity and Identity in Detention: Punishment and Society in a Global Age. *Theoretical Criminology* 16: 123–40. [CrossRef]

Bosworth, Mary. 2019. Immigration Detention, Punishment and the Transformation of Justice. *Social and Legal Studies* 28: 81–99. [CrossRef]

Brandariz, José Ángel. 2021. An expanded analytical gaze on penal power: Border criminology and punitiveness. *International Journal for Crime, Justice and Social Democracy* 10: 99–112. [CrossRef]

Brandariz, José Ángel, and Cristina Fernández-Bessa. 2020. A changing and multi-scalar EU borderscape: The expansion of asylum and the normalisation of the deportation of EU and EFTA citizens. *International Journal for Crime, Justice and Social Democracy* 9: 21–33. [CrossRef]

Bulman, May. 2021. Immigration Detention Centre Forced to Close due to Covid Outbreak. *The Independent*. Available online: www.independent.co.uk/news/uk/home-news/immigration-detention-centre-closed-covid-outbreak-home-office-b1784499.html (accessed on 18 April 2021).

Campesi, Giuseppe. 2013. *La detenzione Amministrativa degli Stranieri: Storia, Diritto, Politica*. Roma: Carocci.

Campesi, Giuseppe. 2015. Hindering the Deportation Machine: An Ethnography of Power and Resistance in Immigration Detention. *Punishment & Society* 17: 427–53.

Caprioglio, Carlo, and Enrica Rigo. 2020. Le Restrizioni alla Libertà di Movimento ai Tempi del Covid-19. *Questione Giustizia*. Available online: www.questionegiustizia.it/articolo/le-restrizioni-alla-liberta-di-movimento-ai-tempi-del-covid-19_30-03-2020.php (accessed on 9 April 2021).

Carretero, Leslie. 2020. Coronavirus: En Belgique, "l'Etat ne fait rien pour protéger les migrants". *InfoMigrants*. Available online: www.infomigrants.net/fr/post/23785/coronavirus-en-belgique-l-etat-ne-fait-rien-pour-proteger-les-migrants (accessed on 9 April 2021).

Cassidy, Jane. 2020. Alison Thewliss Urges Release of Immigration Detainees. *The National*. Available online: www.thenational.scot/news/18375848.alison-thewliss-urges-release-immigration-detainees/ (accessed on 12 April 2021).

Contrôleur Général des Lieux de Privation de Liberté (CGLPL). 2020. Les Droits Fondamentaux des Personnes Privées de Liberté à l'épreuve de la Crise Sanitaire: 17 Mars au 10 Juin 2020. Available online: www.cglpl.fr/wp-content/uploads/2020/07/CGLPL_Rapport-COVID.pdf (accessed on 9 April 2021).

Chew, Vivienne, Melissa Phillips, and Min Yamada Park, eds. 2020. *COVID-19 Impacts on Immigration Detention: Global Responses*. Sydney: International Detention Coalition and HADRI/Western Sydney University, Available online: Idcoalition.org/wp-content/uploads/2020/10/COVID-19-Impacts-on-Immigration-Detention-Global-Responses-2020.pdf (accessed on 16 April 2021).

Cies No. 2020. Ante el Coronavirus, Exigimos la Libertad para las Personas Internas en los Centros de Internamiento de Extranjeros. Available online: Ciesno.wordpress.com/2020/03/13/ante-el-coronavirus-exigimos-la-libertad-para-las-personas-internas-en-los-centros-de-internamiento-de-extranjeros/ (accessed on 13 April 2021).

Coalizione Italiana Libertà e Diritti Civili (CILD). 2020. Detenzione Migrante ai Tempi del Covid. Available online: https://cild.eu/wp-content/uploads/2020/07/Dossier_MigrantiCovid.pdf (accessed on 21 April 2021).

Commissioner for Human Rights. 2020. Council of Europe. Commissioner Calls for Release of Immigration Detainees While Covid-19 Crisis Continues. Available online: www.coe.int/en/web/commissioner/thematic-work/covid-19/-/asset_publisher/5cdZW0AJBMLl/content/commissioner-calls-for-release-of-immigration-detainees-while-covid-19-crisis-continues?inheritRedirect=false&redirect=https%3A%2F%2Fwww.coe.int%2Fen%2Fweb%2Fcommissioner%2Fthematic-work%2Fcovid-19%3Fp_p_id%3D101_INSTANCE_5cdZW0AJBMLl%26p_p_lifecycle%3D0%26p_p_state%3Dnormal%26p_p_mode%3Dview%26p_p_col_id%3Dcolumn-1%26p_p_col_count%3D1 (accessed on 9 April 2020).

Connor, Phillip. 2020. *More than Nine-in-Ten People Worldwide Live in Countries with Travel Restrictions Amid COVID-19*. Washington, DC: Pew Research Centre, Available online: www.pewresearch.org/fact-tank/2020/04/01/more-than-nine-in-ten-people-worldwide-live-in-countries-with-travel-restrictions-amid-covid-19/ (accessed on 14 April 2021).

Conxicoeur, Christian. 2020. Coronavirus Covid-19: Le Centre de rétention Administrative de Lyon Presque Entièrement évacué. France Info. Available online: https://france3-regions.francetvinfo.fr/auvergne-rhone-alpes/rhone/lyon/coronavirus-covid-19-centre-retention-administrative-lyon-presque-entierement-evacue-1805022.html (accessed on 9 April 2021).

Coppens, Marc. 2020. 200 illegale personen op vrije voeten als gevolg van coronacrisis. *HLN*. Available online: www.hln.be/binnenland/200-illegale-personen-op-vrije-voeten-als-gevolg-van-coronacrisis~{|a1b17321/?referer=https%3A%2F%2Ft.co%2FKoFwOrmDFr%3Famp%3D1 (accessed on 9 April 2021).

Cossé, Eva. 2020. Greece Again Extends Covid-19 Lockdown at Refugee Camps. *Human Rights Watch*. Available online: www.hrw.org/news/2020/06/12/greece-again-extends-covid-19-lockdown-refugee-camps (accessed on 9 April 2021).

Council of Europe. 2020. Spain's Authorities Must Find Alternatives to Accommodating Migrants, Including Asylum Seekers, in Substandard Conditions in Melilla. Available online: www.coe.int/en/web/commissioner/-/spain-s-authorities-must-find-alternatives-to-accommodating-migrants-including-asylum-seekers-in-substandard-conditions-in-melilla (accessed on 15 April 2021).

D'Ancona, María Ángeles Cea. 2016. Immigration as a threat: Explaining the changing pattern of xenophobia in Spain. *Journal of International Migration and Integration* 17: 569–91. [CrossRef]

De Giorgi, Alessandro. 2010. Immigration control, post-Fordism, and less eligibility: A materialist critique of the criminalization of immigration across Europe. *Punishment & Society* 12: 147–67.

Dehm, Sara. 2020. The Entrenchment of the Medical Border in Pandemic Times. *Border Criminologies*. Available online: www.law.ox.ac.uk/research-subject-groups/centre-criminology/centreborder-criminologies/blog/2020/07/entrenchment (accessed on 7 April 2021).

Detention Action. 2020. Covid-19: People Must Be Released from Detention. Legal Challenge and Petition. Available online: Detention.org.uk/covid-19-people-must-be-released-from-detention-legal-challenge-and-petition/ (accessed on 12 April 2021).

DLA Piper. 2021. A Global Analysis of Prisoner Releases in Response to COVID-19. Available online: www.dlapiper.com/en/france/news/2021/03/swift-targeted-action-to-reduce-prison-population-during-covid-19/ (accessed on 31 May 2021).

European Committee for the Prevention of Torture (ECPT). 2021. Report to the Maltese Government on the Visit to Malta Carried Out by the European Committee for the Prevention of Torture and Inhuman or Degrading Treatment or Punishment (CPT) from 17 to 22 September 2020. CPT/Inf (2021) 1. Available online: https://rm.coe.int/1680a1b877 (accessed on 12 April 2021).

European Council on Refugees and Exiles (ECRE). 2020. Information Sheet 5 May 2020: Covid-19 Measures Related to Asylum and Migration across Europe. Available online: www.ecre.org/wp-content/uploads/2020/05/COVID-INFO-5-May-.pdf (accessed on 9 April 2020).

European Migration Network (EMN). 2020. Special Annex to the 30th EMN Bulletin. EU Member States & Norway: Responses to COVID-19 in the Migration and Asylum área. January—March 2020. Available online: https://ec.europa.eu/home-affairs/sites/default/files/00_eu_30_emn_bulletin_annex_covid_19.pdf (accessed on 20 April 2021).

European Migration Network (EMN). 2021. Inform #5—Impact of Covid-19 Pandemic on Voluntary and Forced Return Procedures and Policy Responses. Available online: https://ec.europa.eu/home-affairs/sites/default/files/docs/pages/00_eu_inform5_return_en.pdf (accessed on 20 April 2021).

Erfani, Parsa, Nishant Uppal, Caroline Lee, Ranit Mishori, and Katherine Peeler. 2021. COVID-19 Testing and Cases in Immigration Detention Centers, April-August 2020. *JAMA* 325: 182–84. [CrossRef] [PubMed]

Esposito, Francesca, Emilio Caja, and Giacomo Mattiello. 2020. "No one is Looking at Us Anymore." Migrant Detention and Covid-19 in Italy. Border Criminologies. Available online: www.law.ox.ac.uk/sites/files/oxlaw/no_one_is_looking_at_us_anymore_1.pdf (accessed on 4 May 2021).

Europa Press. 2020a. Interior abre la Puerta Liberar a Internos en CIE tras Analizar 'caso por caso' Posibilidades de Retorno. Europa Press. Available online: www.europapress.es/epsocial/migracion/noticia-interior-abre-puerta-liberar-internos-cie-analizar-caso-caso-posibilidades-retorno-20200319192419.html (accessed on 13 April 2021).

Europa Press. 2020b. Los dos centros de internamiento de extranjeros de Canarias ya están vacíos. ElDiario. Available online: www.eldiario.es/canariasahora/365-dias-de-migraciones/centros-internamiento-extranjeros-canarias-vacios_132_1211080.html (accessed on 13 April 2021).

European Commission. 2017. Commission Recommendation of 7 March 2017 on Making Returns More Effective When Implementing the Directive 2008/115/EC of the European Parliament and of the Council. C(2017) 1600 Final. Available online: https://ec.europa.eu/home-affairs/sites/default/files/what-we-do/policies/european-agenda-migration/20170302_commission_recommendation_on_making_returns_more_effective_en.pdf (accessed on 19 April 2021).

European Commission. 2020a. Communication from the Commission. Covid-19: Guidance on the Implementation of Relevant EU Provisions in the Area of Asylum and Return Procedures and on Resettlement. C(2020) 2516 Final. Available online: https://ec.europa.eu/info/sites/info/files/guidance-implementation-eu-provisions-asylum-retur-procedures-resettlement.pdf (accessed on 20 April 2021).

European Commission. 2020b. Communication from the Commission to the European Parliament, the Council, the European Economic and Social Committee and the Committee of the Regions on a New Pact on Migration and Asylum. COM(2020) 609 Final. Available online: https://eur-lex.europa.eu/resource.html?uri=cellar:85ff8b4f-ff13-11ea-b44f-01aa75ed71a1.0002.02/DOC_3&format=PDF (accessed on 19 April 2021).

European Commission. 2021. Member States' Notifications of the Temporary Reintroduction of Border Control at Internal Borders Pursuant to Article 25 and 28 et seq. of the Schengen Borders Code. Available online: https://ec.europa.eu/home-affairs/sites/default/files/what-we-do/policies/borders-and-visas/schengen/reintroduction-border-control/docs/ms_notifications_-_reintroduction_of_border_control.pdf (accessed on 6 April 2021).

Expresso. 2020. Carta aberta. Covid-19 e os Centros de Detenção em Portugal: 41 associações e mais de 100 cidadãos pedem libertação dos Migrantes. Expresso. Available online: https://expresso.pt/opiniao/2020-04-09-Carta-aberta.-Covid-19-e-os-Centros-de-Detencao-em-Portugal-41-associacoes-e-mais-de-100-cidadaos-pedem-libertacao-dos-migrantes (accessed on 12 April 2021).

FARR. 2020. Stoppa Utvisningarna av våra Medmänniskor Omedelbart! Available online: www.mynewsdesk.com/se/farr/pressreleases/stoppa-utvisningarna-av-vaara-medmaenniskor-omedelbart-2982462 (accessed on 12 April 2021).

Fernández, Soraya. 2021. Interior reabre el Desvencijado CIE de Algeciras tras Gastar más de un millón en reformas. *ABC*. Available online: https://sevilla.abc.es/andalucia/cadiz/sevi-interior-reabre-desvencijado-algeciras-tras-gastar-mas-millon-reformas-202101230944_noticia.html (accessed on 13 April 2021).

Fernández-Bessa, Cristina. 2021. *Los Centros de Internamiento de Extranjeros: Una Introducción Desde las Ciencias Penales*. Madrid: Iustel.

Fernández Bessa, Cristina, and José Ángel Brandariz. 2018. 'Profiles' of Deportability: Analyzing Spanish Migration Control Policies from a Neocolonial Perspective. In *The Palgrave Handbook of Criminology and the Global South*. Edited by Kerry Carrington, Russell Hogg, John Scott and Máximo Sozzo. London: Palgrave, pp. 775–95.

Fialho, Christina, and Nacho Hernández Moreno. 2020. In the Age of COVID, Spain Offers the World a Pathway to Detention Abolition. *Immprint*. July 7. Available online: https://imm-print.com/in-the-age-of-covid-spain-offers-the-world-a-pathway-to-detention-abolition/ (accessed on 31 May 2021).

Fundamental Rights Agency (FRA). 2020a. Migration: Key Fundamental Rights Concerns—Quarterly Bulletin 3—2020. Available online: https://fra.europa.eu/en/publication/2020/migration-key-fundamental-rights-concerns-quarterly-bulletin-3-2020 (accessed on 21 April 2021).

Fundamental Rights Agency (FRA). 2020b. Migration: Key Fundamental Rights Concerns—Quarterly Bulletin 4—2020. Available online: https://fra.europa.eu/en/publication/2020/migration-key-fundamental-rights-concerns-quarterly-bulletin-4-2020 (accessed on 21 April 2021).

García Hernández, César Cuauhtémoc. 2014. Immigration Detention as Punishment. *UCLA Law Review* 61: 1346–414.

García Hernández, César Cuauhtémoc. 2017. Abolishing Immigration Prisons. *Boston University Law Review* 97: 245–300.

Global Detention Project (GDP). 2020. Country Report: Immigration Detention in Belgium: Covid-19 Puts the Brakes on an Expanding Detention System. Available online: www.globaldetentionproject.org/immigration-detention-belgium-2020 (accessed on 21 April 2021).

Genschel, Philipp, and Markus Jachtenfuchs. 2021. Postfunctionalism reversed: Solidarity and rebordering during the COVID-19 pandemic. *Journal of European Public Policy* 28: 350–69. [CrossRef]

Gibney, Matthew. 2008. Asylum and the Expansion of Deportation in the United Kingdom. *Government and Opposition* 43: 146–67. [CrossRef]

Gobierno de España. 2020. El Ministerio de Inclusión alcanzará las 7.000 plazas propias de acogida en siete nuevos espacios en Canarias. In *Gabinete de Comunicación. Ministerio de Inclusión, Seguridad social y Migraciones*; November 20. Available online: https://prensa.inclusion.gob.es/WebPrensaInclusion/noticias/ministro/detalle/3935 (accessed on 2 June 2021).

Hafezi, Parisa. 2020. Iran Temporarily Frees 85,000 from Jail Including Political Prisoners. *Reuters*. March 17. Available online: www.reuters.com/article/us-health-coronavirus-iran-prisoners-idUSKBN21410M (accessed on 19 April 2021).

Hall, Ben, Guy Chazan, Daniel Dombey, Sam Fleming, Davide Ghiglione, Miles Johnson, Sam Jones, and Victor Mallet. 2020. How Coronavirus Exposed Europe's Weaknesses. *Financial Times*. Available online: www.ft.com/content/efdadd97-aef5-47f1-91de-fe02c41a470a (accessed on 16 April 2021).

Harger, Rachel. 2020. Immigration Detention and the Politics of COVID-19. *Red Pepper*. Available online: www.redpepper.org.uk/immigration-detention-and-the-politics-of-covid-19/ (accessed on 12 April 2021).

Hasselberg, Ines. 2016. *Enduring Uncertainty: Deportation, Punishment and Everyday Life*. New York: Berghahn.

Hawks, Laura, Steffie Woolhandler, and Danny McCormick. 2020. COVID-19 in Prisons and Jails in the United States. *JAMA Internal Medicine* 180: 1041–42. [CrossRef] [PubMed]

Home Office. 2020. Statistics Relating to COVID-19 and the Immigration System, May 2020. Available online: https://assets.publishing.service.gov.uk/government/uploads/system/uploads/attachment_data/file/887808/statistics-relating-to-covid-19-and-the-immigration-system-may-2020.pdf (accessed on 12 April 2021).

Home Office. 2021. Guidance for Immigration Removal Centres (IRCs), Residential Short-Term Holding Facilities (RSTHFs) and Escorts during the COVID-19 Pandemic: Version 5.0. Available online: https://assets.publishing.service.gov.uk/government/uploads/system/uploads/attachment_data/file/957918/detention-and-escorting-services-guidance-during-covid-19-v5.0.pdf (accessed on 12 April 2021).

Hooks, Gregory, and Bob Libel. 2020. *Hotbeds of Infection: How ICE Detention Contributed to the Spread of COVID-19 in the United States*. Geneva: Global Detention Network, Available online: www.detentionwatchnetwork.org/sites/default/files/reports/DWN_Hotbeds%20of%20Infection_2020_FOR%20WEB.pdf (accessed on 19 April 2020).

Hooks, Gregory, and Wendy Sawyer. 2020. *Mass Incarceration, COVID-19, and Community Spread*. Northampton: Prison Policy Initiative, Available online: www.prisonpolicy.org/reports/covidspread.html (accessed on 8 April 2021).

Human Rights Watch (HRW). 2020. Spain: Respect Rights of People Arriving by Sea to Canary Islands. Ensure Adequate Reception Conditions, Accedd to Information and Asylum. Available online: www.hrw.org/news/2020/11/11/spain-respect-rights-people-arriving-sea-canary-islands (accessed on 2 June 2021).

International Commission of Jurists (ICJ). 2020. The Impact of COVID-19 Related Measures on Human Rights of Migrants and Refugees in the EU: Briefing Paper. Available online: www.icj.org/wp-content/uploads/2020/06/Covid19-impact-migrans-Europe-Brief-2020-ENG.pdf (accessed on 21 April 2021).

InfoMigrants. 2020. Deportations from Germany Halved During Pandemic. *InfoMigrants*. Available online: www.infomigrants.net/en/post/25997/deportations-from-germany-halved-during-pandemic (accessed on 19 April 2021).

Inquest. 2020. Powerful Coalition of Organisations Call on Government to Immediately Reduce Number of People in Detention Settings. Available online: www.inquest.org.uk/covid-19-letter (accessed on 12 April 2021).

Ironmonger, Jon. 2020. Coronavirus: UK Detention Centres 'Emptied in Weeks'. *BBC*. Available online: www.bbc.com/news/uk-525600932020 (accessed on 12 April 2021).

Jesuit Refugee Service (JRS). 2021. Covid-19 and Immigration Detention: Lessons (Not) Learned. Available online: https://jrseurope.org/en/resource/covid-19-and-immigration-detention-lessons-not-learned/ (accessed on 21 April 2021).

Kassie, Emily, and Barbara Marcolini. 2020. How ICE Exported the Coronavirus. The Marshall Project. Available online: www.themarshallproject.org/2020/07/10/how-ice-exported-the-coronavirus?utm_medium=social&utm_campaign=share-tools&utm_source=twitter&utm_content=post-top (accessed on 14 April 2021).

Kerwin, Donald. 2020. *Immigration Detention and Covid-19: How a Pandemic Exploited and Spread through the US Immigration Detention System*. New York: Center for Migration Studies, Available online: https://cmsny.org/wp-content/uploads/2020/08/CMS-Detention-COVID-Report-08-12-2020.pdf (accessed on 19 April 2021).

Kluth, Andreas. 2021. For the EU to Survive, It Can't Keep Failing. *Bloomberg*. Available online: www.bloomberg.com/opinion/articles/2021-03-04/the-european-union-is-failing-to-protect-its-own-citizens (accessed on 16 April 2021).

Knews. 2020a. NGOs Raise Alarm over Inhumane Conditions at Overcrowded Migrant Camp. *Knews*. Available online: https://knews.kathimerini.com.cy/en/news/ngos-raise-alarm-over-inhumane-conditions-at-overcrowded-migrant-detention-camp (accessed on 9 April 2021).

Knews. 2020b. Mass Deportations Underway in Cyprus. *Knews*. Available online: https://knews.kathimerini.com.cy/en/news/mass-deportations-underway-in-cyprus (accessed on 19 April 2021).

Knews. 2021. Officials Weigh in on Pournara Brawl. *Knews*. Available online: https://knews.kathimerini.com.cy/en/news/officials-weigh-in-on-pournara-brawl (accessed on 19 April 2021).

Kucukgocmen, Ali. 2020. *Turkish Parliament Passes Bill to Free Thousands from Prison Amid Coronavirus*. Toronto: Reuters, Available online: www.reuters.com/article/us-turkey-security-prisoners-idUSKCN21V241 (accessed on 19 April 2021).

La Cimade. 2020. Enfermement en Rétention Malgré la Situation Sanitaire et des Frontières Fermées aux Expulsions. Available online: www.lacimade.org/enfermement-en-retention-malgre-la-situation-sanitaire-et-des-frontieres-fermees-aux-expulsions/ (accessed on 9 April 2020).

Lasciateentrare. 2020. Associazioni e avvocati di tutta Italia scrivono al Ministro, alle Prefetture e ai Questori. *Lasciateentrare*. Available online: www.lasciatecientrare.it/emergenza-coronavirus-bloccare-gli-ingressi-nei-cpr-e-procedere-alla-progressiva-chiusura-dei-centri/ (accessed on 9 April 2020).

Lecadre, Renaud. 2020. Coronavirus: Le Conseil d'Etat refuse la fermeture des centres de retention. *Libération*. Available online: www.liberation.fr/france/2020/03/27/coronavirus-le-conseil-d-etat-refuse-la-fermeture-des-centres-de-retention_1783367/ (accessed on 9 April 2020).

Leerkes, Arjen, and Dennis Broeders. 2010. A case of mixed motives? Formal and informal functions of administrative immigration detention. *The British Journal of Criminology* 50: 830–50. [CrossRef]

Leerkes, Arjen, and Mieke Kox. 2017. Pressured into a Preference to Leave? A Study of the "Specific" Deterrent Effects and Perceived Legitimacy of Immigration Detention. *Law & Society Review* 51: 895–929.

Lindberg, Annika, Anna Lundberg, Sofia Häyhtiö, and Elisabet Rundqvist. 2020. Detained and Disregarded: How COVID-19 Has Affected Detained and Deportable Migrants in Sweden. Border Criminologies. Available online: www.law.ox.ac.uk/research-subject-groups/centre-criminology/centreborder-criminologies/blog/2020/07/detained-and (accessed on 12 April 2021).

Lopez, William, Nolan Kline, Alana LeBrón, Nicole Novak, María Elena De Trinidad Young, Gregg Gonsalves, Ranit Mishori, Basil Safi, and Ian Kysel. 2021. Preventing the Spread of COVID-19 in Immigration Detention Centers Requires the Release of Detainees. *American Journal of Public Health* 111: 110–15. [CrossRef]

López-Riba, José María. 2020. La gestión policial de la crisis sanitaria. Ctxt. Available online: https://ctxt.es/es/20200401/Politica/31731/Jose-Maria-Lopez-Riba-policia-coronavirus-confinamiento-estado-alarma.htm (accessed on 14 April 2021).

Lopez-Sala, Ana. 2021. Luchando por sus derechos en tiempos de Covid-19. Resistencias y reclamaciones de regularización de los migrantes *Sinpapeles* en España. *REMHU, Revista Interdisciplinar da Mobilidade Humana* 29: 83–96. [CrossRef]

Loran, Charlie. 2020. Riots at the CETI Centre in Melilla Come to an End, But How Long for? *EuroWeekly News*. Available online: www.euroweeklynews.com/2020/08/27/riots-at-the-ceti-centre-in-melilla-come-to-an-end-but-how-long-for/ (accessed on 19 April 2021).

MacGregor, Marion. 2021. New Migrant Camps in the Canary Islands. *InfoMigrants*. Available online: www.infomigrants.net/en/post/29909/spain-new-migrant-camps-in-the-canary-islands (accessed on 15 April 2021).

Macmadu, Alexandria, Justin Berk, Eliana Kaplowitz, Marquisele Mercedes, Josiah Rich, and Lauren Brinkley-Rubinstein. 2020. COVID-19 and mass incarceration: A call for urgent action. *The Lancet Public Health* 5: E71–E72. [CrossRef]

Majcher, Izabella, Michael Flynn, and Mariette Grange. 2020. Introduction: Harmonising, Institutionalising, Normalising: How the "Crisis" Became an Opportunity for Expanding Immigration Detention Regimes. In *Immigration Detention in the European Union: In the Shadow of the 'Crisis'*. Edited by Izabella Majcher, Michael Flynn and Mariette Grange. Cham: Springer, pp. 1–13.

Majkowska-Tomkin, Magda. 2020. Countries Are Suspending Immigration Detention Due to Coronavirus. Let's Keep It That Way. *Euronews*. Available online: www.euronews.com/2020/04/29/countries-suspending-immigration-detention-due-to-coronavirus-let-s-keep-it-that-way-view (accessed on 8 April 2021).

Martín, María. 2020. Los Centros de Internamiento de Extranjeros se vacían por primera vez en tres décadas. *El País*. Available online: https://elpais.com/espana/2020-05-06/se-vacian-los-centros-de-internamiento-de-extranjeros-por-primera-vez-en-tres-decadas.html (accessed on 12 April 2021).

Martín, María. 2021. Tension Spreads Through Migrant Shelters in Spain's Canary Islands. *El País*. Available online: https://english.elpais.com/spanish_news/2021-02-08/tension-spreads-through-migrant-shelters-in-spains-canary-islands.html (accessed on 15 April 2021).

Martínez, Daniel, Jeremy Slack, and Ricardo Martínez-Schuldt. 2018. The Rise of Mass Deportation in the United States. In *The Handbook of Race, Ethnicity, Crime, and Justice*. Edited by Ramiro Martínez Jr., Meghan Hollis and Jacob Stowell. Hoboken: Willey Blackwell, pp. 173–201.

Mitsilegas, Valsamis. 2015. *The Criminalisation of Migration in Europe: Challenges for Human Rights and the Rule of Law*. New York: Springer.

Moffette, David. 2018. *Governing Irregular Migration: Bordering Culture, Labour, and Security in Spain*. Vancouver: UBC Press.

Mucchielli, Julien. 2020. Les centres de rétention se vident, l'administration persiste. *Dalloz actualité*. Available online: www.dalloz-actualite.fr/flash/centres-de-retention-se-vident-l-administration-persiste#.YHB0eT9pqUl (accessed on 9 April 2021).

Muñoz, Lucía, and Jairo Vargas. 2020. Interior reabre de inmediato y en plena segunda ola los CIE cerrados por la pandemia. *Público*. Available online: www.publico.es/sociedad/reapertura-cie-interior-reabre-inmediato-plena-segunda-ola-cie-cerrados-pandemia.html (accessed on 13 April 2021).

NOS. 2020. Vreemdelingen vrijgelaten uit detentie vanwege coronacrisis. *NOS*. Available online: https://nos.nl/artikel/2328839-vreemdelingen-vrijgelaten-uit-detentie-vanwege-coronacrisis.html (accessed on 12 April 2021).

Observatoire de l'enfermement des étrangers (OEE). 2020. Face à la crise sanitaire, l'enfermement administratif des personnes étrangères doit immédiatement cesser. Available online: https://observatoireenfermement.blogspot.com/p/communiques-de-presse.html (accessed on 9 April 2021).

Orejudo, Patricia. 2020. Los centros de internamiento de extranjeros ante la situación del Covid-19. *Otrosí*. Available online: www.otrosi.net/analisis/los-centros-internamiento-extranjeros-ante-la-situacion-del-covid-19 (accessed on 14 April 2021).

Piser, Karina. 2020. The End of Immigration Detention Doesn't Mean the End of Fortress Europe. *Foreign Policy*. Available online: https://foreignpolicy.com/2020/07/31/coronavirus-asylum-end-immigration-detention-spain-france-end-of-fortress-europe/ (accessed on 16 April 2021).

Refugee Rights Europe. 2020. The Invisible Islands: Covid-19 Restrictions and the Future of Detention on Kos and Leros. Available online: https://refugee-rights.eu/wp-content/uploads/2020/05/RRE_TheInvisibleIslands.pdf (accessed on 9 April 2021).

Roman, Emanuela. 2020. Rethinking Immigration Detention During and After Covid-19: Insights from Italy. Border Criminologies. Available online: www.law.ox.ac.uk/research-subject-groups/centre-criminology/centreborder-criminologies/blog/2020/06/rethinking (accessed on 3 April 2021).

Rosenberger, Sieglinde, and Carla Küffner. 2016. After the Deportation Gap: Non-Removed Persons and their Pathways to Social Rights. In *Migration and Integration: New Models for Mobility and Coexistence*. Edited by Roland Hsu and Cristoph Reinprecht. Wien: Vienna University Press, pp. 137–50.

Sainz, Pablo 'Pampa'. 2020. El Defensor del Pueblo confirma la liberación de internas de los CIE. *El Salto*. Available online: www.elsaltodiario.com/coronavirus/defensoria-del-pueblo-confirma-la-liberacion-de-internas-del-cie (accessed on 13 April 2021).

Saiz, Eva. 2020. Los centros de extranjeros se han vaciado por la pandemia y no ha habido una hecatombe. *El País*. Available online: https://elpais.com/espana/2020-06-18/los-centros-de-extranjeros-se-han-vaciado-por-la-pandemia-y-no-ha-habido-una-hecatombe.html (accessed on 18 April 2021).

Sánchez, María. 2020a. Vuelven el sufrimiento y la incertidumbre con la reapertura de los CIE en plena pandemia. *Cuarto Poder*. Available online: www.cuartopoder.es/derechos-sociales/2020/10/24/vuelven-el-sufrimiento-y-la-incertidumbre-con-la-reapertura-de-los-cie-en-plena-pandemia/ (accessed on 13 April 2021).

Sánchez, María. 2020b. El año en el que se cerraron los CIE (y se volvieron a abrir). *Cuarto Poder*. Available online: www.cuartopoder.es/sociedad/2020/12/28/el-ano-en-el-que-se-cerraron-los-cie-y-se-volvieron-a-abrir/ (accessed on 14 April 2021).

Shah, Silky. 2021. The Immigrant Justice Movement Should Embrace Abolition. *The Forge*. March 4. Available online: https://forgeorganizing.org/article/immigrant-justice-movement-should-embrace-abolition (accessed on 31 May 2021).

Sharma, Damini, Weihua Li, Denise Lavoie, and Claudia Lauer. 2020. Prison Populations Drop by 100,000 During Pandemic. The Marshall Project. Available online: www.themarshallproject.org/2020/07/16/prison-populations-drop-by-100-000-during-pandemic (accessed on 8 April 2021).

Shenker, Jack. 2021. Locked in Barracks with Covid Running Rampant: Is This Any Way to Treat Asylum Seekers? *The Guardian*. Available online: www.theguardian.com/commentisfree/2021/jan/27/locked-covid-asylum-seekers-napier-barracks-kent (accessed on 19 April 2021).

Solidarité Sans Frontières (SSF). 2020. Coronavirus: Des mesures de protection pour tout le monde. Available online: www.sosf.ch/fr/sujets/asile/informations-articles/appel-aux-autorites.html (accessed on 12 April 2020).

Stuber, Lea, and Christian Zeier. 2021. Neue Vorwürfe an Betreiberin nach massivem Corona-Ausbruch. *Berner Zeitung*. Available online: www.bernerzeitung.ch/neue-vorwuerfe-an-betreiberin-nach-massivem-corona-ausbruch-622541895066?fbclid=IwAR3QY1FX-vbXkdHSDst-S0RFqibTV345zjYWIKYD98I4iekF42Pmf8HDC0A (accessed on 18 April 2021).

Taylor, Diane. 2020a. Coronavirus: Call to Release UK Immigration Centre Detainees. *The Guardian*. Available online: www.theguardian.com/world/2020/mar/14/coronavirus-call-to-release-uk-immigration-centre-detainees (accessed on 12 April 2020).

Taylor, Diane. 2020b. Home Office Accused of Pressuring Judiciary over Immigration Decisions. *The Guardian*. Available online: www.theguardian.com/politics/2020/may/06/home-office-accused-of-pressuring-judiciary-over-immigration-decisions (accessed on 12 April 2021).

Tosh, Sarah, Ulla Berg, and Kenneth Sebastian León. 2021. Migrant Detention and COVID-19: Pandemic Responses in Four New Jersey Detention Centers. *Journal on Migration and Human Security* 9: 44–62. [CrossRef]

Trandum Supervisory Board. 2021. Tilsynsrådet for Politiets utlendingsinternat, Trandum: Årsmelding 2020. Available online: www.regjeringen.no/contentassets/e19229021ca74bee9f678d1b52b70f4b/arsmelding-trandum-2020.pdf (accessed on 12 April 2021).

Tribune de Genève. 2020. Des détenus libérés de détention administrative. *Tribune de Genève*. Available online: www.tdg.ch/suisse/detenus-liberes-detention-administrative/story/13892640 (accessed on 12 April 2021).

Turnbull, Sarah. 2017. Immigration Detention and Punishment. *Oxford Research Encyclopedia. Criminology and Criminal Justice*, 1–24. [CrossRef]

United Nations Working Group on Alternatives to Immigration Detention (UNWGATD). 2020. COVID-19 & Immigration Detention: What Can Governments and Other Stakeholders Do? Available online: https://migrationnetwork.un.org/sites/default/files/docs/un_network_on_migration_wg_atd_policy_brief_covid-19_and_immigration_detention_0.pdf (accessed on 20 April 2021).

Vargas, Natalia. 2020. El juez de control del CIE de Barranco Seco ordena la libertad de los internos por razones de salud pública. *El Diario*. Available online: www.eldiario.es/canariasahora/365-dias-de-migraciones/cie-barranco-seco-libertad-internos_132_1220191.html (accessed on 13 April 2021).

Vargas, Natalia. 2021. El brote de COVID-19 en Hoya Fría afecta a 21 personas y vuelve a evidenciar las carencias del CIE. *El Diario*. February 3. Available online: www.eldiario.es/canariasahora/migraciones/cie-hoya-fria-brote-tenerife-covid_1_7191231.html (accessed on 18 April 2021).

Vaughan-Williams, Nick. 2015. *Europe's Border Crisis: Biopolitical Security and Beyond*. Oxford: Oxford University Press.

Weber, Leanne. 2020. Could a Pandemic Kickstart the Re-Bordering of the World? Border Criminologies. Available online: www.law.ox.ac.uk/research-subject-groups/centre-criminology/centreborder-criminologies/blog/2020/07/could-pandemic (accessed on 3 April 2021).

WHO. 2020. UNODC, WHO, UNAIDS and OHCHR Joint Statement on COVID-19 in Prisons and Other Closed Settings. Available online: www.who.int/news/item/13-05-2020-unodc-who-unaids-and-ohchr-joint-statement-on-covid-19-in-prisons-and-other-closed-settings (accessed on 16 April 2021).

WHO Europe. 2020a. Preparedness, Prevention and Control of COVID-19 in Prisons and Other Places of Detention: Interim Guidance. 15 March 2020. Available online: https://apps.who.int/iris/bitstream/handle/10665/336525/WHO-EURO-2020-1405-41155-55954-eng.pdf?sequence=1&isAllowed=y (accessed on 8 April 2021).

WHO Europe. 2020b. Pandemic Fatigue: Reinvigorating the Public to Prevent COVID-19: Policy Considerations for Member States in the WHO European Region. Available online: https://apps.who.int/iris/bitstream/handle/10665/335820/WHO-EURO-2020-1160-40906-55390-eng.pdf?sequence=3&isAllowed=y (accessed on 18 April 2021).

Widra, Emily. 2021. How much have COVID-19 releases changed prison and jail populations? *Prison Policy Initiative*. Available online: www.prisonpolicy.org/blog/2021/02/03/january-population-update/ (accessed on 8 April 2021).

Wille, Christian, and Rebekka Kanesu, eds. 2020. *Bordering in Pandemic Times: Insights into the COVID-19 Lockdown*. Luxembourg and Trier: UniGR-Center for Border Studies, Available online: https://ubt.opus.hbz-nrw.de/opus45-ubtr/frontdoor/deliver/index/docId/1428/file/UniGR-CBS_Borders+in+Perspective_thematic+issue_Vol.+4.pdf (accessed on 16 April 2021).

Wonders, Nancy. 2017. Sitting on the fence—Spain's delicate balance: Bordering, multiscalar challenges, and crimmigration. *European Journal of Criminology* 14: 7–26. [CrossRef]

Ybarra, Megan. 2021. Site Fight! Towards the abolition of immigrant detention on Tacoma's Tar Pits (and everywhere else). *Antipode: A Radical Journal of Geography* 53: 36–55. [CrossRef]

Zedner, Lucia. 2016. Penal subversions: When is a punishment not punishment, who decides and on what grounds? *Theoretical Criminology* 20: 3–20. [CrossRef]

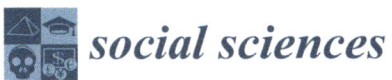

Article

Governing Migration through COVID-19? Dutch Political and Media Discourse in Times of a Pandemic

Maartje Van Der Woude * and Nanou Van Iersel

Van Vollenhoven Institute for Law, Governance & Society, Leiden Law School, P.O. Box 9520, 2300 RA Leiden, The Netherlands; n.van.iersel@law.leidenuniv.nl
* Correspondence: m.a.h.vanderwoude@law.leidenuniv.nl

Abstract: This article explores the political and media discourse in The Netherlands around COVID-19 and migration. In so doing, it asks to what extent the dynamics of 'governing COVID-19 through migration' are visible in this discourse. By asking this question, the article builds upon the theoretical frameworks of 'governing through crime' and 'governing through migration control'. Both theoretical frameworks place a strong emphasis on the role of discourse in framing certain social phenomena as a threat, concern or risk. By carrying out a discourse analysis on Dutch political and media debates around COVID-19 and migration in the period 1 January 2020–1 November 2021, the article illustrates that despite the linking of migration and crime not only being very visible but also seemingly normalized in this discourse, the links made between COVID-19 and migration were much more nuanced. Furthermore, although COVID-19 and migration were discussed together, the discourse does not show any evidence of governing COVID-19 through migration by using the pandemic to push for very restrictive migration laws targeting only 'vagabonds' while still allowing the mobility of 'tourists').

Keywords: governing through migration; COVID-19; crimmigration; The Netherlands; discourse

1. Introduction

In the acknowledgement of his seminal work "Governing Through Crime: How the War on Crime Transformed American Democracy and Created a Culture of Fear" Jonathan Simon (2007) observes how 'crime and crime control have become one of the fundamental challenges to democratic governance that the developed world faces'. In his thesis Simon illustrates how crime has become the dominant frame through which a broad variety of social problems are presented, and therefore also seen. As he illustrates in 'Governing through Crime', this framing of, for instance, teen pregnancy as a possible future crime problem (as single mothers will most likely raise delinquent children), leads to the criminalization of behaviors that should not fall under the realm of the criminal law. A year after Simon's book was published, Bosworth and Guild (2008) used his 'governing through crime' thesis to call attention to what they called 'governing through migration control'. In their article, the authors illustrated how, in the context of the United Kingdom, discursive metaphors and practices of punishment have spilled over into public spheres beyond the criminal justice system, in particular into the realm of migration control (Bosworth and Guild 2008, p. 704). For instance, they note how there has been a growing tendency to lump together quite disparate groups of non-citizens in media and political discourse, from asylum seekers to so-called 'economic migrants' to foreign nationals in prison, effectively erasing differences between them (Bosworth 2008, 2016). Whereas much has been written about the criminalization and securitization of migration, the authors move beyond this dominant angle that had characterized much of the criminological analysis of border control until then, and instead highlight the governmental role of boundary reinforcement during insecure times. Apart from highlighting the preferred use by the UK government of highly flexible administrative processes in dealing with migration matters, the authors call attention to the discourse that is being used to frame and build support for the development of a fine-grained system of migration control and boundary making. By taking the case of The Netherlands, a country that is often portrayed as 'tolerant' and very 'open', as a focal point in this article, we aim to shed light on the question of to what extent Dutch political and media discourse seems to imply a link between COVID-19 and migration and therefore seems to imply the necessity of border-tightening in response to potentially sick or virus-spreading migrants. In other words, we want to analyse whether the political and media discourse in The Netherlands is using COVID-19 in such a way that it might be setting up the introduction of repressive migration and border control measures like the 'fine-grained' system that Bosworth and Guild (2008) talked about.

2. A Quick Glance at the Wider Discourse on COVID-19 in Europe

The image of the migrant as a threat to public health is not new; the narrative that migrant populations around the globe carry a wide array of communicable diseases, and therefore pose a threat to public health in destination communities, is a strong one and tends to resurface in moments of crisis. In 2018 the World Health Organization published the report 'No Public Health Without Refugee and Migrant Health' to counter this narrative in the context of the European continent (WHO 2018). Yet, the COVID-19 crisis has illustrated that the urge for scapegoats in times of global turmoil caused by a pandemic trumps scientific reports and more nuanced debates. According to Hungarian President Victor Orbán it is "(...) primarily foreigners who brought in the disease, and that it is spreading among foreigners."[1] Poland's prime minister, Mateusz Morawiecki, furthermore stated that most cases of COVID-19 in Europe are "imported, in the strict sense of the word," either by foreigners or by Poles returning from abroad. His message is that the Polish nation is clean and pure, and would not experience the current crisis if it were less involved in freedom of movement.[2] Greece's nationalist New Democracy government, meanwhile, has cited the risk of coronavirus infection as a reason for pressing ahead with its controversial plan to build "closed" camps—detention centres, in other words—for asylum seekers trapped by European policies on the Aegean islands of Lesbos and Chios. In France, Marine Le Pen has used the spread of the coronavirus to make a renewed call to close France's frontier with Italy, effectively suspending the Schengen agreement on open borders. Leaders of far-right parties in Germany and Spain have echoed the sentiment.[3] Furthermore, populist Eurosceptic Nigel Farage, whom many credit with making Brexit happen, tweeted about a "Covid crisis in Dover," baselessly claiming that a boat carrying migrants had landed in southeast England, "with 12 on board and they all tested positive for the virus."[4] These and other developments led the UN Secretary General in May 2020 to issue a public statement in which he warned of the fact that the 'pandemic continues to unleash a tsunami of hate and xenophobia, scapegoating and scare-mongering'. In order to counter this, he calls on political leaders 'to show solidarity with all members of their societies and build and reinforce social cohesion' and on the media 'to do much more to flag and, in line with international human rights law, remove racist, misogynist and other harmful content'.[5]

Looking at these responses to the spread of the pandemic by various political figures in the European Union, they seem to fit in with a larger trend of anti-immigration and pro-nationalist sentiment on the continent that became especially visible in response to the so-called 2015 migration crisis. In that year, large numbers of refugees made their way to Europe in response to the Syrian war and the violence that erupted as a result. Scholars of border criminology have discussed how national responses to the so-called European migration crisis have also shown how some of the world's most seemingly open and wealthy societies feel the need to restrict mobility and, as Barker states, in so doing "'undo their own historical, albeit complex, trajectories towards equality, democratization and individual liberty'" (Barker 2017, p. 442). This urge to restrict mobility is reflected by a growing nationalist public and political discourse in which asylum seekers in particular, but definitely not exclusively, are being portrayed as dangerous and 'crimmigrant' others whose presence will threaten the national identity and the cultural fabric of society. As a result, there has been an increased focus all throughout Europe on developing mechanisms that can distinguish between 'good' and 'bad' mobilities, or what Bauman terms 'tourists' and 'vagabonds' (Bauman 1998; also see Weber and Bowling 2008). This development—that only seems to have been amplified and intensified by the pandemic—puts the right of free movement for all who are inside the European Union to the test (Van Der Woude et al. 2017).

3. A Closer Look at Simon's 'Governing through Crime' Thesis

As mentioned in the introduction, in his work, Simon points out the connection between discourse—understood as the language beyond the sentence and thus including power dynamics—and policy. Both influence each other: discourse can spark policy change and vice versa. Without wanting to unravel the complex relation between the two, Simon highlights the problems of, as he sees it, an institutional tendency to approach societal issues through a military lens. This is problematic, he contends, because the rhetoric of securitization conflates societal issues with matters of national security. Since a central government and its institutions are the sole legitimate actors to respond to threats to national security, a state maintains and extends its own purpose by securitizing complex societal challenges. One of the ways in which this dynamic manifests is through discourse. In an earlier publication, Simon notes that the use of military language in non-military policy domains can be indicative of governing through crime (Simon 2001). To illustrate this, one might think of expressions like 'The fight or battle against COVID-19', 'Nurses and doctors at the frontline', and 'Healthcare workers as frontline workers'. This is exactly what Simon is talking about: military language (visible in words like fight and frontline) moving from one domain (namely, a military domain) to another policy domain (namely, public healthcare). This is not to say that anyone who has used such statements falsely treats COVID-19 as a matter of national security. Rather, it shows that language can be indicative of wider dispositions towards securitization.

Moreover, since our discourse analysis will be concerned with the dynamics of governing *through* crime (and migration), it becomes equally important to demarcate this from (simply) governing crime. Simon offers two points of departure for this differentiation, namely, proximity and proportionality (Simon 2007, p. 5). To start with proportionality, governing through crime often manifests in policy responses that are disproportionate to the harms they seek to address. In turn, such disproportionality raises questions about whether a certain policy response is aimed to mitigate or solve a certain harm, or whether it serves ulterior motives. As Simon also notes: "we can expect people to deploy the category of crime to legitimate interventions that have other motivations" (Simon 2007, p. 4). This tendency has also been described by Garland in the context of what he calls the political strategy of 'acting out': The act of showing force in response to complex and difficult-to-manage security problems by using strong language and far-reaching measures in order to give the impression that the problem is taken seriously, while knowing that the proposed measures will most likely not actually lead to a proper solution to the problem as they do not address its root cause(s) (Garland 2001).

Besides proportionality, there is the notion of proximity. This refers to whether a given societal issue is sufficiently related to (national) security to approach it as such, and more generally whether it is reasonable to connect two given policy domains to one another. Although the Dutch language does not distinguish between safety and security—an interesting observation in itself—this distinction does have an effect in policy. Security incidents, by definition, are purposefully caused or facilitated by mal-intended people (e.g., theft or terrorism). Contrary to this, safety incidents take place without anyone being fully responsible for them (e.g., earthquakes or unintended accidents). This difference demonstrates why securitization tends to come with scapegoats; indeed, there is no securitization without someone or some group to blame for it. In other words, proximity reminds us that when two policy areas are linked (both in discourse and in policy), the relationship between them should be judged for logical consistency and desirability. Together with proportionality, these notions can also be employed to differentiate between governing migration and governing *through* migration.

To concretize this with an example, on 20 April 2021, a plenary debate on minors that went missing after entry into The Netherlands took place. Several members of the Dutch parliament critiqued the Secretary of State for the Ministry of Justice and Security for her lack of effort to trace these missing children. One member of parliament suggested the following: "We cannot imagine the miseries these children have experienced. If the Secretary of State truly wishes to protect these children, she must close the borders. She must close our borders and she should not let those children in here anymore."[6] While it is true that closing the borders may decrease the numbers of unaccompanied minors that go missing in the long term, this policy measure is neither proximate nor proportionate; the policy proposed (closing the borders) is not straightforwardly connected to the harm that is discussed (missing unaccompanied alien children). Consequently, it is questionable whether such a proposal is in fact aimed at resolving this harm, or if the harm is used to justify and operationalize underlying sentiments such as xenophobia.

To also illustrate a counterexample, we do *not* consider the following statements to be 'governing through migration and/or crime': During the pandemic it has been frequently discussed whether refugee camps on the islands of Lesbos and Chios should receive (additional) humanitarian support from, among others, the Dutch government. There were fears of outbreaks of COVID-19 and of its consequences for the already appalling conditions in the camps. In this case, a discourse is forming that indeed links migrant groups such as refugees on the one hand and the potential outbreak of COVID-19 on the other. Nevertheless, the connection is correct in this context; (the living conditions in) refugee camps are causally related to the risk of spread. All in all, the distinction between 'governing' and 'governing through' is facilitated by Simon's proximity and proportionality principle, but it is fair to say that discourses always have borderline cases—a caveat that we will explain further when explaining the research method for discourse data collection and interpretation.

4. The Netherlands: A Beacon of Tolerance Gone Dim?

Several countries in Northern Europe have the international reputation of being leading examples on inclusion, equality and tolerance. With strong welfare systems in place, countries such as Norway, Sweden and The Netherlands, are seen as countries that in general are taking good care of their citizens. Besides the aspect of social welfare, having relatively mild and humane penal climates also seems to be part of this grand narrative of hospitality and inclusion. Dutch criminal justice polices have long been characterized as "tolerant", lenient and liberal: permissive towards many vices, foreigner-friendly and blessed with a mild penal climate, and generally perceived to be a beacon of moderation (Downes 1988). The centrality of tolerance and humanity in matters of criminal justice in The Netherlands seems to coincide with a strong emphasis on human rights. With Norway and Sweden, The Netherlands is often depicted as a so-called gidsland ("guiding country") and thus seen as the 'conscience of the world' by setting moral standards in international relations and guiding other countries in the proper direction (Dahl 2006; Engh 2009; Herman 2006). The Netherlands is an interesting case as the country is historically known to be a 'gidsland'—a guiding country—for the implementation of human rights and often praised for its tolerance (Franko et al. 2019). Yet, more recent history has shown a different face of The Netherlands as a country where, upon taking a closer look, immigration law and criminal law are becoming increasingly intertwined (Van Der Woude et al. 2014) and in which political parties that actively and openly claim to be anti-Islam and racist are gaining a foothold (Van Der Woude 2020). The tweet by Geert Wilders, party leader of the anti-Islam and Euro-sceptic right wing party "Party for Freedom" (PVV) in response to the COVID-19 crisis is illustrative in that sense. In October 2020, when COVID-19 cases were soaring in The Netherlands he tweeted: "So the treatments and surgeries of "Henk" and "Ingrid" [two quintessential Dutch names to refer to the native, white Dutch population,

AUTHOR.] who are suffering from cancer, heart failure or other illnesses have to, yet again, be postponed because our IC units are predominantly being occupied by "Mohammed" and "Fatima" who do not speak our language and who don't care about the restrictions?". Not only is he stigmatizing Dutch citizens of Moroccan descent as not being able to speak Dutch and abusing our healthcare system, he is also presenting them as a risk to public health for not following the rules. Despite an overall loss in the total number of seats in parliament compared to the previous elections, the Party for Freedom (PVV) did come out as the third largest political party in the Dutch elections of March 2021.

5. Research Approach

As explained in the previous paragraph, the Dutch case is an interesting case to take a closer look at in light of the central aim of this article, which is to see to what extent Dutch political and media discourse can be qualified as instigating the governance of COVID-19 through migration. In this section we clarify our research approach by discussing the method of discourse analysis, our data collection and our data analysis.

5.1. Method: Discourse Analysis

The term 'discourse analysis' refers to a method for investigating the construction of social reality. Meanings we give to words and images depend on cultural assumptions and help to maintain cultural assumptions. Cultural values are linked to events. Language or images about certain events have a socio-cultural value, which in turn produces socio-cultural effects. The system of communication expressions related to a wider social and cultural network is called 'discourse'. (McDonald 2003) There are many ways to study discourse, ranging from the more to less rigid and/or critical in approach. Several theorists, therefore, rightly point out the lack of clarity surrounding the analysis of discourses (cf. McDonald 2003; Garrett and Bell 1998; Van Dijk 1998; Said 1974).

For this research we have taken inspiration from Carol Bacchi's 'What's the Problem Represented to Be' (WPR) analysis of policy discourse (Bacchi 2009). Bacchi's approach draws heavily on a Foucaudian perspective in suggesting that we are governed by problematizations. Bacchi therefore does not distinguish between policy and policy proposals, because both are part of the broader discourse that influences the degree of social attention to a problem. In this way, administrators not only respond to existing social problems (which would be 'for the taking' for administrators); administrators play an active role in constructing these problems through the discourse they form in proposing and discussing policy. Both policy and policy proposals are aimed at addressing and solving problems; however, all policies rest on specific interpretations and presentations of 'the problem'. To return to the example we gave earlier, the proposal of a PVV member to close the borders in response to unaccompanied minors going missing shows that this member has a very specific problem view. The problem, according to him, does not seem to lie with the fact that these children are going missing, but with the presence of these children. In addition, policy and policy proposals are also shaped by (unspoken) 'self-evident' assumptions. For example, it can be assumed that the meaning of certain concepts is universal—think, for example, of the concept of the 'illegal' migrant—where in reality this is controversial. In this way we are partly governed by the ways in which certain things are problematized (as well as the way in which other matters are regarded as unproblematic). The aim of Bacchi's WPR approach is to identify and critically study the problematizations underlying a specific policy document or proposal and to uncover the (implicit) assumptions on which a problem interpretation rests.

It is important to note that a discourse analysis does not yield neutral or objective conclusions, as any scientific result is influenced by, among other things, the selection and execution of a method and the positionality of the researcher(s). Bacchi also emphasizes that applying the WPR approach does not guarantee homogeneous results. Not only do the personal interests, analytical focus and assumptions of the researcher(s) play a role in the selection of a relevant policy document or proposal, but their interpretation will also differ per researcher. Despite the systematic consideration of proximity and proportionality (in order to consistently differentiate between governing through migration and governing migration), there are many in-between cases; expressions which are neither fully governing through migration nor governing migration (or expressions which are both). In that respect, it is important to note that our analysis of public and political discourse is an impression of debates in Dutch society rather than an exact reflection of them. Finally, the political sensitivity of this analysis should also be acknowledged, as well as the risk that our personal political beliefs may influence conclusions. To make the analysis as neutral as possible, we will consistently state political colors from a party or other source, and we always work from the principle of charity, i.e., presenting other people's arguments in their strongest form.

5.2. Data Collection

This study focuses on the timeframe of 1 January 2020-1 November 2020.This timeframe is related to our specific focus on the impact of COVID-19 on discourses about migration. Although COVID-19 spread before 2020, the implications of this for The Netherlands were first discussed around January 1st. In the context of this article, under 'political discourse' we understand the text and talk of professional politicians or political institutions, such as presidents and prime ministers and other members of government, parliament or political parties, both at the local, national and international levels to include both the speaker and the audience. We chose to combine an analysis of political discourse with an analysis of media discourse, as political discourse is increasingly mediatized and media discourse increasingly politicized. To grasp public and political discourse, we have respectively focused on national and local media as well as parliamentary and governmental debates in The Netherlands. The choice of parliamentary debates and reports, and of news articles, is not based on a reductive understanding of political and public discourse; in contrast, it is inherent in discourse analysis to work with sources that, while indicative of the bigger picture, are not fully representative. In addition, it should be noted that although we now seem to suggest a strict separation between media and political discourse, as already mentioned, in reality these discourses are intertwined.

All the sources were open access available; for the parliamentary and governmental debates in The Netherlands the national database www.officielebekendmakingen.nl was consulted, a database that gives access to the transcripts of all governmental, parliamentary and other debates by political institutional actors and committees. Within the scope of our timeframe, we have collected and stored every document that mentions COVID-19 (or any variation thereof, like pandemic or corona). This led to a selection of 564 documents. These documents have been checked manually to see if they contained one or more of the following search terms: (labor) (im)migration, (labor) (im)migrant(s), alien(s), border(s), asylum(seeker; process; application), refugee(s), healthcare, crime and integration. This led to a final selection of 137 documents for the political discourse (all of which thus discuss both COVID-19 and one or more of the aforementioned search terms).

The sources for the media analysis were obtained through the NexisUni news database that is freely accessible through our University Library. In the selection of national newspapers and magazines we have paid attention to political diversity, and we have prioritized larger media platforms; for local newspapers, we have included all available newspapers within our timeframe[7]. Obviously, this approach leaves out an important domain where discourse happens nowadays, that is, social media. However, for this article we chose to limit ourselves to official media resources. For the media discourse the initial collection of media outings counted 408 and, after a similar check as described for the political discourse, we included a total of 84 articles.

5.3. Data Analysis

We converted both final selections to Atlas.ti, a computer program for data analysis in qualitative research that helps to structure the process of coding and analysis. This means that we have two Atlas.ti files (one for political discourse and one for media discourse) in which all our data (respectively 137 and 84 documents) have been stored and coded manually. In our endnotes, we refer to document numbers (e.g., D1, 2, 3), which are based on our documentation system in the database. By adding a P or an M we distinguished between the political discourse and the media discourse. DP1, for example, refers to document 1 on political discourse in Atlas.ti, whereas DM1 refers to document 1 on media discourse. In the Appendices A and B we provide an overview of the various documents, so that they can be traced back to their original source.

Our codes consist of a combination of the above search terms (migration, border, asylum, etc.) and any variation of COVID-19. Using these codes as a guideline, we were able to quickly identify paragraphs and sentences in our data that were discussing both migration and COVID-19. After that, each set of codes was manually reviewed to see if a link was made between COVID-19 and migration, and if so, what the nature of this link was. This means that we looked at specific sentences as well as at short paragraphs (usually about five sentences long). Also, sentences and paragraphs are always viewed in the context of the entire source; after all, with many codings, it was necessary to read both backwards and forwards to understand the nature of any particular link between COVID-19 and migration. For example, an isolated sentence or paragraph often does not provide a definitive answer about how a statement is intended and/or how it will be received by a possible audience.

Furthermore, we assessed each alleged link between COVID-19 and migration for proximity, proportionality, the perceived (implicit and/or explicit) underlying problematization, and any unspoken assumptions. This process was guided by questions like 'how is migration / how are [various groups of] migrants being problematized in the light of COVID-19?', 'how are [various groups of] migrants being framed?', 'what are the underlying assumptions?', 'are the linked entities sufficiently related to one another for them to be connected like this?', 'is the link logically consistent?', and 'are proposed countermeasures proportionate and proximate to the harm they seek to address?'. On the basis of our answers to these guiding questions, we were able to group together paragraphs and sentences into categories like 'Governing migration through COVID-19' and 'Governing migration and COVID-19'.

6. Results

Our primary objective has been to identify the extent to which governing migration through COVID-19 manifests in media and political discourse. In other words, we have not only sought to examine whether the rhetoric of governing through migration is prevalent in discourse, but also whether COVID-19 plays a role in this rhetoric. We will start by discussing the role of COVID-19, after which we will turn to some more general observations on the ways migration and migrants are represented in media and political discourse.

7. Political Discourse

Starting with political discourse, it is important to note that the results are diverse, and ought to be treated with nuance. Generally, it can be concluded that while governing migration through COVID-19 manifests in debates, this rhetoric is also frequently challenged and critiqued in parliament, government, or both.

7.1. Problematizing Migrant Communities inside and outside The Netherlands through COVID-19

Overall, out of 134 documents, 42 contained one or multiple expression(s) which are indicative of governing migration through COVID-19.[8] As mentioned in the introduction, the narrative that migrant populations around the globe carry a wide array of communicable diseases and, therefore, pose a threat to public health in destination communities, is a strong one and tends to resurface in moments of crisis. This narrative, in which migrants are perceived as carriers of disease, only comes up occasionally in the 2020 political discourse. The rhetoric of governing migration *through* COVID-19 is more diverse than we initially expected; it also manifests through discussions on border policies, humanitarian aid for refugee camps, economic hardship, and governmental compensations for overdue asylum processes during COVID-19.

To start with the narrative that migrants could bring and spread COVID-19, there are but a few examples of this in political discourse. For example, in response to several questions in parliament, the Ministry of Justice and Security declares that "approximately fifty aliens have been denied entrance into The Netherlands to mitigate the spread of COVID-19 since 19 March 2020".[9] In this example, COVID-19 seems to justify the specific rejection of aliens. Another example relates to labor migrants. The Minister of Health, Welfare and Sport expresses the following during a debate about COVID-19 outbreaks in workplaces:

"Is it possible to test more goal oriented? The answer to that question is "yes". I mentioned slaughter houses as one of the examples of which you know: there are many labor migrants there. Perhaps the cooling conditions, the working conditions, also play a role (...)"[10]

This example is perhaps more subtle in its assumption that labor migrants would spread COVID-19. Nonetheless, the Minister appears to assume that the presence of labor migrants is among the factors that led to an outbreak in slaughterhouses. Only on second thought does he seems to consider the labor conditions.

More commonly, governing migration through COVID-19 manifests in broader discussions. For example, in debates on border policies, two political parties stand out in their appeal to governing migration through COVID-19, namely, the Party for Freedom (PVV) and the Forum for Democracy (FvD). These parties are respectively characterized as nationalist right-wing populist and conservative right-wing populist; both are Eurosceptic and anti-immigration. These parties have urged the current Dutch government to close the borders, similar to some other member states of the European Union. To illustrate their stances, a member of PVV expresses the following during a parliamentary debate:

"Because other countries have closed their borders due to corona measures, their asylum influx has almost completely dried up. With 270 asylum migrants in April, the lowest number in at least twenty years, there lies a unique opportunity to prevent the asylum influx from increasing again."[11]

Here, it is clear that COVID-19 is treated as a legitimation to close the Dutch borders, with the specific aim of averting migrants. At the same time, it is worth highlighting that the government itself explicitly counters this form of governing migration through COVID-19. The government frequently expressed its discontent regarding the reintroduction of internal border controls in the European Union, and writes:

"(...) the introduction of internal border control to counter the influx of asylum into The Netherlands is not the government's preference."[12]

Besides border policies, we have identified some mild expressions of governing migration through COVID-19 in debates surrounding the Dutch Immigration and Naturalization Services (IND). This organization is responsible for asylum processes, and is legally required to process any request within six months. If this term is exceeded, the Dutch government is obliged to financially compensate asylum seekers in the form of penalty payments. While the IND deals with structural backlogs, and as COVID-19 has only amplified rather than caused the backlogs, the costs of these payments has exceeded 70 million euros. In light of this, a temporary amendment of the law has been approved, as a result of which the Dutch government is no longer required to pay compensation for overdue asylum processes. While this suspension is not a direct result of COVID-19, it is at least remarkable that asylum seekers and migrants are being cut off financially for overdue governmental work within the timeframe of this pandemic. In other words, COVID-19 seems to have facilitated momentum to cut back on asylum processes.

A final context in which governing migration through COVID-19 manifests is that of economic hardship in combination with insufficient public healthcare facilities and supplies. Regarding migrant communities outside The Netherlands, the scarcity of medical supplies is an argument to refrain from humanitarian aid for refugee camps. This argument exclusively comes from party members of PVV and FvD. As a member of PVV expresses it:

> "I would like to object to the fact that we will be sending some 15,000 relief goods to Greek islands (...) whilst the number of corona cases in The Netherlands has doubled in comparison to Tuesday. Then we are not going to send relief supplies to Greece that we desperately need for our own peoples here, are we? Have we gone completely crazy?".[13]

With regard to migrant communities inside The Netherlands, these too are occasionally held accountable for inadequate medical care. Another member of PVV contends:

> "If we had not fired 75,000 healthcare workers, if billions had not been spent on asylum seekers, and if that money had instead been invested in healthcare, then the crisis—really—would have been smaller."[14]

7.2. Problematizing the Impact of COVID-19 on Migrant Communities within and outside The Netherlands

While varying expressions of governing migration *through* COVID-19 are present in political discourse, there are just as many documents in which the specific vulnerabilities of migrant communities inside and outside The Netherlands are stressed. Out of 134 documents, 55 documents contain one or multiple expression(s) which stress the impact of COVID-19 on migrant communities.[15] Members of the political party DENK have been particularly vocal about this:

> "The virus does not discriminate. We can all get it and it is impossible to predict what the effects will be. However, certain groups suffer more than others. While one Dutch person wonders whether there is a food package left at the food bank, another is upset, because he cannot drink his beer in the village café. And there is a clear difference in consequences for the elderly and the young, people with and without work, and people with and without a migration background. For example, statistics indicate that the excess mortality among people with a migration background is 48%, and without 38%."[16]

DENK has a left-wing political orientation, and statements like this are broadly shared as well as put forward by parties with left-wing and centrist political orientations. Similarly, several outbreaks of COVID-19 among labor migrants in The Netherlands have resulted in an increase in governmental support. While these migrants have sometimes been accused of disobedience in respect of the measures against COVID-19, the pandemic has mostly shed light on their poor working and living conditions. Consequently, a task force was set up for the protection of labor migrants in May 2020. The objective of this was to mitigate outbreaks of COVID-19, as well as to strengthen the position of labor migrants in the long term.[17]

With regard to migrant communities outside of The Netherlands, we can see that while COVID-19 is used to restrict humanitarian aid for refugee camps, the reverse is also true; COVID-19 is also cited as a reason to increase humanitarian aid flows for refugee camps. For example:

> "We still see that all over the world, vulnerable refugee children are suffering from the corona crisis in refugee camps. Who cares for them?"[18]

7.3. Problematizing Migrants for Other Things than COVID-19

Having elaborated on our results in relation to COVID-19, we will now turn to some more general observations on the ways in which migrants are represented in political discourse. First of all, governing migration through COVID-19 is merely one of the ways in which governing through migration manifests. Migrants are also linked to, if not blamed for, a lack of affordable housing in The Netherlands and carbon dioxide emission in relation to climate change. Out of 134 documents, 11 contain one or multiple expression(s) of this.[19] To start with affordable housing, a quote by a member of PVV is quite illustrative of this rhetoric:

> "Immigration swiftly increases the housing shortage; construction workers cannot compete with the enormous growth of immigrants."[20]

This rhetoric belongs to the domain of governing through migration because it falsely implies a causal link between housing shortages and immigration. In a similar vein, members of FvD argue that the admittance of migrants leads to higher carbon dioxide emissions, leading to an overall intensification of climate change.[21]

7.4. Not Problematizing the Connection between Migration and Crime

Since PVV and FvD are generally considered populist parties, their engagement in these forms of governing through migration is not too surprising. More remarkable is the frequency with which migration and migrants are linked to crime by a wide array of political parties (including liberal, socialist, Orthodox–Calvinist and Christian–democratic ones). Out of 134 documents, 35 contain one or multiple expression(s) of crimmigration.[22] Currently, the biggest party in The Netherlands is a liberal one: the People's Party for Freedom and Democracy (VVD). After PVV and FvD, this party most regularly links migration to crime. For example, when a member of PVV requested a plenary debate between government and parliament to discuss high crime rates among asylum seekers, the Secretary of State for the Ministry of Justice and Security (VVD) shared his concerns. This Secretary of State, who is responsible for the implementation of migration policies, has responded to this by '*lik-op-stuk-beleid*', meaning that minor violations and incidents among asylum seekers are immediately punished. Such punishments come in the form of withholding living allowances, transfer to high-surveillance locations, and restraining orders.[23] During this same debate, the Secretary of State concludes:

> "The figures in this incident overview are indeed worrying and nuisance in any form is unacceptable. They are alarming messages indeed. I agree with Mister Hiddema [member of FvD, NI] on that. But at the same time, we must see the following. Like Mister Emiel van Dijk [member of PVV, NI] has put forward, we would prefer to close the borders and not let them in here. But we have an asylum system and that means that . . . We are a constitutional state: anyone who comes here to ask for asylum, will get a procedure. (...) We do our utmost to ensure that this runs as smoothly as possible, that no shoplifting takes place and that indeed all other organizations work well together to ensure that nuisance is limited as much as possible."[24]

Besides this, crime rates are also linked to the presence of migrant communities. The following expressions are examples of this; both come from the Reformed Political Party (SGP), which is a conservative Orthodox–Calvinist party.

> "(...) is the urban unrest [referring to drug-related crime, NI] not also an integration problem?"[25]

> "Noting that crime figures continue to show a worrying overrepresentation of people with a non-Western migration background; calls on the government to recognize and investigate this problem and to develop a targeted approach to reduce crime in these groups as well as in total."[26]

8. Media Discourse

The media discourse showed some similarities, but also some differences compared to the political discourse. In line with the political discourse, an oft-discussed topic in the various news articles was the situation in the various refugee camps located in different locations on the outskirts of the European Union.

8.1. Problematizing Refugees as Victims and/or a Potential Threat to Public Health

Of the 84 articles that were included in our analysis of media discourse, 30 addressed matters around refugees.[27] The majority of these articles spoke of the various refugee camps at the external borders of the European Union, in particular the Canary Islands and Italy, but with an emphasis on the situation on the Greek islands of Samos and Lesbos. It was on the latter island where a destructive fire broke out in an encampment called 'Moria'. A close read of the articles reveal two main problematizations: on the one hand, as illustrated by the deplorable and inhumane circumstances under which asylum seekers have to 'live' in the encampments, the lack of 'care' for the health of asylum seekers amidst a global pandemic was problematized. As vividly described based on first hand experiences and observations by NGO workers, the amount of people packed together in the encampments without access to personal protective equipment and without the possibility of taking necessary hygienic measures is a 'humanitarian disaster' in the making.[28] Several articles indeed mention outbreaks of COVID-19 among asylum seekers.[29]

At the same time, there are articles that discuss how the global pandemic, given the inequalities between the Global North and the Global South in the distribution of medical equipment (and later on also the vaccine), might also spark more migration from the Global South to the Global North. What this shows is how the problematization of the asylum seeker, or more broadly the migrant, as the victim of inhumane circumstances is closely intertwined with a less explicit problematization of the asylum seeker as a potential risk to public health because of the very same circumstances that support the problematization of the asylum seeker as the victim. We also see the problematization of migration sparked by COVID-19 in general, as in "COVID-19 will lead to migration pressure on Europe's external borders due to the growing instability in vulnerable countries".[30] This begs the question to what extent calls for financial and medical support for the Global South are driven by true humanitarian motives or moreso by the self-interest of European member states in the Global North?[31] How, moreover, should this wish to provide help in the Global South be seen in light of observations by Doctors without Borders (MSF) who, based on the actions of several European member states located at the external borders of Europe, state that "European countries are now using COVID-19 to obstruct humanitarian aid".[32] The NGO is addressing actions by the Italian authorities as a result of which the boat *Sea Watch 4*, the search and rescue ship run by Sea-Watch and MSF, could not provide help to boat refugees drowning in the Meditarreanean.

A topic that seemed more prominent in media discourse than in political discourse is the extent to which different migrant communities in The Netherlands were hit harder by the COVID-19 crisis and what the cause of this could be.

8.2. Problematizing Migrant Communities in The Netherlands as Victims and/or a Potential Threat to Public Health

A substantial number of articles (35) in our final selection of media discourse centered around the extent to which migrant communities in The Netherlands were, as in countries such as the US and the UK, disproportionately affected by the virus. In those articles, as in the articles discussing the situation of refugees and asylum seekers outside of the country, two narratives—or two problematizations—come to the fore: (a) the migrant as a victim of social and economic circumstances that will increase their risk of contracting COVID-19 or being seen as scapegoats, and (b) the potentially hazardous migrant who is more likely to spread the virus due to their religious and cultural practices or general lack of respect for and compliance with COVID-19 restrictions in The Netherlands.[33] The first narrative in many ways can be seen as a counter narrative to the more xenophobic and especially Islamophobic second narrative.

To start with the second narrative, migrant communities as potential spreaders of the virus, this narrative seemed to especially take flight after a head doctor from the Amsterdam University Medical Hospital Intensive Care Unit mentioned in an interview that there were many people with a migrant background hospitalized in the intensive care units.[34] Although the doctor states that there are most likely many reasons contributing to this, his statement was used by anti-Islam politician Geert Wilders to send his earlier quoted tweet about Mohamed and Fatima taking up beds that should go to autochthonous Dutch people. Following Wilders' Tweet the Chairman of the Dutch catering industry association stated that research had shown that 'COVID-19 outbreaks among migrant communities' were more problematic than the risk of contracting COVID-19 in a restaurant or a cafe.[35] There are several articles that indeed seem to problematize some cultural and religious practices that are associated with different migrant communities in The Netherlands, with a clear emphasis on the Moroccan and Turkish communities but also with mentions of the Surinamese and Ghanese community. An important aspect of concern are large gatherings in the context of religious activities—a concern that is especially voiced around the month of Ramadan.[36] It has to be mentioned that religious gatherings *in general* have been problematized in the context of the pandemic, not just those of Muslims. Besides this, another cause for concern, outside of the context of religion, is gathering with friends, family and community members more generally,[37] as well as not being upfront about having COVID-19 out of a sense of shame of having contracted the disease.[38] These dynamics would, according to the articles, be more present within migrant communities than within native Dutch communities.

The problematization of migrant communities as spreaders of COVID-19 is not unique to The Netherlands. Several pieces illustrate not only the scapegoating mechanism that almost automatically seems to kick in when countries are faced with an intangible threat, but also illustrate how in various other countries different migrant communities have been targeted because of it.[39]

The second problematization that is clearly visible in the media discourse seems to be a direct response to the one that was just discussed. While taking the notion of migrant communities as reluctant to respect the COVID-19 restrictions as a point of departure, these articles paint a much more nuanced picture. The articles address the complex mix of social and economic factors as a result of which migrant communities are not in a privileged situation where they are able to work from home, to self-quarantine or socially distance themselves from family or community members who have tested positive, or to homeschool or home entertain their children. Combined with higher levels of obesity and diabetes in these communities, these circumstances make clear how the virus 'discriminates'. The virus, as is communicated clearly in these pieces, has led to a further deterioration of the already vulnerable living situation in which migrant communities often find themselves.[40] These articles also point out that migrant communities are not the only communities facing that reality; lower class, lower educated white Dutch communities are in the same boat. What is further questioned is the extent to which the government has been clear and inclusive in its communication on COVID-19 and the measures around it. The call to use 'unusual suspects' and 'unusual leaders' in connecting with different communities—Imams, athletes, musicians, etc.—is echoed in these contributions as well.[41] Thus, all in all, this problematization can be seen more as a problematization of the current state of affairs in Dutch society, in which the socio-economic gap between various groups has grown tremendously over the past decades and in which polarization and fear of 'the other' seem to have become more and more common.

9. Conclusions

Actions speak louder then words, but words do set the stage for possible further actions. The Dutch political and media discourse shows a two-sided picture: on the one hand, migration and migrant communities in The Netherlands are problematized in the light of COVID-19; on the other hand, the analysis of both political and media discourse also shows that pushback is indeed being offered against the 'pandemicization' of migrants, especially as far as migrant communities in The Netherlands are concerned. When it comes to discussions on asylum-seekers and refugees, the pushback is less visible and all parties express concern about the situation in refugee camps and the implications for the country if the people living in these camps were to in fact make their way to The Netherlands. Interestingly enough, despite these concerns and contrary to many other European countries, The Netherlands has never closed its borders by reinstating permanent border checks. Although problems are observed in the way in which different groups of people comply with the COVID-19 rules, the causes that are identified to explain this non compliant behavior are very diverse. For example, the higher numbers of Dutch people with a migrant background in the ICU, and also the higher mortality rates among this group, are not exclusively sought in that background. Indiscriminate governing of COVID-19 'through' migration seems to be mostly absent. With the exception of the parties that have an explicit anti-migration, anti-Islam and anti 'open' borders agenda—Forum for Democracy and the Party for Freedom—the other coalition and opposition parties are reluctant to explicitly link COVID-19 to migration or to propose stricter anti-migration policies on that basis. The reasons for the limited presence of 'governing COVID-19 through migration' in the Dutch discourse are not clear, and somewhat unexpected. In our opinion at least, the absence of that clear link does not immediately give rise to too much optimism. This somewhat skeptical attitude is reinforced by the extent to which the linking of migration and crime—and thus the assumption of a causal relationship between the two phenomena—seems to have become normalized in the discourse, with neither government nor opposition parties questioning it. The interlinking of crime and migration has been widely problematized by scholars studying the process of crimmigration (Stumpf 2006; Van Der Woude et al. 2014), who have illustrated how this process can lead to the creation of a penal subsystem focused on territorial exclusion of the national social body instead of reintegration which has been crafted for the non-citizen (Aas 2013, 2014; Bosworth et al. 2018; Bowling and Westenra 2020). Franko refers to this penal subsystem as a form of 'bordered penality', indicating how the absence of formal citizenship status crucially affects the procedural and substantive standards of justice afforded to non-members and leads to the creation of two parallel penal systems: one for citizens and one for non-citizens. The fact that the link between crime and migration—with all its underlying assumptions—is normalized all over the political spectrum is cause for concern.

It should be also noted that the analysis presented in this article focuses on the first phase of the pandemic in The Netherlands; the collected data include the first and part of the second wave. There have now been a third and fourth wave, and there are concerns about a possible fifth wave. In other words, uncertainty persists and, most likely, will affect the overall discourse. Both Bauman and Beck point out that in times of uncertainty, the most visible groups of 'others' will eventually be identified as being (partly) responsible for the underlying problem (Beck 1986; Bauman 1998). It will also be interesting to see how the pandemic will influence thinking about mobility in general. To stay with Bauman, the question is to what extent tourists (postmodern westerners) and vagabonds (refugees, asylum seekers, illegal immigrants or dissidents) will both be able to move around the world again or whether there will be (even more) attempts to limit the mobility of vagabonds and the 'crimmigrant other' (Franko 2020). While according to Bauman it was already the case before the pandemic that the light was green for tourists to move freely around the world, while the light for vagabonds was red, it is expected that this last light will turn a darker red due to the pandemic. After all, if tourists want to travel safely, the vagabonds have to give way. Illustrative of the latter is the development of the European Travel Information and Authorization System as part of a broader development towards 'smarter' border control. The description of ETIAS states that it concerns a "largely automated IT system created to identify security, irregular migration or high epidemic risks posed by visa-exempt visitors traveling to the Schengen States, whilst at the same time facilitate crossing borders for the vast majority of travelers who do not pose such risks."[42] Irregular migration here is lumped together with safety and health risks as a risk against which member states must be protected, but which should not affect tourists.

Author Contributions: Collection, M.V.D.W. and N.V.I.; data analysis, M.V.D.W. and N.V.I.; writing of the contribution, M.V.D.W. and N.V.I. All authors have read and agreed to the published version of the manuscript.

Funding: This research was funded Leiden University Fund/ Schim van der Loeff Foundation, grant number W20407-4-51.

Conflicts of Interest: The authors declare no conflict of interest.

Appendix A. Political Discourse Documents (Indicated in the Text as DocumentPolitical DP + Number)

1. Plenair debat 02.06 (2)
2. Plenair debat 02.06
3. Plenair debat 06.07
4. Plenair debat 15.06
5. Plenair debat 16.06 (2)
6. Plenair debat 01.04
7. Plenair debat 01.07
8. Plenair debat 01.09
9. Plenair debat 02.07 (3)
10. Plenair debat 02.07 (8)
11. Plenair debat 02.09 (3)
12. Plenair debat 03.06
13. Plenair debat 03.09 (4)
14. Plenair debat 03.09 (5)
15. Plenair debat 03.09 (6)
16. Plenair debat 03.09
17. Plenair debat 04.06 (5)
18. Plenair debat 08.04
19. Plenair debat 09.09 (4)
20. Plenair debat 09.09 (5)
21. Plenair debat 09.09
22. Plenair debat 10.06 (3)
23. Plenair debat 10.06 (4)
24. Plenair debat 12.03 (3)
25. Plenair debat 14.05
26. Plenair debat 14.07 (2)
27. Plenair debat 16.04
28. Plenair debat 16.09
29. Plenair debat 17.06 (2)
30. Plenair debat 17.09 (2)
31. Plenair debat 17.09
32. Plenair debat 18.03
33. Plenair debat 18.06 (4)
34. Plenair debat 18.06
35. Plenair debat 19.08
36. Plenair debat 20.05 (2)
37. Plenair debat 20.05
38. Plenair debat 22.04
39. Plenair debat 22.09
40. Plenair debat 24.06 (2)
41. Plenair debat 24.06
42. Plenair debat 25.06 (2)
43. Plenair debat 26.03
44. Plenair debat 26.05
45. Plenair debat 28.05 (2)

46. Plenair debat 28.05
47. Plenair debat 30.06 (2)
48. Vragenuur 19.05
49. Verslag mondeling overleg 01.07
50. Verslag mondeling overleg 16.06
51. Voorstel van wet 06.10
52. Verslag schriftelijk overleg 03.07 (7)
53. Verslag schriftelijk overleg 07.10
54. Verslag schriftelijk overleg 11.06
55. Verslag schriftelijk overleg 12.06
56. Verslag schriftelijk overleg 15.06
57. Verslag schriftelijk overleg 24.08
58. Verslag schriftelijk overleg 26.05
59. Verslag schriftelijk overleg 29.09 (2)
60. Verslag van de vaste commissie 03.07 (6)
61. Verslag van de vaste commissie 09.06 (2)
62. Verslag van de vaste commissie 13.10
63. Verslag van de vaste commissie 24.04 (3)
64. Verslag algemeen overleg 06.05
65. Verslag algemeen overleg 06.10
66. Verslag algemeen overleg 07.10
67. Verslag algemeen overleg 08.04
68. Verslag algemeen overleg 10.07 (3)
69. Verslag algemeen overleg 12.05 (2)
70. Verslag algemeen overleg 12.05 (3)
71. Verslag algemeen overleg 12.05
72. Verslag algemeen overleg 12.06
73. Verslag algemeen overleg 13.05 (2)
74. Verslag algemeen overleg 13.05 (3)
75. Verslag algemeen overleg 13.05
76. Verslag algemeen overleg 16.07 (3)
77. Verslag algemeen overleg 16.09 (3)
78. Verslag algemeen overleg 16.09
79. Verslag algemeen overleg 16.10
80. Verslag algemeen overleg 24.07 (4)
81. Verslag algemeen overleg 24.09 (2)
82. Verslag algemeen overleg 24.09 (3)
83. Verslag algemeen overleg 25.09
84. Verslag algemeen overleg 28.07 (5)
85. Verslag algemeen overleg 29.07 (6)
86. Verslag algemeen overleg 30.04
87. Verslag algemeen overleg 31.07 (2)
88. Verslag algemeen overleg 31.07 (4)
89. Verslag algemeen overleg 31.07 (5)
90. Verslag algemeen overleg 31.07
91. Verslag notaoverleg 17.06
92. Verslag voorstel van wet 05.10
93. Verslag schriftelijk overleg 05.06
94. Verslag schriftelijk overleg 07.10
95. Verslag schriftelijk overleg 08.05 (3)
96. Verslag schriftelijk overleg 08.05 (4)
97. Verslag schriftelijk overleg 08.10
98. Verslag schriftelijk overleg 10.04 (2)
99. Verslag schriftelijk overleg 10.04 (3)

100. Verslag schriftelijk overleg 10.06
101. Verslag schriftelijk overleg 11.06 (3)
102. Verslag schriftelijk overleg 12.05 (4)
103. Verslag schriftelijk overleg 15.05 (2)
104. Verslag schriftelijk overleg 16.04
105. Verslag schriftelijk overleg 16.07
106. Verslag schriftelijk overleg 16.10
107. Verslag schriftelijk overleg 17.06 (3)
108. Verslag schriftelijk overleg 17.06
109. Verslag schriftelijk overleg 18.06
110. Verslag schriftelijk overleg 19.05 (2)
111. Verslag schriftelijk overleg 19.05 (3)
112. Verslag schriftelijk overleg 19.05 (6)
113. Verslag schriftelijk overleg 20.08 (2)
114. Verslag schriftelijk overleg 21.07 (2)
115. Verslag schriftelijk overleg 22.04
116. Verslag schriftelijk overleg 23.03
117. Verslag schriftelijk overleg 23.04 (2)
118. Verslag schriftelijk overleg 23.04 (3)
119. Verslag schriftelijk overleg 24.04 (2)
120. Verslag schriftelijk overleg 24.06 (7)
121. Verslag schriftelijk overleg 26.03
122. Verslag schriftelijk overleg 26.05 (3)
123. Verslag schriftelijk overleg 28.08 (6)
124. Verslag schriftelijk overleg 29.04 (5)
125. Verslag schriftelijk overleg 29.05 (3)
126. Verslag schriftelijk overleg 29.05
127. Verslag schriftelijk overleg 30.03
128. Verslag vragen en antwoord 02.07
129. Verslag vragen en antwoord 06.10
130. Verslag vragen en antwoord 16.06 (2)
131. Verslag vragen en antwoord 16.06 (4)
132. Verslag vragen en antwoord 17.06 (2)
133. Verslag vragen en antwoord 17.06
134. Verslag vragen en antwoord 18.06
135. Verslag vragen en antwoord 27.10 (2)
136. Verslag vragen en antwoord 27.10
137. Verslag vragen en antwoord 29.10

Appendix B. Media Discourse Documents (Indicated in the Text as DocumentMedia DM + Number)

1. Vluchteling op Samos wanhopig
2. Afrika vergeten in coronacrisis is niet in ons belang
3. Bosbrand bij overvol vluchtelingenkamp op Grieks eiland Samos
4. Wij leven hier al jaren tussen ratten en kakkerlakken.
5. Wordt het ooit weer normaal: NRC peilt de stemming in elf Nederlandse buurten
6. 69 nieuwe coronadoden gemeld in Nederland, 44 ziekenhuisopnames
7. Alles beter dan 'dat daar';De Polen oordelen over vijf jaar sociaal-nationalisme
8. 'Als er één besmet raakt, krijgen we het allemaal'
9. 'Amsterdamse Ghanezen hebben vaker corona-antistoffen in bloed'
10. Arts op de Sea-Watch 4: een droom om moedeloos van te raken
11. Artsen zonder Grenzen waarschuwt voor corona in Griekse vluchtelingenkampen
12. Corona Nieuws VN vrezen xenofobie
13. Artsen zonder Grenzen hervat migranten missie op Middellandse Zee

14. Bij Ventimiglia willen vluchtelingen grens over
15. 'Blijf positief en vertrouw op Allah'
16. Buurtsuper en moskee moeten helpen om iedereen te bereiken met corona campagne
17. Corona houdt de Bijlmer in zijn greep
18. Corona in kamp gevluchte Rohingya
19. Corona in kamp Moriazal catastrofale gevolgen hebben
20. 'Corona is niet iets om geheim te houden'
21. Corona is niet kleurenblind, onderzoek wel
22. Corona Jihad
23. Coronavirus duikt op in Rohingya-vluchtelingenkamp in Bangladesh
24. COVID-19 en geweld Libi_ dwingen migrant naar Canarische eilanden
25. 'De kaarten zijn in de lucht gegooid';Mensenrechten in tijden van corona
26. De noodzaak van vaccinsolidariteit boven vaccinnationalisme is groot
27. De overheid greep redelijk snel in en de toeristen bleven weg
28. De vader en moeder van BNT162b2;Een vaccin en zijn politieke context
29. De volgende brand hangt in de lucht
30. 'Deze ramadan maakt extra indruk'
31. Discrimineert het coronavirus Het heeft er alle schijn van
32. Een keizer zonder kleren;Precaire beroepen Het romantische beeld van Europa
33. Eerste 25 van de honderd kwetsbare Griekse vluchtelingen in Nederland aangekomen
34. Eerste coronadode in Grieks migrantenkamp
35. Empathie
36. Evacueer vluchtelingen op Griekse eilanden, nu
37. Geen brasa in de Bijlmer waarom slaat corona hier zo hard toe
38. 'Gevaarlijke situatie' in azc's door tekort hulpmiddelen
39. Gran Canaria gaat meer tentenkampen bouwen
40. Grenscontrole Duitsland rond arbeidsmigranten
41. Grieken bouwen een muur tussen Lesbos en Turkije
42. Griekse migratie kwestie blijft zorgelijk
43. 'Harteloos en xenofoob';Nederland laat jonge asielzoekers in de steek
44. Heel Parijs binnen, behalve het uitschot
45. Hekken rond de wijk corona _n het nieuwe corona beleid treffen vooral de armsten
46. Het plein van de Al-Haram Moskee in Mekka is leeg, zoals ook het Sint-Pietersplein in Rome leeg is
47. Hoop in tijden van misère
48. 'Hulp aan Afrika is in ons belang'
49. IC-chef Girbes: fout om patiënten om etniciteit anders te behandelen
50. Imam: Corona Besmetting wordt soms verzwegen
51. In de Randstad liggen corona-IC's vol migranten
52. In de Randstad liggen de corona-IC's vol migranten
53. In Moria zitten vluchtelingen klem
54. Investeer juist nu in armoedebestrijding
55. Kunnen de rechts-populistische partijen binnen Europa electoraal munt slaan uit de ziekte-uitbraak
56. Maduro vluchtelingen zijn virusdragers
57. Migranten als zondebok de woestijn in sturen Ik denk niet dat wij daar als samenleving beter van worden.
58. Migranten sterven relatief vaker aan coronavirus
59. Niet iedereen kan verantwoordelijkheid voor gezondheid aan;Commentaar
60. Offerfeest op 1.5 meter inmiddels weten de gelovigen hoe het werkt
61. Ongezonder, lager geschoold, niet altijd thuis kunnen werken; Corona Besmettingen
62. Ook de ramadan is even anders
63. Op elkaars lip in plastic tenten
64. Op Lesbos is de chaos compleet 12,000 mensen op straat, terwijl corona rondwaart

65. Opvallend veel migranten onder Britse coronadoden
66. Opvang asielzoekers zit weer propvol;Opvang in Nederland zit vol
67. Overal extra corona controles, maar fruitkweker Ren Simons vreest ze niet
68. Relatief veel migranten sterven door coronavirus
69. Stampvol vluchtelingenkamp Lesbos kansloos bij besmetting coronavirus
70. Stroom bootmigranten uit Libië zwelt weer aan
71. Tegen elke prijs;Essay Vluchtelingen en Europa
72. Veel coronapatienten met migratieachtergrond op ic's: Taalproblemen kunnen rol spelen
73. 'Verplaats vluchtelingenop Lesbosnaar lege hotels'
74. Vluchtelingen betalen hoge prijs voor pandemie miljoenen mensen krijgen niet de hulp die ze nodig hebben
75. Vluchtelingen op Lesbos in gevaar na besmetting
76. Vluchtelingen op Lesbos willen niet opnieuw in een kamp, ook al is het splinternieuw
77. Volk van buiten;Column
78. Voor je het weet zit er 30 man in de huiskamer; Tijdens het Offerfeest; Corona Verslapping
79. Voor vluchtelingen is corona slechts een van de problemen
80. Wie zijn hier de verliezers
81. Wordt de ene bevolkingsgroep harder geraakt door corona dan de andere
82. Zondebok
83. Zorg dat we in deze crisis geen groepen vergeten
84. Zwakke groepen zijn immuun voor corona beleid

Notes

[1] https://www.france24.com/en/20200313-hungary-s-pm-orban-blames-foreign-students-migration-for-coronavirus-spread (last accessed 12 March 2021)

[2] https://ecfr.eu/article/commentary_europe_and_the_virus_the_battle_of_narratives/ (last accessed 12 March 2021)

[3] https://www.theguardian.com/commentisfree/2020/feb/28/coronavirus-outbreak-migrants-blamed-italy-matteo-salvini-marine-le-pen (last accessed 12 March 2021)

[4] https://edition.cnn.com/2021/03/06/europe/europes-next-migrant-crisis-intl-analysis/index.html (last accessed 12 March 2021)

[5] https://www.un.org/press/en/2020/sgsm20076.doc.htm (last accessed 17 May 2021)

[6] https://www.tweedekamer.nl/kamerstukken/plenaire_verslagen/detail/f2e25f66-7044-44f6-814d-b5ae85fec0bc (last accessed 10 May 2021)

[7] The newspapers included are: AD/Algemeen Dagblad, NRC Handelsblad, De Stentor, De Gelderlander, Noordhollands Dagblad, De Telegraaf, Brabants Dagblad, Eindhovens Dagblad, Tubantia, De Volkskrant, Noordhollands Dagblad, de Volkskrant, Dagblad De Limburger, BN/DeStem

[8] DP 1, 3, 6, 7, 17, 20, 22, 24, 26, 27, 28, 31, 32, 35, 38, 42, 43, 45, 46, 50, 61, 62, 69, 82, 85, 90, 91, 93, 96, 98, 104, 112, 114, 115, 116, 117, 121, 122, 124, 126, 135, 137

[9] DP 124

[10] DP 42

[11] DP 1

[12] DP 124

[13] DP 69

[14] DP 6

[15] DP 10, 20, 26, 27, 28, 29, 30, 32, 36, 37, 40, 41, 42, 45, 47, 50, 58, 61, 65, 66, 69, 74, 77, 78, 79, 80, 81, 82, 83, 84, 85, 88, 90, 91, 94, 95, 97, 98, 101, 107, 110, 115, 116, 117, 120, 121, 121, 123, 124, 125, 128, 129, 131, 132, 134, 135

[16] DP 37

[17] https://www.rijksoverheid.nl/actueel/nieuws/2020/06/11/eerste-aanbevelingen-aanjaagteam-bescherming-arbeidsmigranten (Last accessed 12 May 2021)

[18] DP 42

[19] DP 17, 28, 30, 34, 44, 75, 80, 94, 100, 124, 129

[20] DP 3

[21] DP 28

[22] DP 1, 12, 14, 15, 16, 18, 20, 26, 28, 30, 39, 41, 48, 50, 66, 74, 75, 78, 79, 82, 83, 88, 91, 93, 94, 97, 100, 105, 115, 120, 121, 124, 130, 135, 137
[23] DP 48
[24] DP 48
[25] DP 30
[26] DP 30
[27] DM 1, 79, 76, 75, 73, 71, 70, 69, 64, 63, 56, 41, 39, 36, 34, 33, 29, 24, 23, 19, 18, 14, 13, 12, 11, 10, 8, 4, 3, 2
[28] DM 8, 11, 10
[29] DM 75, 64, 34, 18, 19, 14
[30] DM 48, 24
[31] DM 48, 2
[32] DM 13
[33] DM 84, 83, 81, 80, 77, 72, 68, 62, 61, 60, 59, 58, 57, 55, 56, 52, 49, 45, 44, 43, 38, 66, 37, 35, 31, 30, 22, 21, 20, 17, 16, 15, 9, 5
[34] DM 77, 52, 58, 49
[35] DM 57, 82
[36] DM 78, 60, 30, 15
[37] DM 5, 37, 17, 78
[38] DM 20, 50
[39] DM 22, 45, 56, 80, 77
[40] DM 83, 81, 84, 78
[41] DM 84, 72
[42] https://ec.europa.eu/home-affairs/what-we-do/policies/borders-and-visas/smart-borders/etias_en (last accessed 21 May 2021)

References

Aas, Katja. 2013. The ordered and the bordered society: Migration control, citizenship, and the northern penal state. In *The Borders of Punishment: Migration, Citizenship, and Social Exclusion*. Edited by K. F. Aas and M. Bosworth. Oxford: Oxford University Press, pp. 21–39.

Aas, Katja. 2014. Bordered penality: Precarious membership and abnormal justice. *Punishment & Society* 16: 520–41. [CrossRef]

Bacchi, Carrol. 2009. *Analysing Policy: What's the Problem Represented to Be?* London: Pearson Education, Frenchs Forest.

Barker, Vanessa. 2017. Penal power at the border: Realigning state and nation. *TheoreticalCriminology* 21: 441–57. [CrossRef]

Bauman, Zygmunt. 1998. *Globalization: The Human Consequences*. New York: Columbia University Press.

Beck, U. 1986. *Risk Society. Towards a new Modernity*. London: Sage Publications.

Bosworth, Mary, and Maira Guild. 2008. Governing through migration control: Security and citizenship in Britain. *British Journal of Criminology* 48: 703–19. [CrossRef]

Bosworth, Mary. 2008. Border control and the limits of the sovereign state. *Social & LegalStudies* 17: 199–215.

Bosworth, Mary. 2016. Border criminology: How migration is changing criminal justice. In *Changing Contours of Criminal Justice*, 1st ed. Edited by Mary Bosworth, Carolyn Hoyle and Lucia Zedner. Oxford: Oxford University Press, pp. 213–26.

Bosworth, Mary, Aas Katja Franko, and Pickering Sharon. 2018. Punishment. Globalization and Migration Control: 'Get Them the Hell Out of Here'. *Punishment & Society* 20: 34–53.

Bowling, Ben, and Sophie Westenra. 2020. 'A really hostile environment': Adiaphorization, global policing and the crimmigration control system. *Theoretical Criminology* 24: 163–83. [CrossRef]

Dahl, Ann-Sofie. 2006. Sweden: Once a Moral Superpower, Always a Moral Superpower? *Canada's Journal of Global Policy Analysis* 61: 895–908. [CrossRef]

Downes, David. 1988. *Contrasts in Tolerance: Post-war Penal Policy in The Netherlands and England and Wales*. Oxford: Clarendon.

Engh, Sunniva. 2009. The Conscience of the World?: Swedish and Norwegian Provision of Development Aid. *Itinerario* 33: 65–82. [CrossRef]

Franko, Katja. 2020. *The Crimmigrant Other: Migration and Penal Power*. Abingdon-on-Thames: Routledge.

Franko, Katja, Maartje van der Woude, and Vanessa Barker. 2019. Beacons of Tolerance Dimmed? Migration, Criminalization, and Inhospitality in Welfare States. In *Contested Hospitalities in a Time of Migration: Religious and Secular Counterspaces in the Nordic Region*. Edited by Synnove Bendixsen and Trygve Wyller. Abingdon-on-Thames: Routledge, pp. 55–75.

Garland, David. 2001. *Culture of Control. Crime and Control in Contemporary Society*. Oxford: Oxford University Press.

Garrett, and Peter en Allan Bell. 1998. Media and Discourse: A Critical Overview. In *Approaches to Media Discourse*. Oxford: Blackwell Publishers, pp. 1–20.

Herman, Joost. 2006. The Dutch Drive for Humanitarianism: Inner Origins and Development of the Gidsland Tradition and Its External Effects. *International Journal* 61: 859–74. [CrossRef]

McDonald, Myra. 2003. *Exploring Media Discourse*. Oxford: Arnold Publishers.

Said, Edward. 1974. An Ethics of Language. *Diacritics* 4: 28–37. [CrossRef]
Simon, Jonathan. 2001. Governing through Crime Metaphors. *Broolkyn Law Review* 67: 1035–70.
Simon, Jonathan. 2007. *Governing through Crime: How the War on Crime Transformed American Democracy and Created a Culture of Fear*. New York: Oxford University Press.
Stumpf, Juliet. 2006. The crimmigration crisis: Immigrants, crime, and sovereign power. *International Organizations Law Review* 56: 356–420.
Van Der Woude, Maarthe. 2020. Euroskepticism, Nationalism, and the Securitization of Migration in The Netherlands. In *Crimmigrant Nations: Resurgent Nationalism and the Closing of Borders*. Chicago: Fordham University Press, pp. 227–48.
Van Der Woude, Maartje, Joanne Van der Leun, and Jo-anne Nijland. 2014. Crimmigration in The Netherlands. *Law and Social Inquiry* 39: 560–79. [CrossRef]
Van Der Woude, Maartje, Vanessa Barker, and Joanne Van Der Leun. 2017. Crimmigration in Europe. *European Journal of Criminology* 14: 3–6. [CrossRef] [PubMed]
Van Dijk, Teun A. 1998. Opinions and Ideologies in the Press. In *Approaches to Media Discourse*. Oxford: Blackwell Publishers, pp. 21–63.
Weber, Leanne, and Ben Bowling. 2008. Valiant beggars and global vagabonds: Select, eject, immobilize. *Theoretical Criminology* 12: 355–75. [CrossRef]
World Health Organization. 2018. Report on the Health of Refugees and Migrants in the WHO European Region: No Public Health without Refugee and Migrant Health. Available online: https://www.euro.who.int/en/publications/html/report-on-the-health-of-refugees-and-migrants-in-the-who-european-region-no-public-health-without-refugee-and-migrant-health-2018/en/index.html (accessed on 1 July 2021).

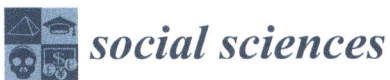

Article

The Exceptional Becomes Everyday: Border Control, Attrition and Exclusion from Within

Regina C. Serpa

Faculty of Social Sciences, University of Stirling, Stirling FK8 4LA, UK; r.c.serpa@stir.ac.uk

Abstract: This article examines processes of migration and border control, illustrating the ways by which everyday housing and welfare services function as mechanisms of exclusion in both direct and indirect ways. Using the thesis of crimmigration, the article demonstrates how border controls have become deeply implicated in systems claiming to offer welfare support—and how a global public health emergency has intensified exclusionary processes and normalised restrictive practices. The article compares border controls in two localities—under the UK government's coercive 'hostile environment' policies (based on technologies of surveillance) and a more indirect 'programme of discouragement' in The Netherlands (based on technologies of attrition). The study demonstrates the role of contemporary welfare states in entrenching inequality and social exclusion (from within), arguing that the exceptional circumstances of the COVID-19 pandemic have facilitated the differential everyday treatment of migrants, revealing a hierarchy of human worth through strategies of surveillance and attrition.

Keywords: COVID-19; welfare; crimmigration; exclusion; surveillance; attrition

Citation: Serpa, Regina C.. 2021. The Exceptional Becomes Everyday: Border Control, Attrition and Exclusion from Within. *Social Sciences* 10: 329. https://doi.org/10.3390/socsci10090329

Academic Editor: Robert Koulish

Received: 11 July 2021
Accepted: 3 September 2021
Published: 4 September 2021

Publisher's Note: MDPI stays neutral with regard to jurisdictional claims in published maps and institutional affiliations.

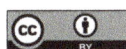

Copyright: © 2021 by the author. Licensee MDPI, Basel, Switzerland. This article is an open access article distributed under the terms and conditions of the Creative Commons Attribution (CC BY) license (https://creativecommons.org/licenses/by/4.0/).

1. Introduction: Bordering Practices in the Contemporary Welfare State

A succession of 'crises' observed in the 21st century—including the rise of terrorism, and more recently, the ongoing COVID-19 pandemic—have reinforced the role of borders as defensive barriers against undesirable influences and external threats, helping to construct the contemporary 'problem' of migration (De Genova and Tazzioli 2016). Ostensibly intended to protect national security and promote peace, freedom and prosperity, physical boundaries have served to strengthen societal divisions through intensifying 'paradigmatic borders'—between inside and outside, citizen and noncitizen—in law, public discourse and everyday human interaction (Krasmann 2007; Paasi 2009). Revealed within these societal divisions is a hierarchy of human worth, maintained by the expanding application of state technologies of control, categorisation, surveillance and punishment in migration governance which regards foreigners or noncitizens as suspect persons, and as such, they are assigned a dual identity of 'criminal' and 'migrant' combined: 'the crimmigrant' (Aas 2013, p. 331). Whilst there is no causal link between crime and migration control, a process of 'crimmigration' (Stumpf 2006) has facilitated a new 'state of exception'— where perceived threats to national security and law and order provide the rationale for creating extraordinary measures (Agamben 2005). In the context of support services, such exclusionary practices have been termed 'welfare penalism' and described as a form of 'benevolent violence' (Barker 2012). This article examines how housing and welfare services have become increasingly implicated in decisions relating to border control and national security and how the COVID-19 pandemic has exacerbated the bordering practices that operate in everyday services (Paasi 2009) to incorporate practices of exclusion from within.

This article is structured as follows: first, the methods are outlined in order to demonstrate the development of crimmigration control, in order to provide the theoretical framing of the research, with a focus on the exceptional and everyday, to analyse the role of the state and civil society in migration securitisation and bordered penality. The article examines how migration governance extends into the contemporary welfare state, through the deployment of technologies of surveillance and attrition. These technologies can be clearly witnessed in the examples of direct and indirect forms of coercion in the UK and The Netherlands, respectively, illustrating the nexus between crimmigration and the use of welfare as a border policing tool. The global pandemic has increased dependency and vulnerability—intensified by processes of attrition (through welfare entitlement) and exclusion from within (via surveillance)—throwing into sharp relief the differential treatment of noncitizens and revealing a hierarchy of human worth.

2. Materials and Methods

This study uses a comparative case study approach to consider the different ways of using welfare provision as a border control tool in two superficially contrasting societies: by comparing punitive features of the 'hostile environment' in the UK and the more indirect coercive control mechanisms of the 'programme of discouragement' in The Netherlands. Comparison is useful in highlighting the contingent nature of phenomena, providing insight into the extent to which pre-existing categories are neither natural nor fixed. A comparative method can challenge orthodox thinking, question assumptions and provide theoretical insight (often using interdisciplinary approaches). As Bloemraad (2013) suggested, comparative study provides fertile ground for an analysis of migration processes involving an analysis of a small number of cases to make sense of 'meaningful, complex structures, institutions, collectives and/or configurations of events' (p. 27). There is additional value in studying these issues from a socio-legal perspective as 'international migration implicates rights and legal status as people cross the borders of sovereign nation-states' (Bloemraad 2013, p. 28). Whilst much research on migration has focused on central government policy and the legal process, this article considers how exceptional circumstances are integrated into everyday practices through the operation of welfare and support policies.

The article thus examines the role of coercion and consent in bordering practices and how exceptional practices of exclusion become normalised under what has been termed 'necropolitics' (Mbembe 2003). The study has two central research questions: What is the relationship between welfare, housing and crimmigration control and how important is context (including relatively stable socio-political conditions and exceptional states of crisis) in the configuration of crimmigration control?

The study draws on examples of crimmigration control from two seemingly distinct localities with different ideological underpinnings, separate administrative systems, contrasting public policies and diverse social practices. The UK is selected as a paradigmatic neoliberal regime, based on explicitly coercive and punitive strategies of surveillance to control migration, supplemented by restrictive, highly conditional welfare systems in which crimmigration control is clearly articulated. In contrast, The Netherlands is a regime noted for its social democratic ethos, a facilitative model of social integration and a welfare system based on the principles of inclusion and consent. At the same time, The Netherlands demonstrates emerging features of crimmigration practice that challenge the assumed opposition between neoliberalism and welfarism (Barker 2018). These two examples can therefore provide insight into both causes and effects of arrangements to control, limit and (in some cases) facilitate the settlement of migrant groups. As the study argues, in practice, the two regimes share many assumptions and principles: concerning border control, the creation of 'in' and 'out' groups and exclusionary practices. More specifically, the article argues that indirect strategies of attrition have become a key mechanism of exclusion. As Bloemraad suggested 'you cannot know what is unique, or common, about a particular case unless you have a comparative point of reference' (p. 42).

Theoretical Framework: Bordering, Crimmigration and Necropolitical Exception

This research is motivated by three pressing trends in western democratic responses to international displacement and global mobility: (1) the development of observable 'crimmigration' control systems that blur the boundaries between immigration and criminal law, (2) deepening inequality and exclusion based on social divisions such as race, class and gender and (3) increasingly conditional and punitive welfare regimes within an environment of retrenchment and financial austerity. More recently, a fourth trend can be observed during the pandemic, which has ushered in a time of hyper immobility (at least temporarily) as borders close and national as well as localised lockdowns become commonplace, normalising a 'state of exception' in the exercise of unprecedented state power to control contagion—on a global scale. The following section offers an overview of the development of crimmigration control, focussing specifically on the extension of migration governance into the contemporary welfare state.

Globalisation in the last half-century has brought greater interdependence of the world's economies, cultures and populations, accompanied and assisted by technological advances which have enabled growing cross-border flows of investment, people and information (Gundhus and Franko 2016). As the distinction between domestic and international domains is increasingly blurred, 'unwanted' forms of migration (whether humanitarian, undocumented or constituted economic migrants) have become emblematic of a hybrid threat—to national security and sovereignty, on the one hand, and safety and order from *within*, on the other (Koulish and van der Woude 2020). In the US and Europe especially, the responses to the perceived 'threat' of migration have broadly centred on intensifying the 'securitization of migration' (Aas 2013; Guia 2013)—an approach often accompanied by an exclusionary and repressive political and social discourse (Koulish 2010; van der Leun and van der Woude 2013). Such processes of securitisation and exclusion—which radically transform state regulation of migration—have been described as 'crimmigration' to explain the intertwining of criminal and migration control with national security, observed in contemporary western democracy (Stumpf 2006; Guia 2013; Aas 2013).

In this article, bordering practice is conceptualised as involving the exercise of social control by 'inclusionary exclusion' (Agamben 2005), whereby the welfare state apparatus (and other civil society institutions) are co-opted by central authorities in the migration control project (Paasi 2009)—a complicity in crimmigration control which is nevertheless often contested and subject to resistance. However, local sites of 'border resistance' (Weber 2019) tend to be fragmented, ambiguous, idiosyncratic and surpassed by the influences of state control: crimmigration, therefore, has a profound effect on the scope and shape of social welfare *vis-à-vis* bordering practices—transforming humanitarian organisations into 'soft cops of the state' (Poulantzas 1969).

The present study applies Agamben (2005) idea of a 'state of exception' as a dominant paradigm of contemporary government, and the research considers how processes used in a period of crisis (whether financial, social or medical) are instituted within day-to-day social interactions. By combining this perspective with Mbembe (2003) analysis of 'necropolitics' which integrates the 'politics of race' and the 'politics of death' (p. 17), the article investigates how essential services have 'the capacity to define who matters and who does not, who is *disposable* and who is not' (Mbembe 2003, p. 27). From the perspective of 'necropolitical exception' (Farmer 2020), we can therefore explore how welfare structures are co-opted to implement migration control via technologies of surveillance and attrition; processes that exclude noncitizens (often racialised minorities and migrants from the postcolonial Global South) from welfare and housing support (Weber 2019). Through the creation of an exceptional space punctuated by dependence and vulnerability that would otherwise be unacceptable for citizens, welfare becomes a 'necropolitical site of violence' where migrant groups are 'kept alive but in a state of injury' (Mbembe 2003, p. 21) through the conditional delivery and denial of essential services.

By drawing on the literature on crimmigration in the UK and The Netherlands, the next sections contrast the bordering practices deployed in the delivery of accommodation and support services for migrant groups—contrasting the use of 'administrative removals' in the UK (through 'Operation Nexus' and 'Everyone In' policies—based on surveillance and coercion) with a 'programme of discouragement' (based on a principle of consent and attrition) in The Netherlands (van der Leun 2003). Whilst crimmigration can be seen as a modality of coercion, it should be noted that not all examples of coercion are evidence of crimmigration[1]. Nevertheless, the study shows how these exclusionary technologies of surveillance and attrition have been affected by the COVID-19 pandemic with welfare agencies complicit in policing the border as 'agents of necropolitical exception' (Farmer 2020) in both direct and indirect ways.

3. Discussion

This section considers the similarities and differences between the UK and The Netherlands. As discussed above, the two countries were chosen on the basis that they represented contrasting approaches to welfare delivery—on the one hand, a regime dominated by neoliberal ideology (UK) and, on the other, one that has adopted an approach influenced by social democracy (Netherlands) which nonetheless limits the inclusionary nature of the welfare state through hard and soft power to preserve a sense of social security for its members (Barker 2018). Given challenges to assumed opposition of neoliberalism and welfarism, this research suggests that the parallel approaches to the policing of the borders through welfare have become accentuated through strategies of attrition, in an unfolding state of exception during a global health crisis.

3.1. UK—Coercion and Technologies of Surveillance

The UK has been extensively criticised for adopting an explicitly punitive approach to migration—for example, by the explicit objective of creating a hostile environment and focusing on immigrant criminality (under Conservative Home Secretaries Theresa May and Priti Patel). Crucially these processes have been extended into welfare policies which have made noncitizens with limited entitlements and precarious legal status increasingly vulnerable to deprivation and homelessness (with rough sleeping used as grounds for removing permission to remain in the UK). As writers such as McKee et al. (2020) have shown, welfare and support agencies (including landlords) have become increasingly recruited in the governance of immigration, using stigma and other forms of power (Tyler 2020) to undermine the legitimacy of claims to migrant rights. These exclusionary processes have been reinforced during the pandemic—as the state of exception (to monitor and limit movement and ensure direct, punitive intervention by the state via information sharing and interagency collaboration) becomes normalised in welfare delivery.

As a consequence of rolling out crimmigration control in the UK since at least 2010 and by enshrining the 'hostile environment' policy in statute within the 2014 and 2016 Immigration Acts, those lacking full citizenship status (particularly those without documented legal status) are increasingly marginalised and excluded from wider society by restricting access to work, welfare and housing. The convergence of criminal and immigration law and its associated exclusionary practices has produced new legal tools available to a range of actors in a variety of institutional contexts, including social welfare providers—amongst others (Bowling and Westenra 2018). Crucially, these social control mechanisms extend far beyond the geographical border to reach deep into civil society, affecting a diverse range of policy areas such as housing, employment, health and education.

Uniquely, within the UK immigration system prior to Brexit, being homeless was the one category into which citizens of countries in the European Union who live in the UK can fall where they are not seen to be exercising their EU member Treaty Rights (as an employee, a jobseeker, a retired person or being economically self-sufficient). The consequence is that, on this basis, a foreign national who ordinarily has the right to live and work in the UK under the European Union's freedom of movement can be subject to administrative removal (deportation) (Serpa 2019). In 2012, 'Operation Nexus'—an interagency collaboration between the police and the Home Office to remove European Economic Area (EEA) nationals without a Right to Reside and/or who have otherwise had encounters with law enforcement—was piloted in London and later rolled out in another six English regions. Between 2012 and 2015, some 3000 'high harm' foreign national offenders (FNOs) were deported under Nexus—many of whom were targeted following engagement with homelessness and support, rather than criminal justice agencies (Griffiths and Morgan 2017). Deportations enforced under 'Operation Nexus' represent a small but significant part of the deportation machine in the UK which ensnares homeless groups along with (alleged and convicted) criminal offenders, contributing to the deportability of the crimmigrant Other. Based on technologies of surveillance, the UK represents a highly coercive and punitive attitude towards the governance of migration, one which clearly articulates the convergence of criminal and immigration law.

These crimmigration processes have been reinforced through proposals in 2021 (under the Nationality and Borders Bill) including suggestions that migrants should be held in an offshore hub; those arriving without permission could be given prison sentences up to four years (from six months under existing legislation) and those guilty of smuggling migrants could face life sentences (rather than 14 years) (Wadhera 2021). Declaring the asylum system as 'fundamentally broken', Patel has proposed new forms of social control to detect, capture, punish and ultimately banish migrant groups (The Home Office 2021). An explicit connection to crimmigration was demonstrated in Patel's speech in May 2021, criticising local group opposition to deportation and defence of local residents—see, for example, the successful action of local community groups in Glasgow Pollokshields to resist the deportation of two local men (Mackie and Brown 2021). Patel's response was as follows:

> I have a message to those who seek to disrupt the efforts of our enforcement officers. They should think about whether their actions may be preventing murderers, rapists and high harm offenders from being removed from our communities—and they should think long and hard about the victims of these crimes.
>
> (The Home Office 2021)

The severity of the rhetoric towards migrants used by Patel and other would-be enthusiastic crimmigration advocates is mirrored in policy. Responses to COVID-19 have resulted in further mechanisms of social exclusion for migrant groups, revealing differential treatment of noncitizens, reflective of a neocolonial logic constituted by a hierarchy of human worth (Mayblin et al. 2020). On 23rd of March 2020, UK Prime Minister Boris Johnson mandated what he described as the 'very draconian measure' of stopping all 'non-essential contact' with others and putting the country into 'lockdown', telling people in a televised statement they 'must' stay at home (UK Government 2020). Three days later, the UK Government implemented the 'Everyone In' policy and instructed local authorities to invest resources in providing accommodation for people sleeping rough during the pandemic. Crucially, migrants with no recourse to public funds (consisting disproportionately of racialised minorities from the Global South—NRPF Network 2021) and European nationals without a Right to Reside were excluded from the 'Everyone In' policy, a fact which some council leaders and migrant rights advocates challenged in the UK courts. On the 3rd of November 2020, the High Court ruled that councils can provide emergency housing during the pandemic to homeless people who would not normally be eligible for support; however, it was left to individual local authority discretion to use alternative powers and funding to assist those with no recourse to public funds (NRPF) who require shelter and other forms of support (Shelter 2021). While there have been no changes to the policy to impose the NRPF, many cash-strapped local authorities continued to exclude ineligible foreign nationals from 'Everyone In', despite the High Court judgement (NRPF Network 2021).

The exclusion of many foreign nationals from emergency homelessness assistance during the ongoing pandemic continues at a time when new immigration rules come into force, providing the UK Government the power to fully roll out an 'Operation Nexus' style programme of removal across the UK. As of the 1st of January 2021, when the Brexit transition period officially ended, rough sleeping has become grounds for refusal, or cancellation of, permission to remain in the UK. Local authorities across England seem well positioned to accommodate a national roll-out: since early 2019, an increasing number of Home Office agents have been embedded in local authority services to monitor advice and assistance offered to homeless migrants (Busby 2019). The implications for rough sleepers are considerable—it is estimated that more than a quarter of all street homeless persons in the UK are foreign nationals (Grierson 2020). Despite pressure from human rights groups to end 'Operation Nexus' and put a stop to expanded plans to deport EU rough sleepers across the UK post-Brexit, Home Secretary Priti Patel defended the policy, issuing a Home Office clarification stating, 'permission may only be refused or cancelled where a person has repeatedly refused suitable offers of support and engaged in persistent anti-social behaviour' (Mellor 2021). Charities have warned that the new immigration rules will deter some rough sleepers from seeking help and could push them into modern slavery and other exploitative work (Lister 2020). It is not yet clear how COVID-19 impacts on the law enforcement side of crimmigration policies that harness housing and welfare services to facilitate deportations; however, it is apparent that homeless foreign nationals—as the only group of rough sleepers excluded from the 'Everyone In' policy—have become much more visible and therefore easily identifiable as candidates for removal.

The effect of such technologies of surveillance and attrition, therefore, is the entrenchment of the criminalisation of migration in the UK by combining civil exclusions (relating to restricting access to homelessness support services) with deportation as an adjunct to criminal penalty (lacking settled status now constituting an illegal stay for EEA nationals in the UK). Deploying interventions based on force and control—and supported by the identification, categorisation and surveillance functions of the welfare state—deportation secures compliance with immigration policy by removing the possibility of choosing not to comply. By excluding many groups of migrants from the 'Everyone In' policy to remove homeless persons from the street, the pandemic (in combination with Brexit) lays the groundwork to intensify and expand such exceptional use of force to deport unwanted foreign nationals. This example not only illustrates how welfare providers have been made complicit by policy in migration control in a UK context but also how such imagining of 'immigrant criminality' is vital to understand the perceived political expediency of instituting a hostile environment for migrants and in general the legitimacy of social exclusion in societies (Franko 2019). In order to provide a contrasting approach, the next section considers how The Netherlands has approached the governance of migration in housing and welfare delivery.

3.2. Technologies of Attrition: The 'Programme of Discouragement' in The Netherlands

The Netherlands has been long commended for adopting a tolerant and humane approach in the treatment of migrants (Van der Woude et al. 2014). However, since the 1990s, Dutch immigration policies have been characterised by restrictive admission policies, increased exclusion of unauthorised migrants and greater pressure for migration control (Engbersen et al. 2006). Increasingly, the trend towards the securitisation and criminalisation of migrants observed in neoliberal regimes (such as the UK and the US) is emerging in The Netherlands and elsewhere in northern welfare states, prompting crimmigration scholars to question the assumed opposition between neoliberalism and welfarism and scrutinise the exclusionary nature of the welfare state's inclusionary logic (Barker 2018; Franko 2019).

Since the 1990s, The Netherlands was among the first countries in the European Union to reform immigration policy specifically targeting irregular migration, set within a context of a (financially and ideologically) pressurised welfare state—diminishing border controls, despite the EU principle of Freedom of Movement (van der Leun 2003; Leerkes et al. 2012). Policies of attrition have been implemented to prevent entry, exclude from social benefits and public assistance and expel irregular immigrants (van der Leun 2006)—this, in combination with increasingly managerialised austere state-run services, has resulted in growing desperation amongst 'unauthorsied' migrant groups. Alongside tightening migration controls, immigration-related penalties (such as deportation) have been introduced for criminal offences—reversing a trend towards limiting penal power in the turn towards crimmigration control. According to Van der Woude et al. (2014), over the 21st century, a 'humane paternalism', historically characteristic of the Dutch criminal justice system, has gradually been replaced with a process of 'managerial instrumentalism', deploying punishment as a 'cultural agent'. This newfound drive towards penalty signalled that 'the Dutch have purged themselves of the misplaced leniency of the past and are no longer afraid to punish' (Downes and Van Swaaningen 2007, p. 66).

Moreover, an association between ethnicity and social problems (especially crime and disorder perceived to be linked with migration from Morocco and the Antilles—Van der Woude et al. 2014) has gained political traction, with broad public support for stricter measures in The Netherlands commonly practiced elsewhere in Europe, such as deportation of immigrants who had committed crimes and 'soft' deportations (Versteegh and Maussen 2012). The punitive turn taken in The Netherlands, amid a backdrop of continuously hardening political and social discourse on immigration (and immigrants), can be traced to the 1980s with the Ministry of Justice white papers *Crime and Society* and *Law in Motion*. These policies have been generally regarded as a turning point in Dutch criminal justice policy, forging an indelible link between concerns about immigration and integration, on the one hand, and crime and safety, on the other, in popular and political imagination (Van der Woude et al. 2014). The sharper end of the crimmigration control system in The Netherlands can be observed in the growing criminalisation of migration (for example, the creation of specific immigration-crime offences including criminalising illegal stays). This 'immigrationalization of criminal law' (Legomsky 2007) includes deportation as an adjunct to criminal penalty, as well as expanding grounds for administrative detention on the basis of an immigrant's criminal background. It is important to note that, although deportation is an 'adjunct to criminal penalty', it is not considered a form of punishment despite having clear punitive consequences for the expelled (Van der Woude et al. 2014).

In response to public perception of the connection between immigration and social disorder, the Dutch government has turned to increased state coercion (Barker 2012). For example, governmental and quasi-governmental services (including welfare departments and social housing providers) are obliged under the 1998 Linking Act to conduct residency checks prior to giving access to certain services and benefits (Leerkes et al. 2012). Although new investigative powers of public sector and non-profit intermediaries have been expanded by the 2000 Aliens Act (amended in 2013 by the Modern Migration Policy and National Visa Acts), the amount of active surveillance of unauthorised migrants performed by civil service organisations in The Netherlands is limited (van der Leun 2003), owing in part to the resistance of relief organisations in policing migration. Rather than embark on a programme to fully converge criminal and immigration control (as is the aim of British migration policies), it would appear the Dutch approach to migration governance is less punitive and more permissive but nonetheless coercive in its exercise of social control and attrition. Given the emerging nature of the law enforcement side of crimmigration policies in The Netherlands, crimmigration is taken as a 'sensitizing concept' (Van der Woude et al. 2014) in understanding the ways in which welfare is used as a border policing tool.

Amid this backdrop of increasing criminalisation of migration, Dutch civil society includes a paradoxical merger of humanitarian care and securitisation imperatives (Kox and Staring 2020). In this context, humanitarian organisations refer to the wide range of agencies that provide relief to alleviate the hardship of migrants—critically, as Kox and Staring (2020) argued, these support organisations do so whilst simultaneously 'reproducing the causes of migrants' suffering and legitimizing restrictive migration policies' (p. 3). As van der Leun and Bouter (2015) demonstrated, internal border controls have rendered migrants without legal status wholly dependent on the (material and non-material) support of humanitarian organisations. Originally established to offer support to groups excluded from state-provided forms of support—many of these agencies emerged from protest movements against restrictive migration policies—these 'emergency relief' organisations now find themselves in the 'ambiguous' position of advocating for migrant rights whilst collaborating with central authorities in migration control (Kox and Staring 2020, p. 3). Whilst there is a measure of organisational resistance to these processes, empirical evidence suggests that unauthorised migrants largely consider these humanitarian organisations to be part and parcel of the Dutch migration control system (Kox and Staring 2020).

Thus, since the 1990s, humanitarian organisations have worked in close collaboration with their respective municipalities, limiting their power to resist central migration policies (Kalir and Wissink 2016). In the Dutch case, such organisations are, in effect, coerced by local municipalities via 'control by compliance' (Baines and van den Broek 2017) into implementing a programme of 'soft deportations' (called Assisted Voluntary Return), which function in addition to (or as a replacement of) state deportations (Leerkes et al. 2012). At the same time, participation in 'migration policing networks' has been contested by multiple acts of 'micro-refusal,' posing a challenge to state-centric bordering practices (Weber 2019; King 2016). Such local resistance to harsh immigration policies was articulated in April 2015 when several Dutch municipalities issued a statement in the daily newspaper *Volkskrant* refusing to cooperate with a decision by the then Dutch cabinet to refuse temporary shelter to failed asylum seekers and instead confirmed their continued commitment to provide '*bed-bad-brood*' arrangements providing shelter, bathing facilities and food relief for unauthorised migrants, rather than 'put or leave rejected asylum seekers out on the street' (Versteegh 2016, p. 366).

Even though central authorities have broadly opposed support for migrants residing in The Netherlands unlawfully, the Dutch government has never signalled an intent to criminalise such support—although there are financial consequences for municipalities that fail to meet state's expectations concerning resource management and policy delivery (Gerard and Weber 2019). Such strategies of attrition mean that, in exchange for support from local municipalities, humanitarian organisations can generally only assist those migrants who meet pre-determined eligibility criteria. The consequence is that only migrants who have a case for legal residency or who agree to voluntarily return to their country of origin are offered support. Emergency relief organisations dependent on municipality support are therefore effectively forced to exclude migrant clients falling outside these criteria (LOS Foundation 2014), demonstrating how indirect control is exercised through systematic withdrawal of services, rather than active intervention. The result is the creation of a 'structurally embedded border' involving 'migration policing networks' (Weber 2013) recruited to have both direct and indirect bordering effects. Denials of service thus create metaphorical but nevertheless powerful borders, leading to differential forms of social, political and economic in/exclusion.

Over the course of the pandemic, this attritional 'control by compliance' has involved 'cutbacks coercion' where state control is exercised through the failure to fund services to adequate levels. In contrast to Hall (2004) definition of coercion, such 'thwarted rights and stunted care' suggest that neglect originates at a systemic level, rather than being arbitrarily imposed, as organisations are under pressure to (reluctantly) act as conduits of control of scarce resources (Baines and van den Broek 2017, p. 142). Such attritional strategies are witnessed in the aforementioned closure and consolidation of several bed-bath-bread facilities over the course of the pandemic, resulting in increased numbers of homeless asylum seekers in desperate need of emergency relief (de Waard 2020). In The Netherlands, where unauthorised migrants are excluded from all formal markets and welfare arrangements (and only allowed essential healthcare, legal aid and primary and secondary education), studies on irregular migration have shown that it has become increasingly difficult to survive without a Dutch residence permit (Burgers and Engbersen 1999; Engbersen et al. 2002; Staring and Aarts 2010). In European states with strong welfare safety nets, such as in Scandinavian countries, the principles of universalism and inclusivity can be sustained, despite treating non-nationals punitively—simply because the 'crimmigrant Other' falls outside the responsibility of the welfare state (Barker 2012; Gundhus 2020). However, the closure of core facilities has intensified these struggles, resulting in deep social exclusion with many becoming dependent on (informal and formal) forms of support, and those lacking resources become vulnerable to exploitation and the possibility of engaging in survival crime (Van der Woude et al. 2014). In this way, the crimmigration–welfare nexus is sustained through an association between migration and extra-legal activities.

4. Conclusions

Despite differences in ideology, emphasis, institutional support and administrative approaches, the article highlights the similarities and differences in approaches to border control in the UK and The Netherlands. Whilst the UK adopts many features of a classic coercive state (dominated by central- and local-level state institutions and governed by technologies of surveillance), the Dutch approach is characterised by indirect coercion (administered increasingly by 'humanitarian' organisations), although underpinned by technologies of attrition. However, the underlying pressures—to reduce resources, limit immigration, control the behaviour of migrant groups, criminalise certain activities and use the agencies of state and civil society to reinforce stigma and social exclusion—are increasingly dominant in the design of welfare systems reflecting a hierarchy of human worth. Indirect coercion has become more apparent in times of crisis, with the effect of increasing dependency and vulnerability simultaneously; technologies of attrition that systematically deny noncitizens access to housing and welfare have therefore become an effective mechanism of exclusion from everyday services, and by extension, quotidian life.

The process of crimmigration implicates housing, welfare systems and other facets of civil society (including educational and healthcare settings) in everyday policing of migration. The use of crimmigration as explicit coercion (in the UK) and as a 'sensitising concept' (in The Netherlands) has potentially severe consequences for noncitizen groups (particularly for those unable to document legal status). The retrenchment of civil and social rights accompanying the extension of crimmigration control across multiple domains of social life (namely, with the introduction of accessorial liability in welfare provision and creating civil exclusions across a range of institutional contexts) has directly contributed to the growing economic and social precarity of migrant groups. For some migrants, the interaction of several systems, such as immigration, labour, welfare and housing markets, creates a reinforcing cycle of poverty that, once trapped, is difficult to escape (Dwyer et al. 2018). Found in a 'Catch-22' situation, socially excluded migrants become unable to afford housing due to low pay or no income, which in itself is a barrier to securing employment (for example, due to costs of travel) necessary to pay for accommodation (Maycock and Sheridan 2012). Migrants facing work and welfare restrictions due to their immigration status have few housing options and in extreme cases can result in homelessness and destitution (Dwyer et al. 2018; Edgar et al. 2004; Fitzpatrick et al. 2013). Engagement in 'survival crime' enhances a post-crimmigration nexus, a process that can legitimate further coercive measures. The COVID-19 pandemic has added to the desperate situation many migrant groups face, as many western democracies respond to an increase in asylum claims by (temporarily) suspending asylum protections, closing emergency relief and shelter provision and, in some instances, extending detention periods leading to the overcrowding of vulnerable adults and children in unsafe and inhumane conditions (Migration Data Portal 2021; Aal et al. 2021). The consequence of these processes is that a strategy of attrition has become more profound, leading to hierarchies of human worth as migrant groups are denied access to core services.

As a mode of social control in the welfare state context, contemporary bordering practices have served to reinforce marginalisation, dependency and destitution—processes that have intensified under a protracted state of exception which has resulted in increased use of indirect strategies of attrition, rather than direct controls through surveillance and explicit coercion. Notwithstanding these processes that render welfare providers complicit in crimmigration control through policy, the case studies presented here also demonstrate a measure of resistance reflected in the legal challenges brought against the UK Government's 'Everyone In' policy and the refusal of relief organisations and municipalities to deny essential services to unauthorised migrants in The Netherlands. Similarly, other research studies have signalled the potential of local-level, multiple, small-scale, temporary but significant strategies to facilitate the emancipatory potential of services through resistance (Weber 2019; King 2016), representing opportunities to create inclusive settlements from within.

Funding: This research was funded by the ESRC, grant number ES/V01210X/1.

Acknowledgments: I want to acknowledge Kim McKee of the University of Stirling, Maartje van der Woude of Leiden University, and the three anonymous referees for their invaluable feedback on this research.

Conflicts of Interest: The author declares no conflict of interest.

Notes

[1] I am grateful to one of the anonymous referees for making this point.

References

Aal, Monty, Grace Linczer Fehrenback, and Mohammad Abu Hawash. 2021. Locked up like animals—Immigrant detention centers in the time of the coronavirus. *Politico*, August 4. Available online: https://www.politico.eu/article/inside-immigrant-detention-centers-coronavirus-times-covid-19-europe/ (accessed on 3 September 2021).

Aas, Katja Franko. 2013. The Ordered and the Bordered Society: Migration Control, Citizenship and the Northern Penal State. In *The Borders of Punishment. Migration, Citizenship, and Social Exclusion*. Edited by Katja Franko Aas and Mary Bosworth. Oxford: Oxford University Press, pp. 21–39.

Agamben, Giorgio. 2005. *State of Exception*. Chicago: University of Chicago Press.

Baines, Donna, and Diane van den Broek. 2017. Coercive care: Control and coercion in the restructured care workplace. *The British Journal of Social Work* 47: 125–42. [CrossRef]

Barker, Vanessa. 2012. Global mobility and penal order: Criminalizing migration, a view from Europe. *Sociology Compass* 6: 113–21. [CrossRef]

Barker, Vanessa. 2018. *Nordic Nationalism and Penal Order: Walling the Welfare State*. London: Routledge.

Bloemraad, Irene. 2013. The promise and pitfalls of comparative research design in the study of migration. *Migration Studies* 1: 27–46. [CrossRef]

Bowling, Ben, and Sophie Westenra. 2018. 'A really hostile environment': Adiaphorization, global policing and the crimmigration control system. *Theoretical Criminology Journal* 24: 163–83. [CrossRef]

Burgers, Jack, and Godfried Engbersen. 1999. *De Ongekende Stad I: Illegale Vreemdelingen in Rotterdam*. Amsterdam: Boom.

Busby, Mattha. 2019. Immigration check outcry sees officers removed by councils. *The Guardian*, February 24. Available online: https://www.theguardian.com/uk-news/2019/feb/24/labour-councils-remove-embedded-immigration-officers (accessed on 3 September 2021).

De Genova, Nicholas, and Martina Tazzioli. 2016. *New Keywords of 'the Crisis' in and of Europe*. New York: Zone Books.

de Waard, Chris. 2020. Leidse bed-bad-broodopvang gesloten: Groep vluchtelingen op straat. *Sleutelstad*, May 1. Available online: https://sleutelstad.nl/2020/05/01/leidse-bed-bad-broodopvang-gesloten-groep-vluchtelingen-op-straat/ (accessed on 3 September 2021).

Downes, David, and Rene Van Swaaningen. 2007. The road to dystopia? Changes in the penal climate of The Netherlands. *Crime and Justice* 35: 31–71. [CrossRef]

Dwyer, Peter James, Lisa Scullion, Katy Jones, and Alasdair Stewart. 2018. The impact of conditionality on the welfare rights of EU migrants in the UK. *Policy and Politics* 47: 133–50. [CrossRef]

Edgar, Bill, Joe Doherty, and Henk Meert. 2004. *Immigration and Homelessness in Europe*. Bristol: Policy Press.

Engbersen, Godfried, Marion van San, and Arjen Leerkes. 2006. A room with a view: Irregular immigrants in the legal capital of the world. *Ethnography* 7: 209–42. [CrossRef]

Engbersen, Godfried, Richard Staring, Joanne van der Leun, Jan De Boom, Peter van der Heijden, and Maarten Cruijff. 2002. Illegale Vreemdelingen in Nederland. In *Omvang, Overkomst, Verblijf en Uitzetting*. Rotterdam: Erasmus University Rotterdam/Risbo.

Farmer, Natalia. 2020. 'I never felt like an illegal immigrant until social work turned up at the hospital': No Recourse to Public Funds as necropolitical exception. *The British Journal of Social Work*, 1–18. [CrossRef]

Fitzpatrick, Suzanne, Glen Bramley, and Sarah Johnsen. 2013. Pathways into multiple exclusion homelessness in seven UK cities. *Urban Studies* 50: 148–68. [CrossRef]

Franko, Katja. 2019. *The Crimmigrant Other: Migration and Penal Power*. London: Routledge.

Gerard, Alison, and Leanne Weber. 2019. Humanitarian borderwork: Identifying tensions between humanitarianism and securitization for government contracted NGOs working with adult and unaccompanied minor asylum seekers in Australia. *Theoretical Criminology* 23: 266–85. [CrossRef]

Grierson, Jamie. 2020. Foreign rough sleepers face deportation from UK post-Brexit. *Guardian*, October 21. Available online: https://www.theguardian.com/uk-news/2020/oct/21/foreign-rough-sleepers-face-deportation-from-uk-post-brexit (accessed on 3 September 2021).

Griffiths, Melanie, and Candice Morgan. 2017. *Deporting High Harm foreign criminals: Operation Nexus*. Policy Briefing 50: Oct 2017. University of Bristol. Available online: http://www.bris.ac.uk/media-library/sites/policybristol/briefings-and-reports-pdfs/2017-briefings--reports-pdfs/PolicyBristol_Briefing_October_2017_operation_nexus_web.pdf (accessed on 3 September 2021).

Guia, Maria Joao. 2013. Crimmigration, securitisation and the criminal law of the Crimmigrant. In *Social Control and Justice: Crimmigration in the Age of Fear*. Edited by Maria Joao Guia, Maartje van der Woude and Joanne van der Leun. The Hague: Eleven International.

Gundhus, Helene. 2020. Sorting out welfare: Crimmigration practices and abnormal justice in Norway. In *Crimmigrant Nations: Resurgent Nationalism and the Closing of Borders*. Edited by Robert Koulish and Maartje van der Woude. New York: Fordham University Press.

Gundhus, Helene, and Katja Franko. 2016. Global policing and mobility: Identity, territory, sovereignty. In *Handbook of Global Policing*. London: Sage.

Hall, Julie. 2004. Restriction and control: The perceptions of mental health nurses in a UK acute inpatient setting. *Issues in Mental Health Nursing* 25: 539–52. [CrossRef]

Kalir, Barak, and Lieke Wissink. 2016. The deportation continuum: Convergences between state agents and NGO workers in the Dutch deportation field. *Citizenship Studies* 20: 34–59. [CrossRef]

King, Natasha. 2016. *No Borders: The Politics of Immigration Control and Resistance*. London: Zed Books.

Koulish, Robert. 2010. *Immigration and American Democracy: Subverting the Rule of Law*. New York: Routledge.

Koulish, Robert, and Maartje van der Woude. 2020. The problem of migration. In *Crimmigrant Nations: Resurgent Nationalism and the Closing of Borders*. Edited by Robert Koulish and Maartje van der Woude. New York: Fordham University Press.

Kox, Mieke, and Richard Staring. 2020. If you don't have documents or a legal procedure, you are out!'Making humanitarian organizations partner in migration control. *European Journal of Criminology*, 1–20. [CrossRef]

Krasmann, Susanne. 2007. The enemy on the border: Critique of a programme in favour of a preventive state. *Punishment & Society* 9: 301–18.

Leerkes, Arjen, Godfried Engbersen, and Joanne van der Leun. 2012. Crime among irregular immigrants and the influence of internal border control. *Crime, Law and Social Change* 58: 15–38. [CrossRef]

Legomsky, Stephen. 2007. The new path of immigration law: Asymmetric incorporation of criminal justice norms. *Washington and Lee Law Review* 64: 469.

Lister, Sam. 2020. Rough sleepers will no longer be helped, instead they'll be deported. *Inside Housing*, October 30. Available online: https://www.insidehousing.co.uk/comment/comment/rough-sleepers-will-no-longer-be-helped-instead-theyll-be-deported-68388 (accessed on 3 September 2021).

LOS Foundation. 2014. *Hulpverlening aan Uitgeprocedeerde Asielzoekers in 2013*. Utrecht: LOS Foundation.

Mackie, Rachel, and Hannah Brown. 2021. Kenmure Street: Police order release of men after deportation raid standoff in Glasgow street where residents blocked UK Border Agency. *The Scotsman*, May 14. Available online: https://www.scotsman.com/news/crime/kenmure-street-police-order-release-of-men-after-deportation-raid-standoff-in-glasgow-street-where-residents-blocked-uk-border-agency-3235341 (accessed on 9 July 2021).

Mayblin, Lucy, Mustafa Wake, and Mohsen Kazemi. 2020. Necropolitics and the slow violence of the everyday: Asylum seeker welfare in the postcolonial present. *Sociology* 54: 107–23. [CrossRef]

Maycock, Paula, and Sarah Sheridan. 2012. *Migrant Women and Homelessness: Key Findings from a Biographical Study of Homeless Women in Ireland*. Research Paper 2. Dublin: School of Social Work and Social Policy and Children's Research Centre, Trinity College Dublin.

Mbembe, Achille. 2003. Necropolitics. *Public Culture* 15: 11–40. [CrossRef]

McKee, Kim, Sharon Leahy, Trudi Tocarzyc, and Joe Crawford. 2020. Redrawing the border through the 'Right to Rent': Exclusion, discrimination and hostility in the English housing market. *Critical Social Policy* 41: 91–110. [CrossRef]

Mellor, Joe. 2021. Damaging post-Brexit immigration rules may push rough sleepers into modern slavery. *The London Economic*, May 7. Available online: https://www.thelondoneconomic.com/n;ews/damaging-post-brexit-immigration-rules-may-push-rough-sleepers-into-modern-slavery-268390/ (accessed on 3 September 2021).

Migration Data Portal. 2021. Migration Data Relevant for the COVID-19 Pandemic. March 10. Available online: https://migrationdataportal.org/themes/migration-data-relevant-covid-19-pandemic (accessed on 3 September 2021).

NRPF Network. 2021. No Recourse to Public Funds Network. Available online: http://www.nrpfnetwork.org.uk/Pages/Home.aspx (accessed on 25 February 2020).

Paasi, Anssi. 2009. Bounded spaces in a 'borderless world': Border studies, power and the anatomy of territory. *Journal of Power* 2: 213–34. [CrossRef]

Poulantzas, Nicos. 1969. The problem of the capitalist state. *New Left Review* 1: 67–78.

Serpa, Regina. 2019. Resisting welfare conditionality. In *Dealing with Conditionality: Implementation and Effects*. Edited by Peter Dwyer. Bristol: Policy Press.

Shelter. 2021. Immigration and Residence Restrictions. Available online: https://england.shelter.org.uk/housing_advice/homelessness/immigration_and_residence_restrictions (accessed on 3 September 2021).

Staring, Richard, and Jose Aarts. 2010. *Jong en Illegaal in Nederland*. Amsterdam: WODC, Ministerie van Justitie.

Stumpf, Juliet. 2006. The the crimmigration crisis: Immigrants, crime, and sovereign power. *American University Law Review* 56: 367–419.

The Home Office. 2021. Home Secretary Priti Patel Speech on Immigration, 24/5/21. Available online: https://www.gov.uk/government/speeches/home-secretary-priti-patel-speech-on-immigration (accessed on 4 July 2021).

Tyler, Imogen. 2020. *Stigma: The Machinery of Inequality*. London: Zed Books.

UK Government. 2020. Prime Minister's Statement on Coronavirus (COVID-19): 23 March 2020. Available online: https://www.gov.uk/government/speeches/pm-address-to-the-nation-on-coronavirus-23-march-2020 (accessed on 3 September 2021).

van der Leun, Joanne. 2003. *Looking for Loopholes: Processes of Incorporation of Illegal Immigrants in The Netherlands*. Amsterdam: Amsterdam University Press.

van der Leun, Joanne. 2006. Excluding illegal migrants in The Netherlands: Between national policies and local implementation. *West European Politics* 29: 310–26. [CrossRef]

van der Leun, Joanne, and Harmen Bouter. 2015. Gimme shelter: Inclusion and exclusion of irregular immigrants in Dutch civil society. *Journal of Immigrant and Refugee Studies* 13: 135–55. [CrossRef]

van der Leun, Joanne, and Maartje van der Woude. 2013. A Reflection on Crimmigration in The Netherlands: On the Cultural Security Complex and the Impact of Framing. In *Social Control and Justice: Crimmigration in the Age of Fear*. Edited by Maria Joao Guia, Maartje van der Woude and Joanne van der Leun. The Hague: Eleven International, pp. 41–60.

Van der Woude, Maartje, Joanne van der Leun, and Jo-Anne Nijland. 2014. Crimmigration in The Netherlands. *Law and Social Inquiry* 39: 560–79. [CrossRef]

Versteegh, L. 2016. About Bed, Bath and Bread: Municipalities as the last resort for rejected asylum seekers. In *Urban Europe: Fifty Tales of the City*. Edited by Virginie Mamadouth and Anne Wageningen. Amsterdam: Amsterdam University Press, pp. 363–68.

Versteegh, Lia, and Marcel Maussen. 2012. *Contested Policies of Exclusion: Resistance and Protest against Asylum Policy in The Netherlands*. Amsterdam: Amsterdam Institute for Social Science Research (AISSR).

Wadhera, Celine. 2021. Priti Patel announces harsher sentences for migrants in bid to deter Channel crossings. *The Independent*, July 5. Available online: https://www.independent.co.uk/news/uk/home-news/priti-patel-illegal-channel-crossing-b1877753.html (accessed on 9 July 2021).

Weber, Leanne. 2013. *Policing Non-Citizens*. New York: Routledge.

Weber, Leanne. 2019. From state-centric to transversal borders: Resisting the 'structurally embedded border'in Australia. *Theoretical Criminology* 23: 228–46. [CrossRef]

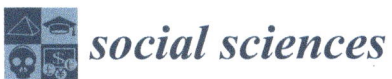

Article

Dealing with the 'Crimmigrant Other' in the Face of a Global Public Health Threat: A Snapshot of Deportation during COVID-19 in Australia and New Zealand

Henrietta McNeill

Department of Pacific Affairs, Coral Bell School of Asia Pacific Affairs, Australian National University, Canberra, ACT 2600, Australia; henrietta.mcneill@anu.edu.au

Abstract: While global travel largely stopped and borders closed during the COVID-19 pandemic, states continued to deport individuals who had been sentenced for committing criminal offences. In Australia and New Zealand, questions over whether and how deportation of migrants during a global pandemic should occur were raised: weighing up arguments of legality, public health, and security. This left many migrants uncertain, isolated in immigration detention waiting for an unknown departure date. The decision was made to continue the deportation process for many, and in some cases breaches of public health restrictions were the basis for deportation. Once deported, mandatory quarantine on arrival under COVID-19 restrictions highlights and exacerbates the challenges that returning offenders normally face. These include extended detention periods; surveillance through detention and monitoring; and securitised discourse by the media and public creating ongoing stigma. This snapshot enables us to understand how states prioritised the removal of 'the crimmigrant other', a securitised threat, while facing the material threat of COVID-19.

Keywords: crimmigration; deportation; immigration detention; return; COVID-19; pandemic; securitisation; threat prioritisation; Australia; New Zealand

Citation: McNeill, Henrietta. 2021. Dealing with the 'Crimmigrant Other' in the Face of a Global Public Health Threat: A Snapshot of Deportation during COVID-19 in Australia and New Zealand. *Social Sciences* 10: 278. https://doi.org/10.3390/socsci10080278

Academic Editor: Nigel Parton

Received: 7 June 2021
Accepted: 19 July 2021
Published: 21 July 2021

Publisher's Note: MDPI stays neutral with regard to jurisdictional claims in published maps and institutional affiliations.

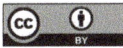

Copyright: © 2021 by the author. Licensee MDPI, Basel, Switzerland. This article is an open access article distributed under the terms and conditions of the Creative Commons Attribution (CC BY) license (https://creativecommons.org/licenses/by/4.0/).

1. Introduction

The COVID-19 pandemic closed borders and created unprecedented restrictions on international travel to mitigate a materialised global public health threat. Naturally, it could be assumed that the worldwide border restrictions would limit deportations too; however, this was not the case, highlighting the precarious and vulnerable nature of migration pathways both into and out of state borders by those deemed 'the crimmigrant other' (Franko 2019). When two 'threats' are faced simultaneously by states—both the material health threat and the constructed threat of criminal non-citizens—how do states act? Which 'threat' becomes prioritised? In this article, I argue that when states have continued to deport 'the crimmigrant other' in the face of a material threat that has affected the world to the extent that COVID-19 has, the securitisation of migration and deportation has clearly been weighted more heavily within a national security risk assessment and taken priority.

Many of us experienced the border closures, restrictions of movement during lockdown, as well as regulations around mask-wearing during COVID-19. At the same time, many migrants were facing deportation. In the United Kingdom, skilled workers working on COVID-19 infection control were refused the right to remain in the country and faced deportation (Townsend 2021). In the United States, immigration authorities used COVID-19 exposure as a threat to asylum seekers to coerce them into accepting deportation (Washington 2021) and US deportations to the Republic of the Marshall Islands have hit record numbers in 2020, despite border restrictions and the full fiscal year not being complete (Johnson 2020). Likewise, Australian criminal deportations for 2019/2020 are the second-highest on record, an increase from the previous two years (Home Affairs 2021a). These examples show that border restrictions and health security threats pose no hinderance to states that intend to remove people they consider a more significant criminal 'threat'.

Australia, New Zealand and neighbouring Pacific Island states and territories make up an area of the world which has been responsive to the health threat of COVID-19 and had comparatively few cases of community transmission. Australia managed borders and lockdowns to stop community transmission; New Zealand has appeared to have successfully eliminated community transmission for sustained periods; and many Pacific Island states never had the virus breach their secured borders. However, with such public and political attention paid to border security and migration to ensure national security when facing such a public health threat, existing issues of securitisation and crimmigration have become amplified. Boon-Kuo et al. (2020, p. 10) found that in Australia 'COVID policing has intensified existing policing practices directed towards the "usual suspects", which disrupts the notion that COVID-19 policing is directed solely towards the legitimate public health objective of preventing contagion'. By having some of the strongest border restrictions within the global context of the COVID-19 pandemic, Australia and New Zealand provide a fascinating microcosm of the application of crimmigration through deportation, and how these securitised approaches have been amplified when faced with a contrasting material public health threat.

This article examines the extent to which states intentionally prioritised constructed threats of convicted non-citizens over material public health threats, arguably operationalised through crimmigration mechanisms and deportation during the COVID-19 global pandemic. As Clapton (2021, p. 138) states, 'in a world of uncertainty and unknowing, unknowns can justify exceptional security actions, rather than clearly identifiable, existential threats'. This article provides an empirical discussion of the balancing of the securitisation of migration against the material threat of COVID-19, using news media reporting (newspaper articles and televised news reports) of Australian deportations and the corresponding New Zealand reception of deportees in 2020 and 2021. This is supported by government documentation (reports, briefing papers, diplomatic cables, and official statistics) detailing New Zealand's own deportations in the period between March 2020 and March 2021, sourced under the Official Information Act 1982 process. Through this analysis, I consider the 'crimmigrant other' as a securitised threat to the state balanced against the material public health threat, and argue that Australia and New Zealand have prioritised the deportation of convicted non-citizens in the face of the very real harm caused by the COVID-19 pandemic.

2. Material vs. Constructed Threats

Health security is understood broadly to be where individuals' and public health interacts with economic security, food security, and the possibility for civil unrest, and therefore is not simply the way in which 'disease may affect military capacity ... and the impact of conflict on health and health care' (McInnes 2014, p. 7). Davies et al. (2015) have shown that states have been paying closer attention to the threat of infectious diseases, within a broader global health security push resulting in increased expenditure and action when outbreaks and health threats (such as anthrax attacks) occurred. A material or objective threat results in actual harm, rather than solely perceived harm. COVID-19 is a prime example of where states acted to combat a materialised health threat due to the large-scale impact on human life, the economy, and national security. To manage the material threat of COVID-19, many states deployed police and military personnel to enforce public health laws and regulations. However, Boon-Kuo et al. (2020, p. 3) found that 'Police do not simply enforce stated public health goals—the extent of discretionary authority awarded to police under COVID strengthens their role in defining *who* and *what* constitutes a health threat' allowing for expanded securitisation during a global pandemic by law enforcement bodies. This enabled law enforcement to pursue their 'usual suspects'—migrants and other vulnerable populations commonly perceived to be a criminal threat—under the guise of a material public health threat (Boon-Kuo et al. 2020, p. 10).

Securitisation is a form of discursive power, whereby expressing the perception of the threat itself constructs that threat and enables an actor to respond in kind. The 'threat' and perception thereof is subjective—perceived as an existential threat by the referent object (that which is threatened). A widely recognised definition is that of eminent Copenhagen School security scholars Buzan and Wæver (2003, p. 491), who state that securitisation is 'the discursive process through which an intersubjective understanding is constructed within a political community to treat something as an existential threat to a valued referent object, and to enable a call for urgent and exceptional measures to deal with the threat'. Therefore, if an issue or entity is constructed as an existential threat to the state as the referent object, then the state can also construct a mandate through which to take extraordinary action. Clapton (2021, p. 132) further explains that 'while securitisation theory's emphasis on the discursive production of security means that threats and referent objects could be anything that actors say they are, this is coupled with a fixed definition and logic of security'.

Over the past two decades, there has been a gradual securitisation of migration, constructing a 'pervasive and insidious connection between migration, crime, and other issues, including national security' (Franko 2019, p. 35). States use increasingly securitised language to describe migrants who have committed criminal offences as a (subjective) threat to national security, through which states have gained a political mandate to take extraordinary action in expelling criminal non-citizens. Crimmigration is a concept which describes states' increasingly harsh legal and policing approaches towards non-citizens, and is a practical representation of the securitisation of migration (Stumpf 2006). Criminal deportation is one of the two 'faces' of crimmigration, describing increasingly harsh approaches taken when those that commit criminal offences in-country are resubjected to migration back to their country of origin (Stumpf 2013). This is particular to migrants, as if a citizen had committed the crime, they would be sentenced, and then released back into the community as a free person, whereas migrants—after serving the same sentence—receive a secondary removal from society: exclusion from the state itself through deportation. Deportation decisions are predominantly intended to reduce the risk to the deporting state. Weber and Pickering (2013) use the terminology 'exporting risk' through return: by returning non-citizens and using political rhetoric against them, the state is portraying the reduction of risk or 'threat' to society from those who are different and could have a negative societal impact through crime. It is this constructed 'threat' of criminal non-citizens and the action of deportation to remove such a threat that I argue is being prioritised over the material threat of COVID-19.

Franko (2019, p. 36) has framed those who are excluded from society on the grounds of crime and immigration, as 'the crimmigrant other'—whose deviance is not just shaped simply by their criminal offending or their non-citizenship, but also by 'another social condition, which distinguishes him or her from other groups of deviants and outsides that have been traditionally portrayed in criminological and sociological literature'. She suggests that 'deportation entails in many respects the production of fear' (Franko 2019, p. 38); therefore, the 'crimmigrant other' framing is part of the discursive power of securitising criminal non-citizens, enabling further extraordinary action against them, such as deportation.

Cooper (2020) found that Australia in particular, has long securitised migration issues. Billings (2019, p. v) claims that Australia is 'at the forefront of crimmigration globally', due to harsh Australian criminal and immigration law enabling large-scale immigration detention and deportation, and prevention of asylum seeker entry by sea. New Zealand too, has been seen to apply crimmigration concepts both in its deportations to Pacific Island states (see McNeill 2021), and in receipt of New Zealanders deported from Australia (see Stanley 2017; McHardy 2021).

Less studied than individual perceived or material threats is when a state faces multiple threats at once, both material and constructed, and how states might address or prioritise these threats. Therefore, proposing how constructed and material threats are balanced when faced simultaneously is this article's original contribution to the literature. Clapton (2021, p. 131) outlines that 'attention must be paid to the ways in which dangers are discursively framed rather than the spatial location of responses to identified dangers or the forms of response that eventuate'. I hypothesize that when faced with multiple simultaneous threats, because a state only has finite resources, how the state frames and securitises such threats and then apportions its security resources on the basis of this framing is therefore indicative of where they consider the greater threat to be. When states have continued to focus on deportation in the face of a material threat that has affected the world to the extent that COVID-19 has, the securitisation of migration and deportation has clearly been weighted more heavily within the risk assessment, and taken priority, including of resourcing. The 'crimmigrant other' is deemed a higher perceived threat than the material threat of a global pandemic, at the expense of migrants' welfare and the potential health risk of detaining people in close proximity and moving people at a time when borders are otherwise closed.

3. Australian Deportations during COVID-19

Australia's migration policy has 'unorthodox and punishing procedures for people appealing against cancellation decisions, prolonged and uncertain periods of immigration detention, and family separation, among other human rights violations' (Billings 2019, p. 12). These practices match Stumpf (2013) two 'faces' of crimmigration: criminalising asylum seekers who come to Australia via boat including their subsequent detention and conditions; and the detention and deportation from Australia of non-citizens with prior criminal convictions or of 'poor character', in an attempt to pre-empt the perceived threat of future criminal activity.

Visa cancellations leading to immigration detention and deportation are a central feature of the immigration framework and manifest in (s)501 of the Migration Act 1958, enabling the cancellation of visas for those perceived to be of poor character, who have association with criminal groups, and those who have been sentenced more than a cumulative 12 months in prison. These elements increase the severity of the law and 'evidencing a political will to crack down on non-citizens who offend, or who might offend' (Billings and Hoang 2019, p. 121). Visa cancellation does not take into account factors other than perceived criminality or character, such as if the non-citizen arrived as a child or was born in Australia, which the courts have claimed creates undue harm to the non-citizen as they do not have any ties to their country of origin: Australia often deports non-citizens who have grown up in Australia and ostensibly have 'learnt' their behaviour in Australia (Billings and Hoang 2019).

Australia has typically deported on average 951 persons per annum under s501 since the 2014 amendments were enacted, deporting an increased 1021 persons during the 2019/20 and another 554 in the six months to 30 December 2020—the year of COVID-19 lockdowns (Home Affairs 2021a). This continuation of deportation during a global pandemic, when borders were otherwise closed, shows a prioritisation of the securitisation of migration over the material health threat of COVID-19. However, deportations are just one indicator of the severe and restrictive conditions faced by migrants during this period.

During the COVID-19 pandemic, migrants in Australia were faced with amplified challenges. Migrants were required to answer questions regarding their nationality and language during the vaccine roll-out, which has been highlighted as possibly creating data that will result in social stigma for particular ethnic groups (Dalzell 2021). Many migrants residing in Australia were not entitled to financial support from the government through the COVID-19 period (and subsequently in the 2021 post-COVID budget the waiting period for migrants to access financial benefits was increased to four years resident in Australia). Therefore, many migrants faced unemployment, underpayment and wage theft due to economic fallout of COVID-19—highlighting the already precarious status of migrants, particularly those in casual or at-risk employment (Aryal Lees and Niner 2021). For example, migrants on temporary student visas had to work multiple casual and/or high-risk jobs and were fearful of admitting to authorities when they had breached public health regulations, likely out of fear for immigration-related repercussions. In one case, a Spanish national on a graduate visa lied to police, during contact tracing during a bout of community transmission of the virus, about working in a second casual job in a pizza shop on top of his quarantine job and being a vector, sparking a three-day lockdown in South Australia.

In many Australian states, not complying with COVID-19 public health regulations became a criminal offence (Boon-Kuo et al. 2020). Therefore, crimmigration-related repercussions occurred: a French national was deported under s501 for organising a party of over 1000 people which did not comply with COVID-19 regulations (Lamb et al. 2021). At the extreme end of this, those who desperately wanted to return home but were restricted by closed borders and limited commercial flights, sometimes resorted to behaving 'inappropriately' to provoke their forced removal by authorities via deportation; however, in one instance 'a [seasonal] worker did not get to return home with his team in the June repatriation flights due to waiting for a pending court case—therefore his actions backfired' (Bailey 2020, p. 71).

During COVID-19, prior to their removal deportees were subjected to even tighter restrictions. In addition to existing motels, hotel apartments, and detention centres, during the COVID-19 period the Department of Home Affairs sought new Alternative Places of Detention including hospitals, aged care homes, and mental health facilities (Eddie 2021). Within detention, people were further isolated from society by having visitors denied (Doran 2020). Their deportations were also delayed and detainees received limited communications from authorities about their deportation dates: for at least one detainee, this delay and uncertainty around his removal had a significant mental health impact and eventuated in suicide (Yu 2020).

The sense of isolation was even more severe for over 200 convicted non-citizens awaiting deportation who were transferred to Christmas Island Detention Centre when it reopened following a 2018 closure unrelated to COVID-19 (Ryan 2020). The August 2020 reopening was blamed upon COVID-19, as the Department of Home Affairs claimed their 'ability to remove unlawful non-citizens from Australia had been curtailed by the coronavirus pandemic' (cited in Karp 2021). However, it appears as though it was inevitable—with the Australian government continuing to spend AUD 23 m on the Christmas Island facility in 2019 when it was empty (Burgess 2019). In addition, critics oppose the government's COVID-19 framing—stating that it was actually reopened to stifle public protests regarding detention (which were criminalised during COVID-19), and remove detainees from public view (Blakkarlay 2020; Boon-Kuo et al. 2020).

Detaining migrants on offshore islands, known as Alternative Places of Detention, creates 'microgeographies of sites in the enforcement archipelagos where these exclusions transpire, where migrants enter into extended periods of spatial, temporal, and legal limbo' (Mountz 2020, p. 60). This is not just exclusion from society once in offshore immigration detention, but more practically detainees are also unable to access vital services: in January 2021, riots erupted when convicted non-citizens awaiting deportation were not given their medication for days at a time, internet access and mobile reception to contact legal representation or families, and were kept inside for 22 h per day (Karp 2021). However, this was not simply about cost: advocates argued that the issue was more than just a restriction of services but instead a bigger issue of 'people in a powerless situation being repetitively treated with disrespect and in an inhumane manner' (Payne cited in Karp 2021). The riots were responded to with rubber bullets and gas cannisters, which further polices and militarises detainees in an already-carceral immigration detention situation. Crimmigration describes an increasingly policed approach to immigration procedures, and this is but one example.

Half of s501 deportations for both character and criminal reasons from Australia are to New Zealand, despite New Zealanders only comprising 10% of the non-citizen population (Billings and Hoang 2019). Under COVID-19, this was higher than usual—with 75% of those deported under s501 between March 2020–2021 of New Zealand citizenship, the next highest nationality of deportation being Vietnamese at 6% (Home Affairs 2021b). The Department of Home Affairs stated that 'removals of non-citizens have not stopped as a result of COVID-19, however have significantly slowed since March 2020 due to the availability of commercial flights and the travel restrictions' (cited in Doran 2020): after ceasing on 16 March 2020, Australia recommenced their deportation programme New Zealand in July 2020 (Home Affairs 2021b). The youngest s501 deportation yet was deported to New Zealand during this period—a solo 15-year-old—showing the extraordinary action Australia was willing to take, and the urgency by which it wanted to be 'rid' of securitised criminal non-citizens.

The Australian government avoided the complexities of limited commercial flights by chartering 'secret' Airbus319s for the purpose, in particular those 'with no markings on its tail except a small Australian flag' (Fabris 2021). The fact that these deportations did not stop, despite almost all other travel being forcibly halted amplifies the securitised nature of these deportations: Australia balanced the risk of criminality (while deportees remained in immigration detention) against the public health threat of COVID-19 transmission through borders and chose to remove non-citizens. The Australian government were willing to take exceptional action against a perceived threat, using their own or a chartered plane to remove those they considered a 'crimmigrant other', in a time when all other travel had been halted.

Australia continued to securitise convicted non-citizens on their deportation during the COVID-19 period. The Department of Home Affairs gave exclusive access to a commercial television channel to interview deportees as they crossed the airport tarmac to their departing flight in March 2021. This was not welcomed by deportees, as the questioning was seen to be confrontational and harassing at the point when those leaving were contemplating the loss of their family and homes—'our country doesn't want you, are you excited to go home?' and 'how does it feel to be kicked out of Australia?' (Fabris 2021). To add to the sensationalism and fear-mongering around deportees, in the same coverage, then-Minister for Home Affairs Peter Dutton described the deporting flight of New Zealanders as 'taking the trash out' (cited in Fabris 2021). While this rhetoric may appear gratuitous, it is perceptibly deliberate and intentional. The discourse further securitises and dehumanises deportees, enabling harsher approaches towards them in efforts to manage them as a threat.

4. New Zealand Reception of Deportations during COVID-19

When Australia introduced harsher deportation legislation in 2014, New Zealand received a five-fold increase in returnees per month and has now receives over 2375 returnees since 2015 (McGowan 2021). This created pressure on the New Zealand Government, who publicly alluded to the deportees' criminality and securitised them. In 2015, the then-Prime Minister referred to criminal deportees from Australia as 'rapists' and 'child molesters', despite the majority of New Zealanders in Australian detention for deportation being held on considerably more minor cannabis charges (Stanley 2017). This discourse shows that deportees are unwanted on both sides of their journey—re-securitised as a threat for their perceived levels of criminality by their state of citizenship. The rhetoric worsened during the COVID-19 period—highlighted as deportees were some of the few able to travel despite the restrictions—but is an example of how deportees have for years been perceived to be criminal offenders forevermore.

Further securitised discourse from New Zealand politicians shows that New Zealand society does not consider that all returnees from Australia to be part of New Zealand society, due to their Australian upbringing. In 2020, New Zealand Prime Minister Jacinda Ardern (cited in Remeikis 2020), when speaking to Australian Prime Minister Scott Morrison, stated:

"You have deported more than 2000 individuals, and among them will be genuine Kiwis who do need to learn the consequences of their actions. But among those 2000 are individuals who are too young to become criminals on our watch, they were too young to become patched gang members, too young to be organised criminals. We will own our people. We ask that Australia stops exporting theirs".

The pressure from the Australian deportation policy and New Zealand's apprehensive reception of deportees, was described as 'corrosive' to the Trans-Tasman relationship (Ardern cited in McGowan 2021). Similarly, in 2021 following the 'trash'-talk by an Australian politician, New Zealand COVID-19 Response Minister Chris Hipkins responded that 'we're receiving them because we're obliged to receive them, but it would be wrong to say we're happy about it' (cited in Doran 2020). Through this exclusionary discourse, deportees are being framed by their state of citizenship as an 'other'; therefore, alongside the perceived ongoing criminality (despite their status as otherwise free citizens), deportees remain a 'crimmigrant other' threat, this time in their state of citizenship.

COVID-19 quarantine for returnees was a convergence of issues that illustrated many of the challenges that deportees to New Zealand face. Instead of arriving and being (relatively) free citizens, returnees under s501 from Australia were kept for 14 days in a separate hotel for returned criminal deportees. Hotel quarantine is something that both New Zealand and Australia have put in place to isolate and quarantine incoming arrivals to create a barrier against the public health threat of COVID-19. Loughnan (2020) has made the comparison between the hotels selected for incoming arrivals, and those used to indefinitely detain refugees and asylum seekers in Australia, and has highlighted the complexities around detention and isolation. Similarly, Nethery and Ozguc (2021) have suggested that Australia's hotel quarantine was well accepted because 'Australians have become somewhat conditioned to accept the idea that liberty—at least the liberty of outsiders—should at times take second priority to the national interest' due to existing immigration detention arrangements for refugees, asylum seekers and deportees. No similar research currently exists for New Zealand, but this analysis shows that the public health threat, and threat of the 'crimmigrant other' are both perceived as both unfavourable to national security and require extraordinary actions to mitigate them.

From March 2020, all arrivals to New Zealand were kept in a 14-day Mandatory Isolation and Quarantine (MIQ) due to the public health threat of COVID-19. Returning deportees—colloquially known as '501s'—were also mandated to quarantine for 14 days on arrival to New Zealand. Initially it was proposed that deportees and general arrivals share hotels; however, there was public pushback against shared facilities—with some members of the public suggesting that returned deportees should be kept on military bases (Holland 2020). This framing is suggestive of a crimmigration lens—where immigration enforcement bodies have the privileges of criminal law enforcement bodies and act similarly.

It was then decided that a specific isolation hotel for deportees would be set up, but the selection of the hotel itself was shrouded in secrecy for fear of 'vigilante justice' being served by members of the public (Block 2021). Ultimately, the selected hotel for deportees was different to that of 'regular' travellers, in that it had extra military and security personnel in place; it was surrounded by a tall black fence to isolate it from the public; and it was next to a police station (Sadler and Cropper 2020). Security guards were placed on all floors, and the windows were screwed shut to prevent escape (Block 2021). The extra costs in such measures show that deportees are still considered a significant 'threat' to the state: the state considers that it is appropriate to spend additional resources on securing this threat, even during a public health emergency. By comparison, a citizen with a comparable criminal record, but who had not been deported from another state, would be able to quarantine like any other member of the public. Despite the description of the hotel, responsible Minister Megan Woods had to remind the public to 'bear in mind this is not a prison' regarding managed isolation facilities for returned deportees (RNZ 2020). The specialist '501' MIQ hotel was ultimately decommissioned and returned to its initial purpose as a general purpose hotel following the opening of the quarantine-free Trans-Tasman Travel Bubble in April 2021. At the time of decommissioning, the MIQ manager stated that 'the hotel has been an excellent facility for these returnees, however it would not currently be suitable for a regular managed isolation facility' (quoted in Block 2021), showing that deportees as a securitised threat were subject to harsher conditions during their isolation simply for the fact that they were deported, compared to 'regular' travellers who posed a material threat of virus contagion.

To get to the hotels, returnees were placed in vans half-filled with police officers who had met them at the airport (Holland 2020). Police and law enforcement meeting returnees on arrival into New Zealand is a normal practise under the Returning Offenders (Management and Information) Act 2015 (hereby referred to as the ROMI Act); however, the police-escorted ride to the hotel is an additional step. Stanley (2017) has described the ROMI Act as 'the ever-expanding creep of crimmigration', whereby in recognising the criminal deportees as 'dangerous' New Zealand has legislated further restrictions upon them, without regard of status, time served or rehabilitation: the state has re-criminalised returning deportees. Restrictions under the ROMI Act include the ability for law enforcement to request biometric information and DNA from all returning criminal deportees, and subjects them to similar conditions to parole in New Zealand for up to five years following arrival, including reporting to a parole officer, housing and accommodation conditions, and may include special geographical restrictions, electronic monitoring and restrictions on substance abuse. By using these conditions, McHardy (2021, p. 3) argues the ROMI Act has been designed to 'mimic domestic parole arrangements' but is 'being implemented in a way that is more restrictive than the regime for domestic offenders'. The receiving state of deportees is in this situation using a crimmigration approach to convey and securitise the 'threat' of returned deportees. New Zealand has continued to undertake this approach in the face of a public health threat, through both the implementation of the ROMI Act conditions and by the strong presence of law enforcement when escorting of returned deportees to their MIQ hotels.

The states' securitised approach played out in the media who reflected and amplified public fears of the deportees' criminality. There was a significant amount of media coverage of their return and sensationalist commentary created stigma against them. In one case, a deportee absconded from quarantine using a sheet to climb out of a hotel window and propel himself down four levels—he was said to be 'on the loose' for eight hours before turning himself in having 'shot off to grab an L&P' [soda drink] (New Zealand Herald 2020; Block 2021). He was later charged with failing to remain in a managed isolation or quarantine facility for a required period under the COVID-19 Public Health Response Act and Order 2020. The coverage of his escape due to the nature of his arrival in New Zealand was widespread, and made it into international media outlets—this is just one example of the excessive and securitised coverage of deportees entering New Zealand during COVID-19 and any perceived 'bad' behaviour. While the nine escapees prior to the escaped deportee case received some (not as much) media coverage, their reason for return was treated more sympathetically (for example, funeral attendance). Such media framing generated significant public discussion about the return of deportees and their perceived immediate non-compliance with New Zealand laws and thus ongoing criminality.

In a twist on the existing forced migration pathway for deportees, New Zealand politicians have called for the deportation of non-citizens who are non-compliant with New Zealand's tight COVID-19 regulations. Opposition leader Judith Collins, when discussing an Australian who refused COVID-19 testing on arrival, said: 'if a New Zealander went to Australia and refused to get tested in a MIQ facility, what do you think would happen to them? They'd be back on a plane to New Zealand' (cited in Kurmelovs 2021). This shows how quickly crimmigration approaches can shift into everyday securitisation rhetoric, particularly when there are extenuating circumstances such as public health threats.

5. New Zealand Deportations during COVID-19

While New Zealand's deportation policy is not as severe as that of Australia's s501 criminal deportation policy, New Zealand too deports those who have committed criminal offences, under s157, s160 and s161 of the New Zealand Immigration Act 2009. Between March 2020–2021, New Zealand deported 232 people to at least 15 countries, most prominently China and India (MBIE 2021). Like Australia, while there were a minimal number of deportations (seven total) in April and May 2020 when lockdowns and strict restrictions on movement were in place, deportations did not completely recommence until June 2020 when 31 people were deported in one month (MBIE 2021). Immigration New Zealand do not differentiate in their data between those who are deported for overstaying their visas and those who are deported for criminal offences, stating that 'criminal offenders may be deported for reasons other than their criminal offending, e.g. individuals who were deported as a result of their unlawful status in New Zealand but who may also be criminal offenders' (MBIE 2021).

Of those 232 people, 171 were deported due to unlawfully being in New Zealand by overstaying their visas—a trend in New Zealand deportations more generally (MBIE 2021). The precarious status of migrants on temporary visas is recognised and has been highlighted during the COVID-19 period. Immigration raids continued in sectors which have employed workers without valid visas, leading to deportation (Xia 2021). In addition, many Pacific Islanders residing in New Zealand have been faced with the prospect of overstaying due to closed borders and limited commercial flights during the pandemic—while visa extensions were made available, there were difficulties. Over 100 Tongans fell prey to fraudulent 'residency for cash' scams where they used private providers to attempt to maintain their legal status; however, once it was realised due to their overstaying status, they became fearful of reporting the scam to authorities for fear of arrest and deportation putting them in an even more precarious situation (Hopgood 2021).

Prior to the COVID-19 pandemic, New Zealand did not regularly undertake immigration detention and does not have purpose-built immigration detention centres like Australia does. Normal practice involves deportees being placed on the first available flight to their state of origin. However, during the COVID-19 pandemic, time detained has risen due to limited access to flights. If a flight cannot be obtained within 96 h of a person's release from prison, Warrants of Commitment are required by law to further detain those who present a flight risk or risk of absconding. Warrants of Commitment can last a maximum of 28 days, before authorities must seek a judge to approve another warrant or enable release under certain conditions (New Zealand Police 2020). During the COVID-19 period, this has meant that 14 people (7 of whom were being deported on criminal grounds) were being kept in immigration detention, the longest being 273 days in Christchurch Women's Prison—a facility normally used for criminal incarceration rather than immigration detention (Cardwell 2020). These extreme circumstances go beyond the initial intention of an otherwise short-term detention clause, showing that New Zealand was willing to go to extraordinary lengths to deal with the constructed threat of 'crimmigrant other'.

The New Zealand Government is aware of the concerns regarding Warrants of Commitment, but framed the response as one to closed borders: 'some countries, including some Pacific Island nations, were unwilling to take back their citizens and have limited capacity to manage returning deportees in isolation facilities' (Cardwell 2020). Deportation during COVID-19 became a documented concern for the New Zealand Government by June 2020, as it was realised that Warrants of Commitment were being extended beyond 'the legal obligation to deport identified individuals as soon as possible following their release' while attempting to balance the 'risk that migrants who are liable for deportation may pose to New Zealand communities' (MFAT 2020). One of the ways that this has been mitigated is by the Parole Board who has been 'empathetic and in many cases has agreed to defer granting parole specifically for the purposes of deportation', thereby keeping the to-be-deportee incarcerated in a criminal prison for longer than they may otherwise have been held (MFAT 2020). The so-called 'empathy' is clearly aimed towards the state rather than the individual incarcerated. An extended carceral state for deportees is another extraordinary securitised measure against the 'crimmigrant other', taken under the auspices of the public health threat but that does not contribute to health outcomes.

While deportations 'have largely been paused' during the COVID-19 period (MFAT 2020), New Zealand Police (2020) reports from May 2020 show that there were 44 people still awaiting criminal deportation to the Pacific region in 2020—with destinations including the small island developing states of Tonga, Samoa, Vanuatu, Kiribati and Tuvalu. This number is building up due to those in prison reaching the ends of their sentences—and it is likely that when deportations are recommenced, there will be large numbers of deportees for small Pacific states to manage. Deportations were eventually made to Tonga and Samoa in June 2020 when seven people were deported, with 18 people deported total deported to both states between April 2020–March 2021 (MBIE 2021). Pacific states are under-resourced to manage reintegration and rehabilitation of deportees, and there are concerns by New Zealand that an 'influx of criminal deportees ... could contribute to the destabilisation of countries facing severe economic crises of their own' due to the impact of COVID-19 (MFAT 2020). The highlighted concern is apt, as it highlights an existing problem that Pacific states are facing—significant numbers of deportees arriving from Australia, New Zealand and the US—in addition to having limited resources to police or socially reintegrate deportees who are culturally and linguistically isolated (McNeill 2021). In addition, the New Zealand Government is balancing criminal deportation places (including police escorts) on planeloads to Pacific states, with the many Pacific peoples who want to return to their home having been stuck during COVID-19 (MFAT 2020). The risk management here is not so much about the public health threat to Pacific states, but an issue of capacity.

6. Conclusions

When states have continued to prioritise deportation even in the face of a material threat that has affected the world to the extent that COVID-19 has, the securitisation of migration and deportation has clearly been weighted as a more pronounced threat to national security. Despite the global pandemic, 'borders are not changing; instead, their violence appears in different forms and is exposed on the same "disposable bodies"' (Ozguc in Sterling-Folker et al. 2021, p. 16). National security resources were already stretched, and yet the policing, incarceration and deportation of migrants was not merely unabated but escalated during the COVID-19 period. Once detained and eventually deported, migrants endured significant isolation and stigmatization, exacerbated by the COVID-19 context. Returned deportees faced even more hurdles on their arrival. Governments too have struggled with providing detainees with the same level of certainty of deportation that they would have received ordinarily, holding deportees in detention for longer than usual, infrequently left 'out of sight and out of mind'.

Ultimately, deportation of the 'crimmigrant other' did continue, despite otherwise closed borders. When faced with two simultaneous threats to national security, the material public health threat of COVID-19 and the constructed threat of crime from criminal non-citizens, Australia and New Zealand chose to continue and extend detention and deportation practices—thereby prioritising the securitised perceived threat over the material threat that is in fact causing harm to the community.

What this says about states' threat perceptions is that they reinforced by their own securitisation, rather than tangible harm. Therefore, once the global pandemic has subsided, we are likely to see the securitisation of migration continue in detention and deportation practices, exacerbated rather than restricted by the events of COVID-19.

Funding: This research received no external funding.

Conflicts of Interest: The author declares no conflict of interest.

References

Aryal Lees, Rosi, and Sara Niner. 2021. *Tracing the Impacts of the COVID Pandemic on Australia's Fastest-Growing Migrant Group*. Clayton: Monash University, Available online: https://lens.monash.edu/@politics-society/2021/04/12/1383007/tracing-the-impacts-of-the-covid-pandemic-on-australias-fastest-growing-migrant-group (accessed on 25 May 2021).

Bailey, Rochelle-Lee. 2020. Border Closures: Experiences of Ni-Vanuatu Recognised Seasonal Employer Scheme Workers. *Oceania* 90: 168–74. [CrossRef]

Billings, Peter. 2019. Introduction. In *Crimmigration in Australia: Law, Politics, and Society*. Edited by Peter Billings. Singapore: Springer, pp. 3–18.

Billings, Peter, and Khanh Hoang. 2019. Characters of Concern, or Concerning Character Tests? Regulating Risk through Visa Cancellation, Containment and Removal from Australia. In *Crimmigration in Australia: Law, Politics, and Society*. Edited by Peter Billings. Singapore: Springer, pp. 119–48.

Blakkarlay, Jarni. 2020. There's more to the Reopening of Christmas Island's Detention Centre, Immigration Experts Say. *SBS News*. August 5. Available online: https://www.sbs.com.au/news/there-s-more-to-the-reopening-of-christmas-island-s-detention-centre-immigration-experts-say (accessed on 25 May 2021).

Block, George. 2021. Covid-19: Isolation Hotel for Australian Deportees Shut Down Due to Trans-Tasman Bubble. *Stuff*. May 8. Available online: https://www.stuff.co.nz/national/health/coronavirus/300302500/covid19-isolation-hotel-for-australian-deportees-shut-down-due-to-transtasman-bubble (accessed on 25 May 2021).

Boon-Kuo, Louise, Alec Brodie, Jennifer Keene-McCann, Vicki Sentas, and Leanne Weber. 2020. Policing biosecurity: Police enforcement of special measures in New South Wales and Victoria during the COVID-19 pandemic. *Current Issues in Criminal Justice*. [CrossRef]

Burgess, Katie. 2019. 'It's a Real Yes Minister Exercise': The Cost of Running an Empty Detention Centre. *The Canberra Times*. August 27. Available online: https://www.canberratimes.com.au/story/6350056/its-a-real-yes-minister-exercise-the-cost-of-running-an-empty-detention-centre/ (accessed on 25 May 2021).

Buzan, Barry, and Ole Wæver. 2003. *Regions and Powers: The Structure of International Security*. Cambridge Studies in International Relations. Cambridge: Cambridge University Press.

Cardwell, Hamish. 2020. Deportees Waiting more than 200 Days behind Bars due to Covid-19 Travel Disruption. *RNZ News*. December 14. Available online: https://www.rnz.co.nz/news/national/432764/deportees-waiting-more-than-200-days-behind-bars-due-to-covid-19-travel-disruption (accessed on 25 May 2021).

Clapton, William. 2021. The exceptionalism of risk: Trump's Wall and travel ban. *European Journal of International Security* 6: 129–47. [CrossRef]

Cooper, Katja. 2020. The Rudd/Gillard Government, Asylum Seekers, and the Politics of Norm Contestation. Doctor of Philosophy Thesis, University of Queensland, Brisbane, Australia.

Dalzell, Stephanie. 2021. Language, Country of Birth to be Recorded during COVID Vaccine and Positive Tests. *ABC News*. March 8. Available online: https://www.abc.net.au/news/2021-03-08/language-country-birth-recorded-covid-vaccine-positive-test/13219288 (accessed on 25 May 2021).

Davies, Sara E., Adam Kamradt-Scott, and Simon Rushton. 2015. *Disease Diplomacy: International Norms and Global Health Security*. Baltimore: John Hopkins Press.

Department of Home Affairs [Home Affairs]. 2021a. Visa Cancellation Statistics. Available online: https://www.homeaffairs.gov.au/research-and-statistics/statistics/visa-statistics/visa-cancellation (accessed on 25 May 2021).

Department of Home Affairs [Home Affairs]. 2021b. *Response to Freedom of Information Request FA21/05/00264*. Canberra: Commonwealth Government of Australia.

Doran, Matthew. 2020. New Zealand Criminals to Be Deported after Months in Coronavirus Lockdown. *ABC News*. July 14. Available online: https://www.abc.net.au/news/2020-07-14/new-zealand-criminals-to-be-deported-after-months-in-coronavirus/12451688 (accessed on 25 May 2021).

Eddie, Rachel. 2021. Home Affairs Using Hospitals, Aged Care Homes as 'Alternative Places of Detention'. *Sydney Morning Herald*. March 15. Available online: https://www.smh.com.au/national/home-affairs-using-hospitals-aged-care-homes-as-alternative-places-of-detention-20210324-p57djt.html (accessed on 25 May 2021).

Fabris, Jordan. 2021. Con Air: The Secret Flights Sending Foreign Criminals Packing. *Nine News*. March 8. Available online: https://www.9news.com.au/national/con-air-serious-criminals-deported-from-australia-on-secret-flights/fea4df40-178f-457e-be68-330826e9eaf9 (accessed on 25 May 2021).

Franko, Katja. 2019. *The Crimmigrant Other: Migration and Penal Power*. New York: Routledge.

Holland, Zoe. 2020. Covid 19 coronavirus: Australian deportees arrive at their 'boutique-style' Auckland isolation facility. *NZ Herald*. July 14. Available online: https://www.nzherald.co.nz/nz/covid-19-coronavirus-australian-deportees-arrive-at-their-boutique-style-auckland-isolation-facility/5NVM7UBJR3FTBZEWD3DTV3VPLI/ (accessed on 25 May 2021).

Hopgood, Sela Jane. 2021. Deportation Stopping Tongan Church Members Filing a Complaint. *RNZ News*. January 27. Available online: https://www.rnz.co.nz/international/pacific-news/435229/deportation-stopping-tongan-church-members-filing-a-complaint (accessed on 25 May 2021).

Johnson, Giff. 2020. US Deportations Likely Up in FY2020. *RNZ News*. October 26. Available online: https://www.rnz.co.nz/international/pacific-news/429192/us-deportations-likely-up-in-fy2020 (accessed on 25 May 2021).

Karp, Paul. 2021. Fresh Disturbance at Christmas Island Detention Centre due to Inhumane Conditions Advocates Say. *The Guardian*. January 10. Available online: https://www.theguardian.com/australia-news/2021/jan/10/fresh-disturbance-at-christmas-island-detention-centre-due-to-inhumane-conditions-advocates-say (accessed on 25 May 2021).

Kurmelovs, Royce. 2021. Calls to deport Australian woman who refused Covid tests in New Zealand hotel quarantine. *The Guardian*. February 23. Available online: https://www.theguardian.com/australia-news/2021/feb/23/calls-to-deport-australian-woman-who-refused-covid-tests-in-new-zealand-hotel-quarantine (accessed on 25 May 2021).

Lamb, Jessica, Amy Sheehan, and Stephanie Borys. 2021. French Tourist Deported by ABF after Breaching Coronavirus Restrictions with Role in illegal NYE Forest Rave. *ABC News*. January 21. Available online: https://www.abc.net.au/news/2021-01-21/french-tourist-deported-by-abf-over-role-in-illegal-nye-rave/13079600 (accessed on 25 May 2021).

Loughnan, Claire. 2020. 'Not the Hilton': 'Vernacular Violence' in Covid-19 Quarantine and Detention Hotels. *Arena Quarterly*. September 3. Available online: https://arena.org.au/not-the-hilton-vernacular-violence-in-covid-19-quarantine-and-detention-hotels/ (accessed on 25 May 2021).

Ministry of Business, Innovation and Employment [MBIE]. 2021. *Official Information Act Response DOIA2021–179*. Wellington: New Zealand Government.

McGowan, Michael. 2021. Deportation of a Minor: How a 'Corrosive' Policy Sank Cosy Relations between Australia and New Zealand. *The Guardian*. March 18. Available online: https://www.theguardian.com/australia-news/2021/mar/18/deportation-of-a-minor-how-a-corrosive-policy-sank-cosy-relations-between-australia-and-new-zealand (accessed on 25 May 2021).

McHardy, Claudia. 2021. Punishment on arrival: New Zealand's Returning Offenders Act 2015. *Punishment & Society*. [CrossRef]

McInnes, Colin. 2014. The Many Meanings of Health Security. In *Routledge Handbook of Global Health Security*. Edited by Simon Rushton and Jeremy Youde. Routledge: New York, pp. 7–17.

McNeill, Henrietta. 2021. Oceania's 'crimmigration creep': Are deportation and reintegration norms being diffused? *Journal of Criminology*. [CrossRef]

Ministry of Foreign Affairs and Trade [MFAT]. 2020. *Official Information Act Response 27007*. Wellington: New Zealand Government.

Mountz, Alison. 2020. *The Death of Asylum: Hidden Geographies of the Enforcement Archipelago*. Minnesota: University of Minnesota Press.

Nethery, Amy, and Umut Ozguc. 2021. Why are Australians so Accepting of Hotel Quarantine? A long History of Confining Threats to the State. *The Conversation*. April 5. Available online: https://theconversation.com/why-are-australians-so-accepting-of-hotel-quarantine-a-long-history-of-confining-threats-to-the-state-155747 (accessed on 25 May 2021).

New Zealand Herald. 2020. Covid 19 Coronavirus: Deportee Who Escaped from Quarantine Hotel Was on the Loose for Eight Hours. *New Zealand Herald*. September 29. Available online: https://www.nzherald.co.nz/nz/covid-19-coronavirus-deportee-who-escaped-from-quarantine-hotel-was-on-the-loose-for-eight-hours/7XSCM6TNOI4WBPEG3BGWB5CDNE/ (accessed on 25 May 2021).

New Zealand Police. 2020. *Official Information Act Response IR-01-20-14208*. Wellington: New Zealand Government.

Remeikis, Amy. 2020. Jacinda Ardern Lashes Scott Morrison for 'Testing' Friendship over Deportations to New Zealand. *The Guardian*. February 28. Available online: https://www.theguardian.com/australia-news/2020/feb/28/jacinda-ardern-lashes-scott-morrison-for-testing-friendship-over-deportations-to-new-zealand (accessed on 25 May 2021).

RNZ. 2020. Man Escaping Managed Isolation not 'Failure of Security'—Megan Woods. *RNZ News*. September 29. Available online: https://www.rnz.co.nz/news/national/427156/man-escaping-managed-isolation-not-failure-of-security-megan-woods (accessed on 25 May 2021).

Ryan, Hannah. 2020. Australian Government to Reopen Christmas Island Detention Centre during Covid-19 Crisis. *The Guardian*. August 5. Available online: https://www.theguardian.com/australia-news/2020/aug/04/australian-government-to-reopen-christmas-island-detention-centre-during-covid-19-crisis (accessed on 25 May 2021).

Sadler, Rachel, and Emma Cropper. 2020. COVID-19: Deported Kiwis Staying at Auckland's Ramada Hotel. *Newshub*. August 14. Available online: https://www.newshub.co.nz/home/new-zealand/2020/07/covid-19-deported-kiwis-staying-at-aucklands-ramada-hotel.html (accessed on 25 May 2021).

Stanley, Elizabeth. 2017. Expanding Crimmigration: The detention and deportation of New Zealanders from Australia. *Australian New Zealand Journal of Criminology* 51: 4. [CrossRef]

Sterling-Folker, Jennifer, Annette Freyberg-Inan, Lauren Wilcox, Umut Ozguc, and Rosemary E. Shinko. 2021. Forum: Thinking Theoretically in Unsettled Times: COVID-19 and Beyond. *International Studies Review*. OnlineFirst. [CrossRef]

Stumpf, Juliet. 2006. The Crimmigration Crisis: Immigrants, Crime, and Sovereign Power. *American University Law Review* 56: 367–420.

Stumpf, Juliet. 2013. Two Profiles of Crimmigration Law: Criminal Deportation and Illegal Migration. In *Globalisation and the Challenge to Criminology*. Edited by Francis Pakes. London: Routledge.

Townsend, Mark. 2021. Specialist Covid Infection Control Scientist Faces Threat of Deportation from UK. *The Guardian*. March 21. Available online: https://www.theguardian.com/uk-news/2021/mar/20/specialist-covid-infection-control-scientist-faces-threat-of-deportation-from-uk (accessed on 25 May 2021).

Washington, John. 2021. ICE Threatened to Expose Asylum-Seekers to Covid-19 if they did not Accept Deportation. *The Intercept*. February 7. Available online: https://theintercept.com/2021/02/06/ice-covid-threat-asylum-deportation/ (accessed on 25 May 2021).

Weber, Leanne, and Sharon Pickering. 2013. Exporting Risk, Deporting Non-Citizens. In *Globalisation and the Challenge to Criminology*. Edited by Francis Pakes. London: Routledge.

Xia, Lucy. 2021. Eight Illegal Workers Detained, Two Deported after Raids on Government-run sites in Auckland. *Stuff*. May 8. Available online: https://www.stuff.co.nz/business/125072532/eight-illegal-workers-detained-two-deported-after-raids-on-governmentrun-sites-in-auckland (accessed on 25 May 2021).

Yu, Andi. 2020. Death of Detainee as Deportations Delayed. *7 News*. December 19. Available online: https://7news.com.au/news/immigration/death-of-detainee-as-deportations-delayed-c-1798483 (accessed on 25 May 2021).

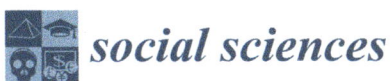

Article

COVID-19 Crisis as the New-State-of-the-Art in the Crimmigration Milieu

Joanna Tsiganou [1], Anastasia Chalkia [2] and Martha Lempesi [3,*]

[1] National Centre for Social Research, 10551 Athens, Greece; jtsiganou@ekke.gr
[2] Faculty of Communication and Media Studies, National and Kapodistrian University, 10562 Athens, Greece; a.chalkia@media.uoa.gr
[3] Center for the Study of Crime, 10559 Athens, Greece
* Correspondence: marthalempesi@yahoo.gr

Abstract: The concept of crimmigration connotes the currently prevailing approach between the different fields of penal, administrative and migration laws. It seems that, progressively, there is an amalgamation of penal law practices with those of civil and administrative law processes in a way creating confusion as to the boundaries of each law discipline and rational. In addition, the protection of public health from COVID-19 interrelates with the above three fields of law while at the same time the measures undertaken for the confrontation of the pandemic are further strengthening the social controls already imposed towards the migrant-refugee populations. Based on the Greek experience, we are particularly interested in mixed migration flows' status of a 'prolonged reception'. We have decided to examine the cases of the 'asylum-seeker' population and the 'undocumented' population who, to a large extent, constitute a large *unseen* category for the national vaccine program implemented to combat the COVID-19 hygiene crisis. The basic idea supported by our present study is that the health field is used as an additive component to crimmigration as it helps the establishment of a concrete screening intensifying the already imposed migration controls. In addition, the official social controls imposed to combat the COVD-19 health crisis contribute to crimmigration through the intensification of the dangerization of mixed migration flows. Currently, the health field, affected by COVID-19, contributes to the intensification of the crimmigration regime and at the same time to a dangerous cul-de-sac.

Keywords: crimmigration; migrants/refugees; COVID-19; vaccination; Greece

Citation: Tsiganou, Joanna, Anastasia Chalkia, and Martha Lempesi. 2021. COVID-19 Crisis as the New-State-of-the-Art in the Crimmigration Milieu. *Social Sciences* 10: 457. https://doi.org/10.3390/socsci10120457

Academic Editor: Robert Koulish

Received: 10 August 2021
Accepted: 12 November 2021
Published: 29 November 2021

Publisher's Note: MDPI stays neutral with regard to jurisdictional claims in published maps and institutional affiliations.

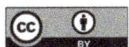

Copyright: © 2021 by the authors. Licensee MDPI, Basel, Switzerland. This article is an open access article distributed under the terms and conditions of the Creative Commons Attribution (CC BY) license (https://creativecommons.org/licenses/by/4.0/).

1. Introduction

The COVID-19 pandemic caused great loss of human life as well as social and economic disruption in Europe and the World. Strict measures have been imposed internationally in order to avoid the spread of the disease and protect public health. The most widespread emergency measures worldwide have been the restrictions on movement (quarantine and lockdown projects), promoting 'social distancing', intense testing, personal hygiene as well as hygiene protection measures and, eventually, a vast vaccination program implemented from 27 December 2020 onwards globally (Escritt 2020).

Marginalized migrant populations living in extremely precarious conditions were prone to be disproportionately affected by the spread of the disease compared to those living in well-arranged environments and being in a position to afford necessary precautions for their health protection. In this regard, our present study examines the Greek public policies implemented to protect asylum-seekers and undocumented migrants against the COVID-19 pandemic, as well as the extent to which they have reached their scope in an efficient and timely manner. The basic hypothesis examined is that said policies helped the amalgamation of penal, administrative and migration law processes facilitating crimmigration rather than alleviate the migration-refugee experience. Our paper supports the idea that public health processes in the era of the COVID-19 pandemic are contributing to the 'dangerization' (Nikolopoulos 2012) of mixed migration populations and have helped the intensification of official controls against them. Given the high visibility of the deviant behavior of migrant perpetrators (Tsiganou et al. 2010), the immigration controls are (re)structured also by means of public health protection processes. Thus, a new field of a manifested and disguised crimmigration emerges.

The literature review reveals that the concept of crimmigration is used to connote the dynamic interplay between the different fields of penal, administrative and migration laws. In some cases, the concept is used to refer to the criminalization of immigration law, or "crimmigration law", (Stumpf 2006) in order to denote the convergence of immigration and criminal law (Stumpf 2006; Guia et al. 2011; Aas and Bosworth 2013; Salamon 2017). In other cases, the concept of crimmigration has been connected broadly with issues such as criminalizatisation (Salamon 2020), border control (Broeders and Hampshire 2013), securitization (Gerard and Pickering 2013), detention (Bourdeau 2019), deportation (Menjivar et al. 2018), exclusion (Rottem 2021) and sovereign bias (Koulish 2016). There are also theoretical and research approaches which witness the infiltration of the crimmigration process within the public health field (Websdale 2020) or have shown "*how COVID-19 has forced new understandings on crimmigration law and politics*" (Koulish 2021). However, public health management in times of pandemics or hygiene crises in conjunction with crimmigration practices needs to be further explored in order to comprehend the dynamic interplay between public health controls and crimmigration processes.

Our study is based on documentary evidence provided through the examination of official documents and news media texts. As already stated, one of our main concerns was to examine whether and to what extent official health policies, even in the emergency occurrence of a pandemic, constitute an additive part of crimmigration. In our undertaking, we have tried to decipher aspects of crimmigration clearly stated, disguised or even hidden throughout our research material, which has been collected through archival research of official documents such as governmental papers, laws and regulations texts, decrees and ministerial decisions, as well as media commentaries and news texts. The research material covers the period from 1 January 2020 to 30 May 2021 when the restrictive measures combating the coronavirus pandemic had been temporarily waved or relaxed.

Our evidence also suggests the reinforcement of the crimmigrant identity through the official management of the health field. As it will be shown, the Greek case bears witness that migrant and refugee populations remain, to a large extent, abandoned without being prioritized in the measures provided to combat the coronavirus pandemic (i.e., hygiene precautions, testing and vaccination). Based on our research material we also argue that such a confrontation has accelerated new forms of mixed migration flows management and control, given the asylum seekers' and undocumented migrants' already existing exclusion from institutional health care. This way, their already established identity as "criminalized subjects"—who do not 'deserve' prioritization in public health care—is reinforced by the state management of the present pandemic inside open/closed 'facilities'.

In the crimmigration context, third-country nationals, as non-citizens, are seen as being always to be blamed and criminalized, their dangerized identity based on the mere fact of their migrant and/or refugee status and the stigma attached to it. Moreover, migrants' and refugees' presence in the 'host' country is perceived as a severe social threat and even as a menace to a society remaining intact before their advent (Salamon 2017). Under the conditions of the present pandemic and the hygiene crisis it has created, migrants and refugees, as non-citizens, are classified not only as (potential) criminals but also as a threat to public health. This way, new negative characteristics are added to their already stigmatized identity so that these populations of non-citizens are confronted and managed not only by means of walls, borders, rules, 'public condemnation' (Stumpf 2006) and 'social closures' (Tsiganou et al. 2010) but also by means of exclusion from assets destined to protect primarily the host country's nationals. Migrants and refugees, as non-citizens, remain excluded once more from access to basic goods—either public or common. As the Greek case testifies, hygiene crises may create new grounds for deepening already existing exclusionary processes.

As the Greek case testifies, under the coronavirus pandemic, migrants and refugees, as non-citizens, remained systematically absent from any prioritization campaign and urgent policy measures to combat the crisis. They have remained, of course, 'quarantined' and systematically untested at their dystopian camps in extreme 'caging' measures for a longer period compared to the native population. It is to be noted that in the official rhetoric, they were represented as being disproportionally not affected by the COVID-19 virus, a justification most handy for the absence of any relevant public care policy. As a result, migrants and refugees, as non-citizens, remained unvaccinated almost half a year after the Greek vaccination plan had been implemented.

Our study concludes by providing a discussion on health discrimination against migrants and refugees, as non-citizens, in a way that creates health and, therefore, societal borders which unavoidably lead to a regime of health 'apartheid' via a vaccination institutional racism that adds new dynamic connotations to 'crimmigrated' identities and the crimmigration conceptualization overall.

2. Methodology

In terms of methodology, we have based the research on to the Critical Frame Analysis originally produced in qualitative research on gender equality policies, having adapted it to our qualitative archival and documentary research of legal documents, administrative decrees, policy texts and media commentaries on immigration. As noted, in the Critical Frame Analysis, *"the concept of frames and framing is presented as a basic concept for the analysis, starting with defining a frame as an interpretation scheme that structures the meaning of reality, and a policy frame as an organizing principle that transforms fragmentary or incidental information into a structured and meaningful policy problem, in which a solution is implicitly or explicitly enclosed. Policy framing then can be seen as the process of constructing, adapting and negotiating policy frames"* (Verloo and Maloutas 2005, p. 2). The Critical Frame Analysis we have followed combines elements from policy theory, discourse analysis and immigration/crimmigration theory. As noted, *"unlike other approaches, frame analysis starts from the assumption of multiple interpretations in policy making, and addresses problems of dominance and exclusion connected to policy making. Implementation of policies is seen as a political process, subject to all mechanisms of political processes. Under conditions of multilevel governance, implementation is a complex process of transfer and translation: unitary concepts or frames, as presented in political decisions and policies at (sub) national and supranational levels contrast with a dynamic reality of multiple frames at national levels. This contrast between an assumed stable unity and a real dynamic diversity is seen as a «black box» of distortions in the implementation of policies. The shifts that occur during implementation often coincide with exclusion processes"* (Verloo 2005, p. 8).

We have thought Critical Frame Analysis as a suitable tool since it enables certain of our research questions to be answered such as the detection of similarities, differences and inconsistencies in the way immigration is perceived or understood as a problem in national and European levels, especially under the urgency of the COVID-19 pandemic circumstances. How are patterns at the national level connected to existing and developing frames at the European Union level? Which processes of exclusion result from dominant frames? What are the consequences of possible inconsistencies detected? We also considered most suitable to our analytic purposes the concepts of policy frames and framing dimensions, since within the Critical Frame Analysis, *"a policy frame is further specified as a specific configuration of positions on the dimensions of diagnosis and prognosis of the policy problem, roles attributed in diagnosis and prognosis and voice given . . . Because not only discursive elements but also attributed roles and voice have an important place in this framework, the approach is labelled Critical Frame Analysis"* (Verloo 2005, p. 20). Whilst we agree with the critique that discourse analysis in general and frame analysis present certain problems for comparisons, especially on how to develop categories that can analyze discourses at various levels that allow for comparison (Van Gorp 2001), and that frame mapping (Riechert 1996) offers no viable alternative as based on frequency and co-occurrence of key terms in text, we felt convinced by the merits of the Critical Frame Analysis, despite the fact that frame analysis needs further methodological development, especially by studying framing in connection to legitimacy and domination (Verloo 2005, p. 20).

Within the Critical Frame Analysis, a policy frame is considered as "an organising principle that transforms fragmentary or incidental information into a structured and meaningful policy problem, in which a solution is implicitly or explicitly enclosed. Hence, policy frames are not descriptions of reality but specific constructions that give meaning to reality and shape the understanding of reality. Research working with these or similar concepts is based on a constructionist approach to reality, where discourse, through its close connection to the construction of truths is seen as having important material and immaterial impacts. In implementation processes, policy frames are the medium, transferred and necessarily adapted from one level to another, from one area to another. Frame analysis is concerned with the (re)construction and negotiation of reality by social/political actors through the use of symbolic tools (Triandafyllidou and Fotiou 1998)—as cited in the original. Framing, then, can be seen as the process of constructing, adapting and negotiating frames (Verloo 2005, p. 20).

Thus, the methodology of the Critical Frame Analysis helps to overcome the above-mentioned problems by analyzing the dimensions of frames rather than constructing a hierarchical set of codes or typologies of frames. These dimensions allow for a comparable description of various positions. Yet, categorizing beforehand can follow a grounded theory approach (Strauss and Corbin 1997). In addition, Critical Frame Analysis helps to "*track the inner (explicit or implicit) logic of processes of policy frames as a crucial element of exclusion and track the discursive histories that are present in the public discourse, within political institutions (like parliamentary debates and documents), civil society (NGOs) and the media. In order to put the accent on power relations involved in policy texts, Critical Frame Analysis therefore will also have to pay specific attention to the role of various actors in framing processes. More specifically, attention for who has voice in defining the problem and who has voice in suggesting suitable courses of action to resolve the problem, is needed, as well as specific focus on the attribution of responsibilities (for causing the problem or for solving the problem)*" (Verloo 2005, p. 22).

Without wishing to duplicate theories and methods, we are following Critical Frame Analysis in that we are framing crimmigration as a policy problem that is a policy frame which has a typical format connected to politics and policy making. We also start according to the critical frame approach from the general assumption that a policy (proposal) will always contain an implicit or explicit representation of a diagnosis of a situation, a phenomenon or a problem, connected to an implicit or explicit prognosis of what is coming and a call for action. In other words, the analysis is based on the assumption that there is a problem, that some solution to this problem is proposed (including ideas on the causes of or responsibilities for the problem, on the ends that can be reached through the use of certain means and on the desirability of certain outcomes) and that it is made clear who has to do something and what has to be done. The key sensitizing questions used to energize the texts are quite similar to the template proposed in the article of Verloo (2005), so there is no need to duplicate its code and categories scheme here. Suffice is to say that the basic structure consists of the dimensions of Diagnosis, Attribution of Responsibility (renamed Roles in Diagnosis), Prognosis and Call for Action (renamed Roles in Prognosis). The dimension of Voice has been also added in our analysis, since policy frames do not always originate in specific actors but also may commence in institutions (administrations, cabinets, committees, etc.) in our case as well. So, on the one hand, theoretical notions from discourse analysis may be used while, on the other, analysis may be facilitated in terms of exclusion/inclusion and power. At a more detailed level, based on discourse analysis, we have also used the sub-element of the Form (form of argumentation, dichotomies, metaphors) within the dimensions of Diagnosis and Prognosis. In addition, the analysis includes within the dimensions of Diagnosis and Prognosis, Carol Bacchi's critique on policy theory, especially her "what's the problem represented to be?" approach (Bacchi 1999). Furthermore, based on Giddens' structuration theory (Giddens 1984), the Critical Frame Analysis is suitable for placing emphasis on the distribution of and access to various resources, next to the rules (interpretations and norms) connected to migration or refugee issues. Thus, normativity maybe separately accessed and highlighted as well as the impact assessment of policies.

3. The Healthcare Aspects of Crimmigration

The COVID-19 pandemic and the measures undertaken to confront it have a tremendous, but to a large extent, differentiated impact on both societies and individuals at a global level, which was dependent on the socioeconomic status of each society and the specific population group. Especially, the identity characteristics of population groups are proven to be crucial towards the protection of the individual members against the pandemic. These characteristics are mainly interrelated with citizenship status and membership. From the beginning of the pandemic, migrants and refugees residing in open/closed facilities became—once more—unseen as the focus of the dominant narrative was the declared and/or implemented policies for the citizen population, contrary to the Commissioner Johannson statement during the Committee on Civil Liberties, Justice and Home Affairs meeting on 2 April. As she has stressed, *"refugee camps, in countries of first asylum, are severely ill-equipped to support a large number of persons who already live in precarious conditions. The spreading of the virus in such contexts may result in a massive humanitarian crisis [. . .] To fight xenophobia, discrimination and racism, and to help vulnerable migrants, I will also make the consultation with civil society, employers, trade unions and other relevant organizations to develop options to protect and support migrants and refugees"* (Johansson 2020).

In Greece, living conditions in open/closed facilities are harsh and inadequate (AIDA-ECRE 2021). In particular, *"social distancing is impossible when 1200 people share a single tap"*. During the first months of 2020, *"over 40,000 refugees are [currently] being detained in five hotspot facilities on Lesvos, Chios, Samos, Leros and Kos"* (Bilgin and Fyssa 2020). Alarming analyses of media stated that evacuated measures for the camps must have taken place and that people living in them were very concerned (Medecins sans Frontieres 2020; Papanicolaou 2020). In addition, the camp at Moria, which was built for 2757 in 2020, accommodated 18,985 persons, which is 6.8 times over its capacity, without taking into account that the majority of refugees are living in olive groves adjacent to the camp in self-made shelters and tents. (Bilgin and Fyssa 2020). Greek Authorities implemented specific measures to the said facilities (Greek Ministry of Migration and Asylum 2020; Mitarakis 2020), but most of them are *"cosmetic in nature"* because they ignore the real existing conditions that can exacerbate the transmission of the disease as the *"general hygienic rules"* were de facto impossible to be followed by the population living therein (Bilgin and Fyssa 2020). This was much more so especially in view of the tangible reality of the *"prolonged reception"* that created a limbo situation for the host migrant-refugee populations and persistently deteriorating living conditions in camps and hotspots (Tsiganou et al. 2020). Furthermore, the social control of migrants has been intensified through a new legislative Act which foresees that the administrative detention can reach up to 36 months (Law 4636/2019). The Act also provides the State can replace the open facilities in force with closed reception and identification centers and create new pre-departure detention establishments (Law 4686/2020). In addition, according to a new controversial but still pending Legislative Order, areas suitable for the establishment of 'closed' detention centers may be requisitioned for reasons of public interest, in order to address the extremely urgent need to avoid endangering public order and public health (Legislative Act, Government Gazette A'28/10.02.2020).

In terms of access to healthcare, in July 2019, the criteria for third-country nationals and European citizens to receive Social Security Number (AMKA) became extremely strict in Greece. It is to be noted that AMKA is necessary for contacting the Greek Administration in the most important occasions as a result, until the advent of COVID-19 in 2020, a large part of the migrant and refugee populations in Greece has ceased to have unimpeded access to public health facilities, following the decision to abolish the AMKA for foreign nationals[1]. Among those who did not have access throughout the reporting period were children and unaccompanied minors (Amnesty International 2019), in violation of the general principles of the World Health Organization, the International Convention on the Rights of the Child and the European Directive 2013/33/EU. During this same period, there was no transitional legal provision until the Joint Ministerial Decision 717/2020 (Government Gazette B 199/31.01.2020) which was issued in the advent of the pandemic and foresees the Temporary Insurance and Health Care Number (PAYPA), which ensures the temporary access of the asylum seekers to the health care system and their potential access to the labor market, six months after their asylum application is submitted. In fact, PAYPA came into force in April 2020, that is almost nine months after the ban of asylum seekers from the healthcare system and four months after the pandemic seized the country and the world (Aggelidis 2020). PAYPA is assigned at the local Asylum Offices/Units, where the relevant application is to be registered. The rejection of the asylum application implies the automatic deactivation of PAYPA, while, on the contrary, in case of acceptance of the application, its AMKA is foreseen. Thus, the populations in question need to have their Special Security Number updated every time their status changes (applicant, claimant, beneficiary) in order to have access to health services. Any obstruction or delay cancels the said access. In addition, in case of a negative decision, their access to health services is nullified.

In any case, the above new legal arrangements make the migrant and refugee populations subject to a regime of constant control, intensified through health provisions since they are being permanently put under Damocles' sword for one of the basic human rights, that of access to health. Additionally, in violation of the principle of non-discrimination, the new conditions arising from the measures implemented to combat COVID-19 pandemic have unjustifiably extended the quarantine measures for the hosted migrant and refugee populations and, therefore, their perpetual exclusion. To mention an example, while the first 'quarantine' period (initial lockdown during March–April 2020) ended for the entire population in Greece, it continued exceptionally only for the migrant-refugee populations 'hosted' in camps, without, however, the measure to be officially justified as based to any 'epidemiological situation' within the camps/reception structures (Fouskas 2020)[2].

4. Vaccine Institutional Racism

In the context of the European Union, the coordination of the European Commission and EU Agencies have supported the development of COVID-19 vaccines to be available promptly to the EU territory (European Commission 2020a). Most Member States launched their national vaccination campaigns in December 2020, and because of the limited supply of vaccines, they identified key priorities in forming their vaccination strategies. Most of the member states pursued the following criteria for prioritizing certain parts of the population (FRA 2021):

- Older people, especially those living in long-term care facilities;
- People with underlying medical conditions who are more likely to develop a severe form of the disease or die if they contract COVID-19;
- Frontline health workers and staff of long-term care facilities.

On the other hand, the Worl Health Organization's (WHO) Strategic Advisory Group of Experts identified low-income migrant workers, irregular migrants, refugees, asylum seekers and those unable to physically distance, including those living in camps and camp-like settings, as priority groups for the allocation of COVID-19 vaccination globally, specifically listing migrants and refugees as groups to be prioritized in stages II and III of the vaccine rollout[3]. In conjunction with the above, medical communities and the relevant literature state that *"globally, refugees and displaced persons must be prioritized to receive vaccines"* (Thomas et al. 2021) and *"that medical institutions need to implement policies that will support and protect refugees, asylum seekers, and displaced persons and reduce any network of transmission"* (Saifee et al. 2021). There is, accordingly, strong international guidance about the prioritization of the migrant-refugee populations to receive vaccination for the sake of the protection of the individuals but also of public health. In other words, there was a global recognition of the precariousness of the said populations and the necessity to be protected receiving priority status.

The explicit rationale of the prioritization of the precarious migrant-refugee populations, as already stated, was not broadly implemented by the EU vaccination plans. Whilst, in 2020, the number of migrants in the EU/EEA (ECDC 2021) (defined as people born in a different country than the one they reside) made up 12% of the total population (453 million people) with the 4% being born in another EU/EEA country or the UK and the other 8% originating from outside the EU/EEA and the UK, more than 3 million refugees and asylum-seekers were registered in 2018, plus fo4ur million undocumented migrants; these groups remained mainly *invisible* for any national vaccine prioritization plan. Especially, concerning persons without legal status or with insecure legal status in the EU only 5 out of 27 Member States have prioritized them in their national vaccination strategies[4]. In addition, key figures about vaccination in the EU, as derived from the European Centre for Disease Prevention and Control (ECDC 2021), do not include any reference to the vaccination of the migrants/refugees populations though other target groups such as residents of long-term care facilities are explicitly mentioned.

Given the initial shortage of vaccines, the criteria for defining who is eligible to receive prioritized vaccination varied among the Member-States' vaccination program as Member States did not take into account the vulnerabilities and the risky living conditions of the precarious populations. Overall, Member States have focused on prioritizing vaccination for older citizens who are disproportionally affected by the COVID-19 virus. However, the age factor, along with the prioritization of other group characteristics, namely, health workers, was not the only variable lying beneath the prioritization scheme. Other 'ghost' factors were to a large extent lurking and set barriers to access to 'healthcare for all', notwithstanding Goal 3 and especially Goal 3.8 of the Sustainable Development Goals of the UN[5] and Article 35 of the Charter of Fundamental Rights of the European Union, which states that health should be ensured without any discrimination[6]. Instead, in the case of the current health crisis, the rollout of vaccination to combat the pandemic has revealed that State-run vaccination plans have been discriminatorily implemented on the basis of the legal status of a person and, particularly, citizenship rights.

According to the latest international research report by the WHO, which seeks to identify how the new coronavirus SARS-CoV-2 (COVID-19) has impacted refugees and migrants around the world, based on their own reported experiences, the following is noted (World Health Organization 2020a):

- Lack of financial means, fear of deportation, lack of availability of healthcare providers or uncertain entitlement to health care were the reasons cited most often for not seeking medical care in case of (suspected) COVID-19 infection.
- Though most refugees and migrants took precautions to minimize the risk of their housing situations, mainly insecure or in crowded camps, the necessity to commute by using public transportation increased the risk of becoming infected.
- Feelings of depression, anxiety and loneliness and increased worries were mainly reported.
- Experiences of perceived discrimination were also reported along with relatively worsening discrimination, especially for those being unemployed.
- Their status concerning work, safety, and financial means have deteriorated.

With respect to the above, the European and Member States' vaccination strategies reveal important deficiencies considering the relevant treatment of migrant and refugee populations, even though the International and Regional Bodies have made a statement for the necessity of inclusive approaches in Member States' health systems (Weekers 2020; ECDC 2020a, 2020b). In addition, European Commission has clearly defined that vulnerable socioeconomic groups and other groups at higher risk, along with groups without physical distance in place, can be defined as priority groups concerning vaccination Member States plans (European Commission 2020b). In addition, the UNHCR (2021a) states that *"by including refugees in their vaccine distribution, they mitigate the risks associated with exclusion and discrimination*. In particular, risk factors for increased exposure to COVID-19 are interrelated with occupational risk (over-representing in public-facing jobs including health and social care, transport, low-skilled jobs, precarious jobs, obliged to work throughout the pandemic, increased use of public transport), overcrowded accommodation (live in poverty and deprived areas, in camps, reception and detention centers, in shared or temporary accommodation, in multigenerational households) and barriers to public health messaging (lack of knowledge of the host country language, vulnerable to misperceptions and misunderstandings) (ECDC 2021). The current hygiene crisis due to the COVID pandemic has shown more clearly than ever that many works in situations of high risk are too often undervalued, i.e., in care facilities, cleaning and agriculture (PICUM n.d.). Even in the period of the highly infectious delta variant, the major vaccination gap for undocumented migrants and refugees is still present[7].

Consequently, the lack of the prioritization or total exclusion of the marginalized migrant-refugee populations from vaccination underlines a State's unwillingness to address an urgent and unprecedented health issue beyond the notion of State sovereignty and indicates the deportation/expulsion of populations management (see Figures 1 and 2). This exclusionary and segregating policy rationale is an endemic part of the crimmigration regime that is currently manifested through a vaccination institutional racism (Stokely et al. 1967) and expresses the unequal distribution of the vaccines between groups because of 'otherness' and lack of citizenship rights.

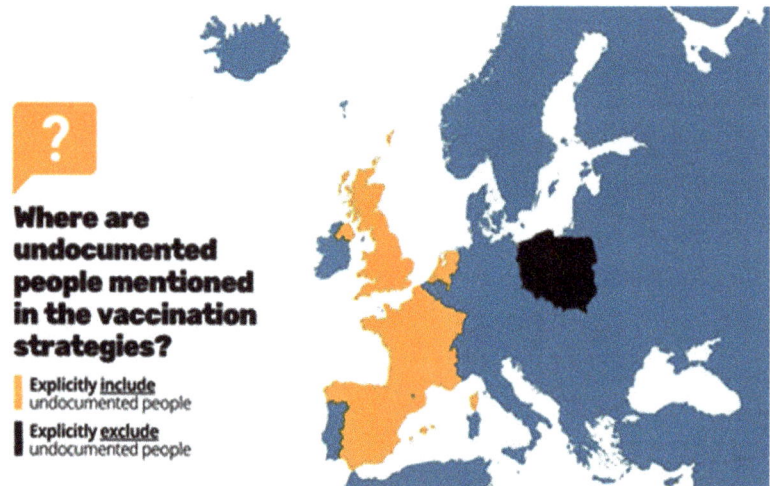

Figure 1. Source: The COVID-19 vaccines and undocumented migrants: What are European countries doing? PICUM (Available online: https://picum.org/covid-19-undocumented-migrants-europe/ (accessed on 1 August 2021).

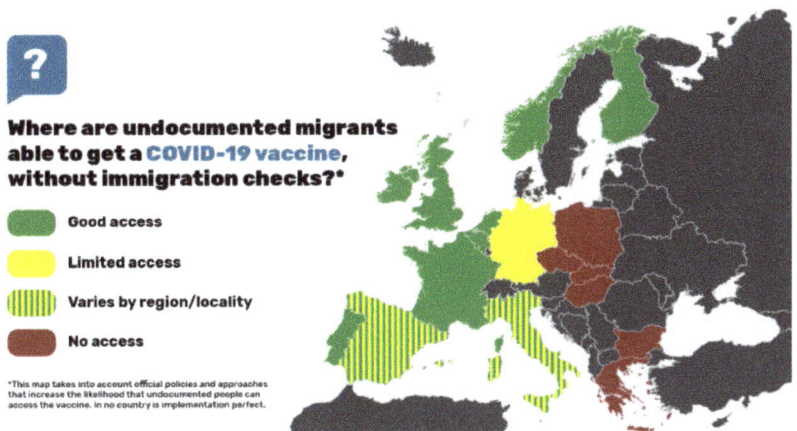

Figure 2. Source: The COVID-19 vaccines and undocumented migrants: What are European countries doing? PICUM (Available online: https://picum.org/covid-19-undocumented-migrants-europe/ (accessed on 15 July 2021)

The Greek Vaccination Plan

The Greek Vaccination Pan, named "Freedom" (Eleftheria) (Greek Government 2021), was launched in December 2020 and initially put in implementation in January 2021. The national booking system operates through a specific website[8] and a mobile application. To register, one needs AMKA and a VAT number (AFM). The site is available in Greek and English and refers only and explicitly to the population group of "citizens". Information in other languages than Greek and English is only provided by the webpage of the UNHCR (2021b).

The Greek vaccination plan consists of three phases with specific identification of the eligible social categories:

1st phase:
- Health and social services workers;
- Residents and staff of nursing homes;
- Residents, patients and staff of care structures for the chronically ill and rehabilitation centers;

2nd phase:
- People 70 years and older (regardless of medical history). Further prioritization:
- People aged 85 and over;
- People aged 80 and over;
- People aged 75 and over;
- People aged 70 and over;
- Patients with diseases that pose a very high risk of COVID-19 disease regardless of age;
- Priority staff for critical functions of the State;
- People 60 to 69 years old (regardless of medical history);
- Patients aged 18 to 59 years with diseases that pose a high risk for disease with COVID-19;
- Priority staff for critical Government functions;

3rd phase:
- People 18 years and older without underlying diseases.

According to the Greek Vaccination Plan, and as also revealed by the FRA (2021) report, in Greece persons without legal status or with insecure legal status did not constitute a priority group for vaccination in the national vaccination strategy. Additionally, in the same FRA report, it is mentioned that migrants and refugees living in 'hotspots' on the Greek islands have not been prioritized for vaccination. Indeed, only six months after the launch of the National Vaccination Plan in Greece, refugees and asylum-seekers living in camps and reception centers started to receive vaccination. Analytically, for the first months of the vaccination plan, only the AMKA holders could be vaccinated. However, the dysfunctional AMKA delivery system blocked access to vaccines and self-tests for tens of thousands of migrants and refugees. In March 2021, Law 4782/2021 provided for the supporting documents and the steps the person without AMKA or PAYPA should follow in order to apply for a temporary AMKA, called PAMKA. The application for PAMKA started to operate in June 2021. It is evident, therefore, that the addition of PAMKA to the state vaccination plan has been invented and implemented only when it was realized that the vaccination rate of Greek citizens was lower than initially anticipated and, therefore, vaccine redundancy was sufficient to cover those previously and mostly excluded (Emmanouilidou 2021). We may detect to this auxiliary vaccination policy the recruitment of an exploitation plan of migrant and refugee populations in order for the much desired 'immunity wall' to be built nationwide.

In practice, the issue of PAMKA requires that a person should have, in addition to the passport, some other identification documents double-crossed by registers kept at public sector bodies. Should the application which a migrant-refugee person has submitted be accepted, s/he receives PAMKA and then s/he could ask for a vaccination appointment. PAMKA is serving solely for arranging a vaccination appointment and the issuance of a vaccination certificate and it does not provide for any other access to the healthcare system for migrant-refugee populations. In May 2021, the Joint Ministerial Decision 2981/2021 (Government Gazette B'2197/26.05.2021) defined more specific categories of beneficiaries of PAMKA issuance, i.e., asylum seekers and unaccompanied minors without PAYPA as well as detained third-country nationals. Receiving access to vaccination becomes, as a result, a very complicated procedure that does not ensure the issue at stake, namely, the creation of an immunity wall and, ultimately, the defense of public health. Thousands of people without legal status are automatically excluded from the vaccination process. This, in turn, implies a direct negative impact on the course of the pandemic. Although there are places with a large concentration of land workers (i.e., the case of Manolada (Generation 2.0 2019)), or cases of places where thousands of undocumented migrants/refugees are living and working, they are not eligible for vaccination even under the conditions of the said current plan (Generation 2.0 2021). Therefore, those without AMKA, PAYPA, PAMKA, or any document from the Greek Authorities do not have access to vaccination. In other words, an administrative issue such as the acquisition of a permanent or a temporary Social Security Number constitutes the insurmountable obstacle to vaccination that excludes migrants/refugees from a core measure of protection against the coronavirus pandemic.

In addition, irrespectively from access to any kind of Social Security Number, migrant/refugees populations kept in camps have remained and still remain unvaccinated. Greek Authorities have justified their non-prioritization by stating that camps do not address "coronavirus morbidity or spread", so staff and residents will be vaccinated "in turn, according to their age cohort according to the regulations applied for the general population"[9]. However, the analysis derived from the public surveillance data indicates that *"compared to the general population the risk of COVID-19 infection among refugees and asylum seekers in reception facilities was 2.5 to 3 times higher (p-value < 0.001). The risk of acquiring COVID-19 infection was higher among refugee and asylum seeker populations in RSs on the Greek mainland (IP ratio: 2.45; 95% CI: 2.25_2.68) but higher still among refugee and asylum seeker populations in RICs in the Greek islands and the land border with Turkey (IP ratio: 2.86; 95% CI: 2.64_3.10), where living conditions are particularly poor. We identified high levels of COVID-19 transmission among refugees and asylum seekers in reception facilities in Greece. The risk of COVID-19 infection among these enclosed population groups has been significantly higher than the general population of Greece, and risk increases as living conditions deteriorate"*

(Kondilis et al. 2021). On the other hand, the official rhetoric avoids the issue of why the first lockdown in Greece (March–May 2020) ended a couple of months later for the migrant/refugee populations residing in camps (Fouskas 2020). By taking into account these controversial accounts, it seems that new exclusionary tactics against the migrant/refugee populations are at stake. In fact, as the Greek case also testifies, institutional policies have not only left out marginalized third-country nationals from the national vaccination plan, in practice, but they have also imposed harsher mobility restrictions against them, highlighting pre-existing inequalities and politics of exclusion, as it is the case elsewhere (Brown 2020; Evershed 2020).

From June 2021 onwards, Greece announced that the National Public Health Organization (EODY) will vaccinate residents in 34 reception centers, 6 Reception and Identification Centers and 8 pre-removal centers (EASO 2021). The vaccines made available in the camps were only selected according to the availability of the three officially approved vaccine brands[10]. However, contrary to the opportunities and choices offered to the Greek citizens, people from third countries who live in precarious conditions are not in a position to decide upon the vaccine brand they wish. In addition, the local authorities of the Lesvos Island have mentioned that *"as the vaccines cannot be left out of the refrigerator for a long time, the vaccinations will be given to a certain number of people, only by appointment and always inside the KYT (the Reception Centre) so as not to burden the vaccination lines of the local community"*[11]. In July 2021, there were no official data for the vaccination progress of those residing in official State camps, but it is estimated that less than 1000 persons have been vaccinated in 3 reception and identification centers at the island's hotspots and 3 host facilities on the mainland[12]. This is not surprising, as the vaccination plan for the camps provides for availability only twice a week[13], and those who have received a second-degree asylum rejection decision are excluded from vaccination (Aggelidis 2021). What is most striking is the highly symbolic gesture of the Greek Authorities that the unused vaccines are to be administered to prisoners and migrant-refugee populations who live in closed facilities (Gakis 2021).

All the above depict not only aspects of discrimination and exclusion but also aspects of migrant and refugee populations' degrading legal status and health conditions. Such procedures reinforce the pre-existing stigma attached to the above populations as if they possess a lower social status. This stigma further affects the already existing and evidenced negative attitudes towards migrants/refugees (Dixon et al. 2019)[14]. Thus, a contradicting social situation emerges which is signifying a *paradox*. On the one hand, those who are perceived as a danger to public health are eligible only to 'leftovers', that is, without sufficient health protection, while, on the other, they are perceived as a danger to public health due to the insufficient protection they receive. This *paradox* serves the perpetuation of the vicious cycle of migrants/refugees' stigmatization, a cycle reinforced by perceptions emanating from the public health field which operates as an additive component to crimmigration. Thus, administrative procedures establish a concrete negative screening and a practice of official controls which disproportionately affect migrant populations and intensify the trajectories of crimmigration. Currently, the health field affected by COVID-19 contributes to the advancement of the crimmigration regime and at the same time to a dangerous cul-de-sac. In addition, the official social controls imposed to combat the COVD-19 health crisis contribute to crimmigration through the intensification of the dangerization of mixed migration flows.

5. Discussion

The COVID-19 pandemic and the measures imposed to confront it have seriously affected daily life and have created a new social reality marked by numerous precautions and restrictions for the total population worldwide. These measures are aimed at both the avoidance of virus spread and broad transmission and the protection of public health. Special groups of the population, due to vulnerability, such as conditions of living (adequate housing, food, access to health services, personal health condition) pose unprecedented challenges for every State in managing the new, urgent and demanding situation, as well as in safeguarding their life and dignity. Especially when national vaccination plans started to be implemented in all EU Member States, third-country nationals who live in precarious conditions were left, to a large extent, less protected, forgotten, abandoned and non-prioritized compared to native citizens and State nationals by most of the Member States' policies.

Studying the relevant official Greek policies through documentary and archival research we realize that the already precarious population of asylum-seekers, refugees and undocumented migrants, under the conditions of the COVID-19 pandemic, continued to reside in crowded facilities, lacking adequate hygiene and being mostly unvaccinated for at least half a year after the national vaccination plan had been launched. Moreover, they have remained quarantined in the same undignified living conditions for a much longer period compared to that provided for the Greek citizens. In addition, the great category of those in camps was 'detained' in crowded spaces, although research evidence showed that it was more likely to be inflicted by the COVID-19 virus. Their segregation and invisibility, or, otherwise, their extended social control and encampment, were the effects of consecutive administrative decisions and legal regulations against all scientific evidence and human rights approaches which truly advocate to the contrary.

Concerning vaccination, marginalized third-country nationals have not been included in the first, second or even the third phase of the Greek National Vaccination Plan, despite the fact that the WHO and other international bodies such as the UNHCR provide guidance for prioritization of those living in harsh conditions. Bureaucratic hindrances such as the issue of a Social Security Number (AMKA) refrained them from being registered to receive a vaccine. The specific administrative provisions provided for the acquisition of a temporary security number (PAMKA) allowed for only part of these populations to be included for vaccination. Yet, migrant and refugee vaccination plans were implemented six months later than the general population vaccination plan and only when it was made clear that the available vaccines were sufficient enough to cover the entire Greek population. Segregation also infiltrated the way migrant and refugee populations had access to a vaccine brand. Their vaccination process was also 'camped' since it could only be operated inside the walls of their residence camp and restricted to twice a week administration of dosages.

Most importantly discrimination, further freedom restrictions and diverse levels of exclusion influenced more deeply the migrant/refugee populations as 'non-citizens'. They were subdued to a life of (a) time restrictions since they have not been prioritized regardless of their harsh conditions which make them more vulnerable to the COVID-19 virus; (b) choice restrictions since they are not offered the opportunity to choose the vaccine brand they wish to be vaccinated with; and (c) place restrictions since those living in camps can only be vaccinated therein. Even the condition of the pandemic was not able to surpass such a systemic space segregation. On the contrary, all freedom restrictions have been further intensified 'for the protection of public health'.

Inferentially, the body (the 'non-citizen body'), the time factor, the place/milieu restrictions and the lack of free choice are merged in a new inequity complex which tends to reinforce the crimmigrated identity of the controlled subject. It could be stressed that harsh living conditions coupled with the above restrictions form new 'normal' cycles of rejections next to other pre-existing ones.

6. Conclusions

Our study reveals that even under the conditions of an emergency, such as the occurrence of a pandemic, the 'crimmigrated' approach of the States concerning the marginalized migrant/refugee populations cannot be annulled or even mitigated. On the contrary, emergency pandemic situations constitute another field for intensifying the dangerization controls, segregation and movement restrictions of various social groups, migrant/refugee populations included. In addition, emergency pandemic situations constitute an extra opportunity in the context of a vaccine institutional racism for further stabilizing the identity of the 'non-citizen crimmigrated' subject as a subject non-liable to prioritized protection. Such a state-of-play provides a 'fertile' ground for new cross-mergers of crimmigration with public health policies. In this sense, the guaranteeing of rights cannot be implemented for all (Arendt 1943), even in situations of great risk and emergency. Although further research is needed, we may validly argue that the way public health policies have been amalgamated with penal, administrative and migration law processes indicates that health field may be used as an additive component to crimmigration as it helps the establishment of a concrete screening intensifying the already imposed migration controls. In addition, the official social controls imposed to combat the COVD-19 health crisis contribute to crimmigration through the intensification of the crimmigration regime and at the same time to a dangerous cul-de-sac.

Author Contributions: J.T. has contributed to the present paper in the sectors of conceptualization, methodology, writing—review and editing; A.C. has contributed to the present paper in the sectors of conceptualization, methodology and writing—review and editing; M.L. has contributed to the present paper in the sectors of conceptualization, methodology and writing—review and editing. All authors have read and agreed to the published version of the manuscript.

Funding: The authors received no financial support for the research, authorship and/or for this article.

Institutional Review Board Statement: Not applicable.

Informed Consent Statement: Not applicable.

Data Availability Statement: Not applicable.

Conflicts of Interest: The authors declare no conflict of interest.

Notes

1. Abolition of the Circular Φ80320/οικ.28107/1857/20-6-2019—as derived from the Joint Ministerial Decision 31547/9662/13.02.2018—by the Circular Φ.80320/οικ.31355/Δ18.2084/11.07.2019 of the Minister of Labor (Decision. For AMKA). The above Joint Ministerial Decision safeguarded access to health services for the migrant population in Greece. See also Aggelidis, Dimitris. The hope for the cancer patient falls into a (legal) vacuum, *Efsyn*, 29 November 2019, available online: https://www.efsyn.gr/ellada/dikaiomata/220998_peftei-se-nomiko-keno-i-elpida-gia-karkinopathi-prosfyga (accessed on 3 August 2021).
2. To Vima, The quarantine continues in host facilities because ... of COVID_19, *To Vima*, 19 July 2020, Συνεχίζεται η απαγόρευση κυκλοφορίας στις δομές φιλοξενίας λόγω ... κορωνοϊού, To Βήμα Online.
3. As explicitly stated, "*sociodemographic groups at significantly higher risk of severe disease or death (depending on country context, examples may include: disadvantaged or persecuted ethnic, racial, gender, and religious groups and sexual minorities; people living with disabilities; people living in extreme poverty, the homeless and those living in informal settlements or urban slums; low-income migrant workers; refugees, internally displaced persons, asylum-seekers, populations in conflict settings or those affected by humanitarian emergencies, vulnerable migrants in irregular situations; nomadic populations; and hard-to-reach population groups such as those in rural and remote areas)*", p. 11, (World Health Organization 2020b).
4. Austria, Croatia, Cyprus, Germany, Romania, (FRA 2021). See also Muscat, Gavin. Asylum seekers and foreigners applying for residency 'denied vaccine'–Only people who 'truly' live in Malta will be vaccinated', *Newsbook*, 1 June 2021.
5. (United Nations n.d.), Sustainable Development Goals, Goal 3: Ensure healthy lives and promote well-being for all at all ages, 3.8 Achieve universal health coverage, including financial risk protection, access to quality essential healthcare services and access to safe, effective, quality and affordable essential medicines and vaccines for all, Health–United Nations Sustainable Development.
6. "Everyone has the right of access to preventive health care and the right to benefit from medical treatment under the conditions established by national laws and practices. A high level of human health protection shall be ensured in the definition and implementation of all the Union's policies and activities." EU Charter of the Fundamental Rights, Article 35 of the Charter, https://eur-lex.europa.eu/legal-content/EN/TXT/PDF/?uri=CELEX:12012P/TXT&from=EN (accessed on 8 August 2021).
7. The Washinghton Post. Europe is racing to vaccinate residents. But in some countries, undocumented immigrants have been left out, *The Washington Post*, 11 July 2021e.
8. Vaccination against COVID-19, Εμβολιασμός κατά της COVID-19, available online: https://emvolio.gov.gr/ (accessed on 1 August 2021).

9   Proto Thema."Mitarakis: Vaccination in the hosting structures starts in early May", Μηταράκης: Αρχές Μαΐου ξεκινάει ο εμβολιασμός στις δομές φιλοξενίας (protothema.gr), 28 March 2021. See also: *"The Greek Minister for Migration Policy stated that Greece planned to start vaccinating residents and staff in refugee camps in May, as epidemiological data did not show particular spread in the camps"*, FRA 2021, p. 21.

10 Efsyn,"Refugee vaccinations on mainland begin on Thursday", Ξεκινούν την Πέμπτη οι εμβολιασμοί προσφύγων στην ενδοχώρα, *Efsyn*, 8 June 2021.

11 Efyn, Twice a week refugee vaccinations in the camps, Δύο φορές την εβδομάδα οι εμβολιασμοί προσφύγων, *Efsyn*, 3 June 2021.

12 Kathimerini, Newsroom, Refugees in camps face a greater risk from the coronavirus, Μεγαλύτερο κίνδυνο από τον κορωνοϊό αντιμετωπίζουν οι πρόσφυγες σε δομές, *Kathimerini*, 1 July 2021.

13 Efsyn, "Twice a week refugee vaccinations in the camps", *Efsyn*, 3 June 2021, ibid.

14 "Most Greeks believe that the effects of immigration are negative, especially in the context of the country's scarce resources [. . .] Overall, 51 percent determine that immigration is ultimately 'bad for Greece, costing the welfare state and draining resources that could be spent on Greeks [..] (Greeks) Anxieties about Islam and Muslims are common [. . .] (and) hold concerns about several aspects of the refugee and migration crisis, including [. . .] Perceptions of disorder and authorities' loss of control of the situation [. . .] Security fears: Concerns about the risk of terrorism and increased crime are present in all segments, but much stronger in the 'closed' groups. Overall, 42 percent of Greeks agree with the proposition that it is too dangerous to let refugees in the country due to the threat of terrorism", (Dixon et al. 2019).

References

Primary Sources

Aggelidis, Dimitris. The hope for the cancer patient falls into a (legal) vacuum, *Efsyn*, 29 November 2019, Πέφτει σε (νομικό) κενό η ελπίδα για καρκινοπαθή πρόσφυγα | Η Εφημερίδα των Συντακτών (efsyn.gr). Available online: https://www.efsyn.gr/ellada/dikaiomata/220998_peftei-se-nomiko-keno-i-elpida-gia-karkinopathi-prosfyga (accessed on 3 August 2021).

Aggelidis, Dimitris. The temporary AMKA for those seeking asylum is being implemented, *Efsyn*, 01 April 2020, Προς εφαρμογή προχωρά ο προσωρινός ΑΜΚΑ για όσους ζητούν άσυλο | Η Εφημερίδα των Συντακτών (efsyn.gr). Available online: https://www.efsyn.gr/node/237498 (accesed on 3 August 2021).

Aggelidis, Dimitris. Survey: Less than 1000 vaccinated refugees, *Efsyn*, 2 July 2021, Έρευνα: λιγότεροι από 1.000 οι εμβολιασμένοι πρόσφυγες | Η Εφημερίδα των Συντακτών (efsyn.gr). Available online: https://www.efsyn.gr/ellada/koinonia/300800_ereyna-ligoteroi-apo-1000-oi-emboliasmenoi-prosfyges (accessed on 3 August 2021).

Decision, For AMKA. Available online: https://www.in.gr/wp-content/uploads/2019/07/%CE%B1%CE%BD%CE%B1%CE%BA%CE%BB%CE%B7%CF%83%CE%B7.pdf (accessed on 1 August 2021).

Efsyn, Refugee vaccinations on mainland begin on Thursday, *Efsyn*, 8 June 2021, Ξεκινούν την Πέμπτη οι εμβολιασμοί προσφύγων στην ενδοχώρα | Η Εφημερίδα των Συντακτών (efsyn.gr). Available online: https://www.efsyn.gr/ellada/ygeia/297612_xekinoyn-tin-pempti-oi-emboliasmoi-prosfygon-stin-endohora (accessed on 3 August 2021).

Efyn, Twice a week refugee vaccinations in the camps, *Efsyn*, 3 June 2021, Δύο φορές την εβδομάδα οι εμβολιασμοί προσφύγων | Η Εφημερίδα των Συντακτών (efsyn.gr). Available online: https://www.efsyn.gr/ellada/ygeia/296859_dyo-fores-tin-ebdomada-oi-emboliasmoi-prosfygon (accessed on 3 August 2021).

Escritt, Thomas. EU states to start COVID-19 vaccinations from Dec. 27, *Reuters*, 17 December 2020. Available online: https://www.reuters.com/article/health-coronavirus-biontech-merkel-idUSKBN28R18W (accessed on 1 August 2021).

Emmanouilidou, Lydia. 2021. In Greece, thousands of asylum-seekers are waiting for the COVID-19 vaccine. *The World*, 11 May 2021. Available online: https://theworld.org/stories/2021-05-11/greece-thousands-asylum-seekers-are-waiting-covid-19-vaccine (accessed on 3 August 2021).

Evershed, Nick. Disadvantaged Areas of Melbourne Hardest Hit in Victoria's Coronavirus Outbreak. *The Guardian*, 25 August 2020. Available online: https://www.theguardian.com/news/datablog/2020/aug/25/disadvantaged-areas-of-melbourne-hardest-hit-in-victoriascoronavirus-outbreak (accessed on 3 August 2021).

Gakis, Giorgos. Κακοκαιρία Μήδεια: Αδιάθετες δόσεις εμβολίων σε ένστολους, Κορυδαλλό και Αμυγδαλέζα, *Newshealth*, 16 February 2021. Available online: https://www.news4health.gr/politiki-ygeias/6513/kakokairia-mideia-adiathetes-doseis-emvolion-se-enstolous-korydallo-kai-amygdaleza (accessed on 3 August 2021).

Joint Ministerial Decision 31547/9662/13-02-2018. Available online: https://www.taxheaven.gr/circulars/28107/k-y-a-ariom-prwt-31547-9662-2018 (accessed on 1 August 2021).

Joint Ministerial Decision 717/2020 (Government Gazette B 199/31.01.2020). Available online: https://www.e-nomothesia.gr/law-news/prosorinos-arithmos-asfalisis-perithalpsis-gia-aitoyntes-asylo.html (accessed on 1 August 2021).

Joint Ministerial Decision 2981/2021 (Government Gazette B'2197/26.05.2021). Available online: https://g2red.org/wp-content/uploads/2021/06/%CE%9A%CE%BF%CE%B9%CE%BD%CE%AE-%CE%A5%CF%80%CE%BF%CF%85%CF%81%CE%B3%CE%B9%CE%BA%CE%AE-%CE%91%CF%80%CF%8C%CF%86%CE%B1%CF%83%CE%B7.pdf (accessed on 1 August 2021).

Kathimerini, Newsroom, Refugees in camps face a greater risk from the coronavirus, *Kathimerini*, 1 July 2021, Μεγαλύτερο κίνδυνο από τον κορωνοϊό αντιμετωπίζουν οι πρόσφυγες σε δομές | Η ΚΑΘΗΜΕΡΙΝΗ (kathimerini.gr). Available online: https://www.kathimerini.gr/society/561418591/megalytero-kindyno-molynsis-apo-koronoio-antimetopizoyn-oi-prosfyges-se-domes/ (accessed on 3 August 2021).

Law 4636/2019. Available online: https://www.e-nomothesia.gr/kat-allodapoi/prosphuges-politiko-asulo/nomos-4636-2019-phek-169a-1-11-2019.html (accessed on 1 August 2021).

Law 4686/2020. Available online: https://www.taxheaven.gr/law/4686/2020 (accessed on 1 August 2021).

Law 4782/2021. Available online: https://g2red.org/wp-content/uploads/2021/06/%CE%9D%CF%8C%CE%BC%CE%BF%CF%82 4782-2021.pdf (accessed on 1 August 2021).

Law and Order. In Korydallos, Amygdaleza, military and police the unavailable vaccines due to snow, military and police, *Law and Order*, 18.02.2021, Σε Κορυδαλλό, Αμυγδαλέζα, στρατιωτικούς και αστυνομικούς τα αδιάθετα εμβόλια λόγω χιονιά, (lawandorder.gr). Available online: https://www.lawandorder.gr/Article/112294/ellada/se-korudallo-amugdaleza-stratiotikous-kai-astunomikous-ta-adiatheta-embolia-logo-chionia (accessed on 3 August 2021).

Legislative Act, Government Gazette A′28/10.02.2020. Available online: https://www.e-nomothesia.gr/law-news/se-phek-praxe-nomothetikou-periekhomenou-gia-tin-epitaxi-ektaseon.html (accessed on 1 August 2021).

Magnesia News. When are those who missed their appointment are going to be vaccinated? Πότε εμβολιάζονται όσοι έχασαν το ραντεβού τους, *Magnesia News*, 18 February 2021. Available online: https://magnesianews.gr/ellada/pote-emvoliazontai-osoi-echasan-to-rantevoy-toys.html (accessed on 3 August 2021).

Muscat, Gavin. Asylum seekers and foreigners applying for residency 'denied vaccine'–Only people who 'truly' live in Malta will be vaccinated', *Newsbook*, 1 June 2021. Available online: https://newsbook.com.mt/en/asylum-seekers-and-foreigners-applying-for-residency-denied-vaccine/ (accessed on 3 August 2021).

Mitarakis. 2020. New package of 6 meters of the Ministry of Immigration and Asylum for the protection from the coronavirus in the KYT Islands and the other hosting structures, Νέα δέσμη 6 μέτρων του Υπουργείου Μετανάστευσης και Ασύλου για την προστασία από τον κορωνοϊό στα ΚΥΤ Νήσων και των άλλων δομών φιλοξενίας-Νότης Μηταράκης, Βουλευτής Χίου, Νέα Δημοκρατία (mitarakis.gr), 27.03.2020. Available online: https://www.mitarakis.gr/gov/migration/1970-dt-yma-nea-desmi-metrwn (accessed on 1 August 2021).

Papanicolaou, Natasha. Moria Corona Virus: "The virus has brought chaos into the camp. There is tremendous stress for something unknown", *PARAPOLITIKA*, 25 March 2020. Available online: https://www.politikalesvos.gr/moria-corona-virus-quot-o-ios-echei-ferei-to-chaos-mesa-sto-kamp-yparchei-tromero-stres-gia-kati-agnosto-quot/ (accessed on 8 August 2021).

Proto Thema: Vaccination in the hosting structures starts in early May", Μηταράκης: Αρχές Μαΐου ξεκινάει ο εμβολιασμός στις δομές φιλοξενίας (protothema.gr), 28.03.2021. Available online: https://www.protothema.gr/greece/article/1108879/mitaraki-arhes-maiou-xekinaei-o-emvoliasmos-stis-domes-filoxenias/ (accessed on 3 August 2021).

The Washington Post. Europe is racing to vaccinate residents. But in some countries, undocumented immigrants have. been left out, *The Washington Post*, 11 July 2021e.

To Vima, The quarantine continues in host facilities because ... of COVID_19, *To Vima*, 19 July 2020, Συνεχίζεται η απαγόρευση κυκλοφορίας στις δομές φιλοξενίας λόγω ... κορωνοϊού-Ειδήσεις-νέα-Το Βήμα Online (tovima.gr). Available online: https://www.tovima.gr/2020/07/19/society/synexizetai-i-apagoreysi-kykloforias-stis-domes-filoksenias-logo-koronoiou (accessed on 3 August 2021).

Published Sources

Aas, Katja Franko, and Maria Bosworth, eds. 2013. *The Borders of Punishment. Migration, Citizenship, and Social Exclusion*. Oxford: Oxford University Press.

AIDA-ECRE. 2021. Conditions in Reception Facilities, Greece. 10 June 2021. Available online: https://asylumineurope.org/reports/country/greece/reception-conditions/housing/conditions-reception-facilities/ (accessed on 1 August 2021).

Amnesty International. 2019. Press Release: *Greece Must Immediately Ensure Free Access to the Public Health System for All Asylum Seekers, Unaccompanied Children and Children of Irregular Migrants*, 14 October 2019. Available online: https://www.amnesty.org/en/documents/eur25/1213/2019/en/ (accessed on 1 August 2021).

Arendt, Hanna. 1943. We Refugees. *The Menorah Journal* XXXI: 69–77.

Bacchi, Carol Lee. 1999. *Women, Policy and Politics: The Construction of Policy Problems*. London: Sage Publications.

Bilgin, Ayata, and Artemis Fyssa. 2020. *Politics of Abandonment: Refugees on Greek Islands during the Coronavirus Crisis*. Eurozine. Available online: https://www.eurozine.com/politics-of-abandonment (accessed on 1 August 2021).

Bourdeau, Philippe. 2019. Detention and immigration: Practices, crimmigration, and norms. *Migration Studies* 7: 83–99. [CrossRef]

Broeders, Dennis, and James Hampshire. 2013. Dreaming of seamless borders: ICTs and the pre-emptive governance of mobility in Europe. *Journal of Ethnic and Migration Studies* 39: 1201–18. [CrossRef]

Brown, Michel. 2020. Foucault's Crows: Pandemic Insurrection in the United States. *Crime, Media, Culture* 17: 7–10. [CrossRef]

Dixon, Tim, Stephen Hawkins, Miriam Juan-Torres, and Arisa Kimaran. 2019. *Attitudes towards National Identity, Immigration and Refugees in Greece*. More in Common. Available online: https://www.moreincommon.com/media/ltinlcnc/0535-more-in-common-greece-report_final_4_web_lr.pdf (accessed on 1 August 2021).

EASO. 2021. COVID-19 Vaccination for Applicants, and Beneficiaries of International Protection, Situational Update, Issue No 1, 31 March 2021. EASO_Factsheet_Landscape_A4 (europa.eu). Available online: https://www.easo.europa.eu/sites/default/files/publications/EASO_Situational_Update_Vaccination31March..pdf (accessed on 1 August 2021).

European Centre for Disease Prevention and Control (ECDC). 2020a. Key Aspects Regarding the Introduction and Prioritisation of COVID-19 Vaccination in the EU/EEA and the UK, Technical Report, 26 October 2020. Available online: https://www.ecdc.europa.eu/sites/default/files/documents/Key-aspects-regarding-introduction-and-prioritisation-of-COVID-19-vaccination.pdf (accessed on 1 August 2021).

European Centre for Disease Prevention and Control (ECDC). 2020b. Covid-19 Vaccination and Prioritisation Strategies in the EU/EEA, Technical Report, 22 December 2020. Available online: https://www.ecdc.europa.eu/sites/default/files/documents/COVID-19-vaccination-and-prioritisation-strategies.pdf (accessed on 1 August 2021).

European Centre for Disease Prevention and Control (ECDC). 2021. Reducing COVID-19 Transmission and Strengthening Vaccine Uptake among Migrant Populations in the EU/EEA, Technical Report, 3 June 2021. Available online: https://www.ecdc.europa.eu/en/publications-data/covid-19-migrants-reducing-transmission-and-strengthening-vaccine-uptake (accessed on 1 August 2021).

European Commission. 2020a. EU Vaccines Strategy. Available online: https://ec.europa.eu/info/live-work-travel-eu/coronavirus-response/public-health/eu-vaccines-strategy_en (accessed on 1 August 2021).

European Commission. 2020b. Communication from the Commission to the European Parliament and the Council, Preparedness for COVID-19 vaccination strategies and vaccine deployment, COM (2020) 680 final, Brussels, 15 October 2020. Available online: https://ec.europa.eu/health/sites/default/files/vaccination/docs/2020_strategies_deployment_en.pdf (accessed on 1 August 2021).

Fouskas, Theodoros. 2020. Migrants, asylum seekers and refugees in Greece in the midst of the COVID-19 pandemic. *Comparative Cultural Studies-European and Latin American Perspectives* 5: 39–58. [CrossRef]

FRA. 2021. Coronavirus Pandemic in the EU-Fundamental Rights Implications: Vaccine Rollout and Equality of Access in the EU, 1 March–30 April 2021, Bulletin #7. Available online: https://fra.europa.eu/sites/default/files/fra_uploads/fra-2021-coronavirus-pandemic-eu-bulletin-vaccines_en.pdf (accessed on 1 August 2021).

Generation 2.0 for Rights Equality and Diversity, *Manolada Watch*, Manolada Watch-Generation 2.0. 2019. Available online: https://g2red.org/manolada-watch/ (accessed on 1 August 2021).

Generation 2.0 for Rights Equality and Diversity, Health is a Fundamental Right, Press Room, 9 July 2021. 2021. Available online: https://g2red.org/health-is-a-fundamental-right/ (accessed on 1 August 2021).

Gerard, Alison, and Sharon Pickering. 2013. Crimmigration: Criminal Justice, Refugee Protection and the Securitisation of Migration. In *The Routledge Handbook of International Crime and Justice Studies*. Criminal Justice, Borders and Citizenship Research Paper No. 2698974. Edited by H. Bersot and B. Arrigo. London: Routledge. Available online: https://ssrn.com/abstract=2698974 (accessed on 1 August 2021).

Giddens, Anthony. 1984. *The Constitution of Society*. Cambridge: Polity Press.

Greek Government. 2021. National Vaccination Operational Plan against COVID-19, ethniko_epiheirisiako_shedio_emvoliasmon_kata_toy_covid-19_v6.1_1.pdf (emvolio.gov.gr). Available online: https://emvolio.gov.gr/sites/default/files/ethniko_epiheirisiako_shedio_emvoliasmon_kata_toy_covid-19_v6.1_1.pdf?t=1 (accessed on 1 August 2021).

Greek Ministry of Migration and Asylum. 2020. 'Coronavirus protection measures at Reception and Identification Centers, accommodation structures and the Asylum Service", Μέτρα προστασίας από τον κορωνοϊό στα Κέντρα Υποδοχής και Ταυτοποίησης, στις δομές φιλοξενίας και στην Υπηρεσία Ασύλου. 17 March 2020. Available online: https://migration.gov.gr/en/metra-prostasias-apo-ton-koronoio-sta-kentra-ypodochis-kai-taytopoiisis-stis-domes-filoxenias-kai-stin-ypiresia-asyloy/ (accessed on 1 August 2021).

Guia, Maria João, Maartie van der Woude, and Joanna van der Leun, eds. 2011. *Social Control and Justice: Crimmigration in an Age of Fear*. The Hague: Eleven International Publishing.

Johansson, Ylva. 2020. Intervention (via video conference) in European Parliament LIBE Committee on the situation at the Union's external borders in Greece, 2 April 2020, Speech, 2 April 2020. Available online: https://ec.europa.eu/commission/commissioners/2019-2024/johansson/announcements/intervention-video-conference-european-parliament-libe-committee-situation-unions-external-borders_en (accessed on 1 August 2021).

Kondilis, Elias, Dimitris Papamichail, Sophie McCann, Elspeth Carruthers, Apostolos Veizis, Miriam Orcutt, and Sally Hargreaves. 2021. The impact of COVID-19 pandemic on refugees and asylum seekers in Greece: A Retrospective analysis of national surveillance data from 2020. Research Paper. *EClinicalMedicine* 37: 100958. Available online: https://www.thelancet.com/action/showPdf?pii=S2589-5370%2821%2900238-8 (accessed on 1 August 2021). [CrossRef]

Koulish, Robert. 2016. Sovereign bias, crimmigration and risk. In *Immigration Detention, Risk and Human Rights*. Edited by Guia Maria João. Cham: Springer, pp. 1–12.

Koulish, Robert. 2021. Special issue Crimmigration in the Age of COVID-19. *Social Sciences* 10: 379.

Medecins sans Frontieres (MSF). 2020. Evacuation of Squalid Greek Camps More Urgent Than Ever over COVID-19 Fears, Press Release, 12 March 2020. Available online: https://www.msf.org/urgent-evacuation-squalid-camps-greece-needed-over-covid-19-fears (accessed on 1 August 2021).

Menjivar, Cecilia, Andrea Gomez Cervantes, and Daniel Alvord. 2018. The expansion of "crimmigration", mass detention, and deportation". *Sociology Compass* 12: 1–15. [CrossRef]

Nikolopoulos, Giorgos. 2012. The criminalization of the migration policy and the new European territorialities of social control. In *The Politics of Criminology. Critical Studies on Deviance and Social Control*. Edited by Stratos Georgoulas. Berlin–Wien–Zürich: LIT Verlag, pp. 185–96.

Platform for International Cooperation on Undocumented Migrants (PICUM). n.d. Covid-19 and the Undocumented Migrants. What Is Happening in Europe? Available online: https://picum.org/covid-19-undocumented-migrants-europe/ (accessed on 1 August 2021).

Riechert, Bonnie Parnell. 1996. Advocacy Group and News Media Framing of Public Policy Issues: Frame Mapping the Wetlands Debates. Unpublished Doctoral dissertation, University of Tennessee, Knoxville, TN, USA.

Rottem, Rosenberg Rubins. 2021. Crimmigration and the 'Paradox of Exclusion'. *Oxford Journal of Legal Studies* gqab025. [CrossRef]

Saifee, Jessica, Carlos Franco-Paredes, and Steven R. Lowenstein. 2021. Refugee Health During COVID-19 and Future Pandemics. *Current Tropical Medicine Reports* 16: 1–4. [CrossRef] [PubMed]

Salamon, Neža Kogovšek. 2017. Mass Migration, Crimmigration and Defiance. *The Case of the Humanitarian Corridor. Southeastern Europe* 41: 251–75. [CrossRef]

Salamon, Neža Kogovšek. 2020. *Causes and Consequences of Migrant Criminalization*. Cham: Springer.

Stokely, Carmichael, Kwame Ture, and Charles Hamilton. 1967. *Black Power: The Politics of Liberation in America*. New York: Vintage Books.

Strauss, Anselm, and Juliet M. Corbin, eds. 1997. *Grounded Theory in Practice*. London: Sage Publications.

Stumpf, Juliet. 2006. The crimmigration crisis: Immigrants, crime, and sovereign power. *The American University Law Review* 56: 367–419.

Thomas, Christine, Mickael Osterholm, and William Stauffer. 2021. Critical Considerations for COVID-19 Vaccination of Refugees, Immigrants, and Migrants. *The American Journal of Tropical Medicine and Hygiene* 104: 433–5. [CrossRef] [PubMed]

Triandafyllidou, Anna, and Anastasios Fotiou. 1998. Sustainability and modernity in the European Union: A frame theory approach to policymaking. *Sociological Research Online* 3. Available online: https://journals.sagepub.com/doi/10.5153/sro.99 (accessed on 1 August 2021).

Tsiganou, Joanna, Labraki Julia, Fatourou Ioanna, and Evaggelos Chainas. 2010. *Migration and Criminality. Myths and Reality*. Athens: EKKE.

Tsiganou, Joanna, Chakia Anastasia, and Martha Lempesi. 2020. Syrian Refugees in Greece. Trajectories of integration. *Koinoniki Politiki* 12: 5–22. Available online: http://eekp.gr/wp-content/uploads/2020/06/PERIODIKO-T12.pdf (accessed on 1 August 2021).

UNHCR. 2021a. UNHCR Calls for Equitable Access to COVID-19 Vaccines for Refugees. *Press Release*, 7 April 2021. Available online: https://www.unhcr.org/news/press/2021/4/606d56564/unhcr-calls-equitable-access-covid-19-vaccines-refugees.html (accessed on 1 August 2021).

UNHCR. 2021b. Help Greece, Vaccination against COVID-19. Available online: https://help.unhcr.org/greece/coronavirus/covid19vaccination/ (accessed on 28 May 2021).

United Nations. n.d. Sustainable Development Goals, Health. Available online: https://www.un.org/sustainabledevelopment/health/ (accessed on 1 August 2021).

Van Gorp, Baldwin. 2001. The Implementation of the Asylum Policy: Which Frame Dominates the Debate? Paper present at the ECPR Joint Sessions, Grenoble, France, April 6–11.

Verloo, Mieke. 2005. Mainstreaming gender equality in Europe. A critical frame analysis approach. In *The Greek Review of Social Research, Special Issue. Differences in the Framing of Gender Inequality as a Policy Problem across Europe*. Edited by Verloo Mieke and Pantelidou Maloutas Maro. Athens: National Centre for Social Research, vol. 117, pp. 11–34.

Verloo, Mieke, and Pantelidou Maro Maloutas. 2005. Editorial: Differences in the framing of gender inequality as a policy problem across Europe. In *The Greek Review of Social Research, Special Issue. Differences in the framing of gender inequality as a policy problem across Europe*. Edited by Verloo Mieke and Pantelidou Maloutas Maro. Athens: National Centre for Social Research, vol. 117, pp. 3–10.

Websdale, Asher. 2020. Crimmigration: A Lens for Public Health Securitisation at the Border? Available online: https://www.law.ox.ac.uk/research-subject-groups/centre-criminology/centreborder-criminologies/blog/2020/06/crimmigration (accessed on 1 August 2021).

Weekers, Jacqueline. 2020. To Be Effective, COVID-19 Vaccination Plans Must Include miGrants, IOM 18 December 2020. Available online: https://weblog.iom.int/fr/node/2399 (accessed on 1 August 2021).

World Health Organization (WHO). 2020a. AparTogetherSurvey, Preliminary Overview of Refugees and Migrants Self-Reported Impact of Covid-19. Available online: https://apps.who.int/iris/bitstream/handle/10665/337931/9789240017924-eng.pdf?sequence=1&isAllowed=y (accessed on 15 July 2021).

World Health Organization (WHO). 2020b. *WHO SAGE Roadmap for Prioritizing Uses of COVID-19 Vaccines in the Context of Limited Supply*. Geneva: WHO. Available online: https://www.who.int/publications/i/item/who-sage-roadmap-for-prioritizing-uses-of-covid-19-vaccines-in-the-context-of-limited-supply (accessed on 1 August 2021).

photo ID with an "Alien Number" by which they would now be known. After a cursory assessment of their immigration and criminal history (when there was any) they exchanged their street clothes for a couple of jumpsuits in one of several colors associated with their custody classification—in my opinion, ill-advised in any settings—and the first departure from correctional practices that I noted that day—blue uniforms for low security, orange uniforms for medium security, and red uniforms for maximum security—and then were assigned to housing units with others in same custody classification.

On the recreation yard, the differences were more pronounced. A large group of men, all of them wearing red uniforms, supposedly to warn others of their violent nature, were supervised by only one detention officer. Some of them were playing a game of horseshoes, tossing real horseshoes around sharpened metal stakes that had been pounded into the ground, as others stood around them and watched. A correctional facility would never release any number of truly dangerous inmates together onto a recreation yard, certainly not a yard enclosed in just a six-foot chain link fence and the one officer in the area, and under no circumstances with heavy metal objects at hand that could—and likely would—be used as weapons if they were violent. When it was time to go back indoors, there was no inventory of the equipment or search of the detainees for contraband. The officer simply escorted them back to their housing unit, through the main corridor where there were a lot of detainees in blue and orange jumpsuits—without incident. The people who ICE has continually characterized as the "worst of the worst," and not trustworthy of being assigned to open housing, and certainly not community supervision under any circumstances, had played by the rules, literally. In fact, most detainees always do.

The vast majority of the people in ICE's custody are contributing members of intact, extended families, with job skills, employment histories, and community ties. They do not want any trouble, only the opportunity to be heard and hopefully, secure relief. Unfortunately, ICE policy and practice is a self-fulfilling prophesy. When the government locks up people who are pursuing civil remedies through the immigration court in jails and prisons, dressed in jumpsuits with their movement monitored moment to moment by uniformed guards, or assigns them to community supervision with an electronic monitoring device tethered to their ankle, we conclude they must be criminals. Why else would the government treat them as such? If ICE were to house migrants on college campuses or in hostels, rectories, training centers and worksites, and similar settings, dressed in street clothes, and had them check in periodically with a coach or an advisor, should any of these provisions actually be warranted, our opinion of them would be as different as the treatment they receive. ICE has never assessed risk correctly or responded proportionately, and despite its unfounded exaggerations as to detainees' dangerousness, many had never been convicted of a crime before they were detained, cause no trouble during their detention, and do not engage in criminal activities of any kind after their release (Schriro 2009).

ICE's oversight and operation of immigration detention is reminiscent of the narrator who misinterpreted the Nacirema's moves and motives as he went about his morning rituals. ICE goes through many of the motions associated with criminal incarceration without an apparent understanding or appreciation of the substantive differences between detainees and inmates, and immigration enforcement's distinctly different role and responsibilities for *civilly* detained individuals in its custody—especially those at heightened risk of serious illness, life-altering complications, and death from COVID-19 during the pandemic. ICE's criminalization of the immigrant deprives all the people in its custody of their rights under international and federal law and absolves Immigration Enforcement of its responsibilities to the detained (Bowling and Westenra 2018).

2. Introduction

Immigration Detention is a patchwork of public and private correctional facilities overseen by ICE, a federal enforcement agency. In June 2021, ICE detained 16,460 adults in 121 facilities in 38 states, frequently alongside pretrial and sentenced inmates and U.S. Marshals Service prisoners, under conditions ICE established in five different sets of

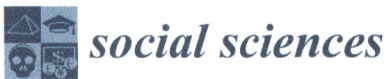

Article

On the Other Side of the Looking Glass: COVID-19 Care in Immigration Detention

Dora Schriro

Independent Researcher, New York, NY 10464, USA; dora.schriro@gmail.com

Abstract: Immigration Detention is a patchwork of public and private correctional facilities overseen by ICE, a federal enforcement agency. In June 2021, ICE detained 16,460 adults in 121 facilities in 38 states, frequently alongside pretrial and sentenced inmates and U.S. Marshals Service prisoners, under varying conditions ICE established with five different sets of detention standards, all of them based on corrections case law and in effect today. Detainees have not fared well in ICE's custody, especially during the pandemic. In CY2020, ICE processed 137,749 detainees, tested only 80,200 for COVID-19 (58%), and recorded 8622 positive cases (11%) at over 100 facilities. Most testing positive for COVID-19—7687 (89%)—contracted the virus in ICE custody, including eight detainees who died. An additional 14,728 detainees (18%) had one or more conditions placing them at high risk for severe illness due to COVID-19 of which ICE only released 5801 (39%). This paper utilizes ICE data and documents on government websites to evaluate ICE's approach to detention management and explore its impact on conditions of detention and how it impeded its readiness and response to the pandemic. It concludes with recommendations that ICE decrease reliance on detention and decriminalize its policies and practices.

Keywords: crimmigration; incarcergration; decriminalization; detention; detention standards; alternatives to detention; conditions of detention; coronavirus

Citation: Schriro, Dora. 2021. On the Other Side of the Looking Glass: COVID-19 Care in Immigration Detention. *Social Sciences* 10: 353. https://doi.org/10.3390/socsci10100353

Academic Editor: Robert Koulish

Received: 31 July 2021
Accepted: 17 September 2021
Published: 23 September 2021

Publisher's Note: MDPI stays neutral with regard to jurisdictional claims in published maps and institutional affiliations.

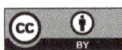

Copyright: © 2021 by the author. Licensee MDPI, Basel, Switzerland. This article is an open access article distributed under the terms and conditions of the Creative Commons Attribution (CC BY) license (https://creativecommons.org/licenses/by/4.0/).

1. Prologue

The Body Ritual among the Nacirema

The Body Ritual Among the Nacirema (Miner 1956) is an anthropological essay, a culture-free description of a man, a Nacirema, which is American spelled backwards. He is standing at the bathroom sink, looking at himself in the mirror while shaving. An observer from another time and place mistakes the mirrored medicine cabinet for a magical box in which many charms and potions are kept, and before which the man chants and sways every morning.

Before joining the U.S. Department of Homeland Security (DHS) to serve as Senior Advisor to DHS Secretary Napolitano on Detention and Removal, I was Warden of a city jail, then Commissioner of two city and two state correctional systems. As I toured the first of many immigration detention facilities operated on behalf of Immigration and Customs Enforcement (ICE), I walked through it as would a newly admitted detainee become acquainted with her place of confinement, starting at the sallyport, then Intake, through the medical area, to the housing units, a combination of 50-bed cellblocks and 100 bunks dormitories in which people were packed, nose to toes, under conditions as severe and secure as high-custody correctional facilities, locked-in as many as 23 h every day. I moved through segregation housing, still operating as it had when it was a prison, then food services, the laundry, law library, visitation, and commissary, onto the recreation yard. This detention center looked like a correctional facility in almost every respect and, initially, appeared to operate as one would (Goffman 1961) and, make no mistake, that would not be a good thing. Detainees surrendered all their personal property at admission along with any semblance of their personal identities; in exchange, each was issued a detention standards it uses and which are based on corrections case law. Detainees do not fare well in ICE's custody, particularly during the pandemic. In calendar year (CY) 2020, ICE processed 137,749 detainees, tested only 80,200 for COVID-19 (58%), and recorded 8622 positive cases (approximately 11%) at over 100 facilities nationwide, including eight detainees who died from the coronavirus while in ICE custody. Among those who tested positive for COVID-19, 7687 (89%) were exposed to the virus while in ICE custody. An additional 14,728 detainees (18%) had one or more conditions that placed them at high risk for severe illness due to COVID-19 of which, ICE released only 5801 high-risk individuals (39%) (GAO-21-414).

I believe ICE can do better. As a matter of law, it must. Immigration detainees are held pending *civil* proceedings in the immigration court. Their detention must not be punitive and their access to healthcare must meet the community standard. ICE has not met either of these requirements.

We are at a flex point. There is need to act, and there is opportunity to do so. One, the pandemic continues to threaten the public's health, particularly in areas of the country where vaccination rates remain low. ICE also reported low rates among detainees nationwide, regardless of the facilities' locations (Melugin 2021). This is not surprising given the state of its healthcare system. Two, the size of the detained population remains relatively low, but it has begun to rise again. Now is the time to eliminate as many beds as possible and change the nature of those that remain. Three, the new Administration is open to the idea of creating a civil, civil system of immigration enforcement.

This paper considers several of the ways in which ICE has misapplied corrections case law, policy and practices to the detriment of the detainees in its custody, particularly during the pandemic. It utilizes ICE data and documents on government websites to consider ICE's approach to detention management, how it has impacted conditions of detention, and impeded its readiness and response to the pandemic. It is recommended that reliance on Immigration Detention is decreased, that it is decriminalized, and ICE is held accountable for its activities and outcomes. In short, this is a brief look in that mirror, at ICE, the aggregated impact of crimmigration law on a quasi-punitive system of immcarceration, and us.

3. COVID-19 and the CDC's Standard of Care for Correctional and Detention Facilities

The U.S. Centers for Disease Control and Prevention (CDC) is the nation's health protection agency (CDC 2019). CDC Guidance is the community standard of healthcare for treating coronavirus, and the CDC Interim Guidance on Management of Coronavirus Disease 2019 (COVID-19) in Correctional and Detention Facilities (CDC Guidance) is the community standard for corrections and immigration detention (CDC 2020). Every detainee in ICE's custody has a right to receive this level of care.

On 11 March 2020, the World Health Organization declared the novel coronavirus (COVID-19) outbreak a global pandemic. On 23 March 2020, the CDC issued its initial CDC Guidance. The CDC has continued to tailor public health responses to coronavirus for incarcerated populations throughout the course of the pandemic.

Chief among its recommendations to prevent the spread of COVID-19 in incarceral settings, the CDC urged correctional and detention facilities to practice extreme social distancing, continual and correct use of personal protective equipment (PPE), and heightened sanitation and vigorous hygiene facility-wide, coupled with cohorting and screening for symptomatic individuals, testing of asymptomatic individuals, quarantine and contact tracing, and when it became available, vaccination. The CDC has never proposed however, that correctional and detention facilities release at-risk persons in their custody, deferring to the executive, legislative and judicial branches of city or county, state, and federal government to make those decisions. Some have been critical of its silence: Instead of centering on public health, it appeared to them that the CDC was preoccupied with the impact of such a recommendation on traditional enforcement priorities (Harvard Law Review 2021).

4. Civil Detention v. Criminal Incarceration

4.1. The Applicable Legal Standard for Immigration Detainees

Convicted prisoners are protected by the Eighth Amendment to the U.S. Constitution, and application to the states by the Fourteenth Amendment, which prohibits the infliction of cruel and unusual punishments on those persons. To establish a violation of the Eighth Amendment, a prisoner must show both a deprivation of a basic human need (Helling v. McKinney 1993) and deliberate indifference (Wilson v. Seiter 1991). In the context of medical or mental health care, she must demonstrate "deliberate indifference to serious medical needs (Estelle v. Gamble 1976).

Pretrial prisoners are protected by the Due Process Clauses of the Fifth and Fourteenth Amendments against any conditions that constitute "punishment (Bell v. Wolfish 1979)". They are afforded at least as much protection as are sentenced inmates regarding medical care (City of Revere v. Massachusetts General Hospital 1983). Deliberate indifference of correctional officials to the serious medical needs of a pretrial prisoner is a violation of her due process.

Immigration detainees are civil detainees held pursuant to civil immigration laws. Their protections are also derived from the Fifth Amendment, shielding persons in the custody of the United States from conditions that amount to punishment (Wong Wing v. United States 1896). ICE may detain non-citizens during the removal process (Fong Yue Ting v. United States 1893) but, because immigration detention is not punishment, its detention must not be excessive in relation to ICE's noncriminal purposes (Zadvydas v. Davis 2001). To do so is improperly punitive, thus unconstitutional (United States v. Solano 1987). Immigration detainees must be afforded the same (Edwards v. Johnson 2000) or superior (Jones v. Blanas 2004, Youngberg v. Romeo 1982) level of protection as are pre-trial prisoners.

4.2. Crimmigration Law and the Quasi-Punitive System of Immaceration

Our blurring of criminal enforcement and immigration control has given rise to a system of crimmigration law. Similarly, our treatment of civilly detained people in immigration proceedings as if they are criminally charged, using criminal incarceration for the purpose of immigration detention, serves to validate public perception and fortify public acceptance of excessive immigration practices, giving way to the quasi-punitive system of immcarceration, with which we grapple today: a random collection of correctional practices with many of its punitive characteristics, unsubstantiated beliefs about deterrence, and none of its due process protections. Preventive justice is neither preventive nor just (Cole 2014). Many detainees seek asylum. Others seek reunification with family members who preceded them. In most cases, migrants are certain that they have no choice but to immigrate, the conditions in the counties of their origin are so detrimental that they are compelled to make the harrowing trip to our borders and surrender themselves thus initiate the process of lawful entry. Their fear for survival has also become ours. Xenophobia informs our policies and procedures and over time, immigration detention has become a deprivation as severe as removal itself (Kalhan 2010).

Immigration enforcement also lacks the criminal justice system's checks and balances, measured practices upon which the disenfranchised depend. Whereas there is considerable discretion distributed across decision-makers in the criminal justice system from the arresting officer, prosecuting attorney, bail bondsman, pre-trial services, and arraignment and trial courts at the front-end to pre-release services, victim advocates, and parole board at the back-end, detain or release decision-making is concentrated primarily within DHS, and controlled largely by Customs and Border Patrol (CBP) and ICE; the focus of their activities along the northern and southern borders, and the interior, respectively. CBP and ICE also regulate the conditions of confinement in CBP patrol stations and ICE detention facilities and operate their respective holding and detention facilities. As CBP and ICE, both immigration enforcement agencies, prefer removal to relief, and detention is an expedited means to that end, one that only they control, they exercise control with impunity. Only the

U.S. Citizenship and Immigration Services (USCIS) within DHS, its charge to adjudicate non-citizens requests for immigration benefits, or the Executive Office for Immigration Review (EOIR) within the U.S. Department of Justice (DOJ), the nation's immigration court system, can change the outcome of immigration cases. Given the disparity in the size, staffing, and status of each of these agencies, it does not happen as often as it should.

In many cases, detention is also mandatory as a matter of law. Mandatory Detention refers to provisions of the Immigration and Nationality Act (INA), § 236(c) and § 235(b), which state non-citizens with certain criminal convictions are not entitled to a bond hearing, they must be detained by ICE, and shall remain detained while removal proceedings are pending against them. As indicated in Table 1, on 14 June 2021, there were 16,460 people in ICE's custody of which, 11,570 (70%) were mandatorily detained although 9510 (58%) had no criminal convictions.[1] ICE refers to this group as "No ICE Threat Level (ICE 2021a). These changes to the INA were made in the 1990's, the same period of time in which Truth-in-Sentencing, Three Strikes, and Juvenile Justice "reforms" were enacted, many of those provisions since reversed. I think it would be worthwhile to reconsider the validity of the assumptions that brought about these amendments as well as beginning with a review of the 28% of detainees who had no convictions and were mandatorily detained nonetheless.[2]

Table 1. Average Daily Threat Level (ICE 2021b).

Facility	ICE Threat Level[1]				ADP Total, all Threat Levels[2]	Mandatory Detention
	Level 1 High Risk	Level 2 Medium Risk	Level 3 Low Risk	No ICE Threat Level No Risk		
TOTALS	4138 (25%)	1460 (9%)	1352 (8%)	9510 (58%)	16,460 (100%)	11,570 (70%)

It is clear that ICE has taken other measures to keep people detained. One notable example is ICE's revision of its Custody Classification detention standard. As developed by the Immigration and Naturalization Services (INS), it was an objective process, an assessment based on facts—whereby an opinion, even informed opinion (based on profiling, familiarity, personal experience, etc.) is different from fact, therefore irrelevant for detainee classification (ICE 2002b)—to a subjective process where "discernable" facts—such as nothing more than a tattoo to establish gang membership—as are acceptable (ICE 2019b). ICE also repeatedly adjusted its risk assessment instrument's algorithm, continually modifying it to raise the custody scores of as many detainees as possible to avoid releasing them (Koulish 2016). When that still did not eliminate as many detainees as ICE believed should remain in custody, ICE revised its already limited range of recommendations in 2018, striking all but one outcome regardless of the detainees' risk score: Detain (Rosenberg and Levinson 2018).

In FFY2019, pre-pandemic (ICE 2019d), ICE's average daily detained population (ADP) reached 50,165 detainees. In FFY2020, mid-pandemic (ICE 2020a), after enforcement activities had been scaled back considerably, the ADP dropped to 19,068 detainees (<62%). ICE's ADP began to rebound and by June 2021, rose to 26,222 detainees (>28%) by mid-June in FFY2021 (ICE 2021a), with the expectation its ADP would continue to increase unless there was a marked change in enforcement policy.

In fact, the pandemic brought about a significant shift in both federal policy and state and local practice. A change in federal public health policy altered CBP's apprehensions of migrants. Another in the courts and correctional systems impacted ICE's arrests. Together, they account for most of the precipitous drop in "book-ins," the combined annual totals of CBP apprehensions and ICE arrests, from 510,854 migrants in FFY 2019 to 182,869 in FFY2020 (<36%) (U.S. ICE 2021).

At the federal level of government, the prior Administration utilized sections 362 and 365 of the Public Health Service Act, 42 U.S.C. §§ 265 and 268, to suspend "the introduction of persons into the United States" beginning in March 2020, purportedly to prevent the introduction of COVID-19 into the country. Named the Migrant Protection Protocols (MPP) but better known as the "Remain in Mexico Policy," its impact was immediate. Pursuant to MPP, most migrants along the southwest border, many of whom sought asylum, must remain in Mexico, currently a year or more, until such time as they are called to appear in immigration court. In August 2021, over 70,000 people seeking asylum were waiting for a date to be heard (Morrissey 2021). Immediately upon taking office in January 2021, the current Administration reversed the MMP. The states of Texas and Missouri sued, seeking its reinstatement, and they prevailed in the federal district court. The Administration petitioned the U.S. Supreme Court to grant a stay, and in August 2021, the Court denied its application (Biden et al. v. Texas et al. 2021) thereby keeping in place MMP for now.

At the state and local levels of government, both the courts were clearing their confined criminal dockets and correctional systems were reducing their jail and prison populations, especially of medical vulnerable individuals, through various release mechanisms. With fewer inmates remanded to correctional facilities, there were also fewer individuals to turn over to ICE and a number of them both pre-trial or pre-plea and sentenced were medically vulnerable. Transferring at-risk individuals, especially those who had neither plead nor proven guilty, from one authority to another was contra-indicated by the Court and the CDC. Nevertheless, ICE continued to take them into their custody upon their release from the criminal justice system although many of them would be released to its ATD program.

It made a measurable difference. In FY 2019, ICE monitored 83,186 adult ATD participants (ICE 2019d); in FY2020, 85,415 adults (>3%) (ICE 2020a); and in FY2021 TD, 103,933 adults (>18%) (ICE 2021a).

Notwithstanding the appreciable decrease in book-ins through the course of the pandemic, COVID-19 more than doubled the time that migrants remain in its custody and under its supervision. Pre-pandemic, delays in the immigration court's detained and non-detained dockets were considerable. Coronavirus compounded both backlogs. The average length of stay (ALOS) in detention rose from 34 days in FY2019 (ICE 2019d), to 63 days in FY2020 (>54%) (ICE 2020a), to 60 days in FY2021 TD (<5%) (2021a). The average length of time in an ATD program (ALIP), was far worse, rising from 352 days in FY2019, (ICE 2019d) to 816 days in FY2020 (>57%) (ICE 2020a), to 788 days in FY2021 TD (<4%) (ICE 2021a).

5. The Immcarceration of Immigration Detention

The shift in immigration policy from "Catch and Release" to "Catch and Remove" in 2005, left ICE scrambling for additional beds to detain the burgeoning non-criminal population. At the ready were thousands of public and private prison beds that had been built the decade before to accommodate the growth in the inmate population brought about by state and federal sentencing initiatives in the 1990's.

ICE acquired many of these beds and did so without the benefit of population forecasting, multi-year capital construction plans, a scope of work with clear selection criteria and agency-specific operating assumptions, or competitive bidding, all of which are widely recognized management tools. Instead, it did what was expedient to meet its mandate: it got those beds by various means to deter and detain. In 2009, when I conducted the nationwide review of immigration detention at the direction of DHS Secretary Napolitano (Schriro 2009), ICE had secured space in over 300 jails and prisons to house as many as 31,000 adults daily, facilities still staffed by correctional personnel, and operating as correctional facilities with all its policies and procedures—counts, controlled movement, searches, shakedowns, and the like—intact. To this, ICE only added the requirement that all facilities housing an average of ten or more detainees would also comply with its detention standards.

ACA Adult Local Detention Correctional Standards v. ICE Immigration Detention Standards

In September 2000, the Immigration and Naturalization Services (INS), consisting of USCIS, CBP and ICE, each of which would become stand-alone agencies within DHS in 2002, promulgated the first detention standards for facilities housing immigration detainees. The INS selected the American Correctional Association (ACA) standards for adult local detention facilities (ALDF), based upon corrections case law for pretrial and locally sentenced prisoners,[3] as the prototype for its 2000 National Detention Standards (NDS) (ACA 2004, 2016). The INS intended detention standards to establish consistent conditions of confinement, program operations, and management expectations within its detention system. Although that was INS' intent, the 2000 NDS made allowances for non-dedicated facilities, merely encouraging them to consider those procedures useful as guidelines, (ICE 2002a). When ICE was formed in 2002, the agency continued to operate immigration detention utilizing the 2000 NDS.

In 2004, the ACA transitioned to performance-based detention standards, and in 2008 ICE published the first of several sets of performance-based National Detention Standards (PBNDS), replicating those of the ACA. As had the ACA, ICE incorporated expected outcomes for each standard and expected practices required to achieve them so as "to improve safety, security, and conditions of confinement for detainees (ICE 2008a)".

In 2011, ICE revised the 2008 performance-based detention standards, incorporating changes made following the release of the 2009 Schriro Report (Schriro 2009) and to address outstanding recommendations. ICE said of the 2011 PBNDS standards, "It represents an important step in detention reform (ICE 2011a)".

In 2016, ICE revised the 2011 detention standards "to ensure consistency with federal legal and regulatory requirements as well as prior ICE policies and policy statements," incorporating provisions of the Prisoner Rape Elimination Act (PREA) and Section 504 of the Rehabilitation Act prohibiting discrimination on the basis of disability, as well as changes to the operation of Special Management Units, expansion of language services, and other ICE and ERO Directives, Memoranda and Policy Statements (ICE 2016a).

In 2019, ICE issued National Detention Standards (NDS) for Non-Dedicated Facilities. Non-dedicated facilities house one or more other populations typically, inmates, often from more than one jurisdiction, occasionally military prisoners, and increasingly U.S. Marshals Service (USMS) prisoners, federal inmates in the temporary custody of the USMS during transport and for criminal court appearances, in addition to detainees, and usually outnumbering them. ICE intended the 2019 NDS would provide the necessary guidance for approximately 45 facilities it had acquired by means of intergovernmental service agreements (IGSA) and had been operating already under the 2000 NDS, approximately 35 USMS facilities that ICE used and inspected against the 2000 NDS, plus approximately 60 facilities (both IGSA and USMS) which did not reach the threshold for ICE annual inspections—generally, those with an average daily population (ADP) of less than 10 detainees (ICE 2019a).

The NDS 2019 represented ICE's most significant departure from any of the preceding detention standards, and in my opinion, has created the most inconsistent conditions under which detainees are held today. In addition to the deference in treatment that INS had introduced in 2000, ICE eliminated 11 of 44 standards, a measure it minimized as merely a "consolidation", but in its place, ICE granted all those providers considerably more latitude in the operation of their facilities, particularly regarding healthcare, the clear consequence of which is even greater disparity in conditions of detention and far fewer protections for detainees in non-dedicated facilities than for those in dedicated facilities. ICE is not concerned, "These are facilities across the country where ICE's state and local law enforcement partners successfully manage their own [criminal] populations under federal, state, and local regulations (ICE 2019a)". Even if this were true, which I do not believe to be the case, applying correctional practices and then superimposing local healthcare policy on many of the facilities that are a part of a national system of immigration detention fails to protect civilly held people who are entitled to more as a matter of law.

As described by ICE, it appeared that the agency intended the 2011 (rev. 2016) PBNDS would replace the 2008 and 2011 Performance-Based National Detention Standards and that the 2019 NDS would replace the 2000 National Detention Standards; however, as indicated in Table 2 that has not been the case. Instead, ICE renamed the 2000 NDS, the 2000 NDS for Non-Dedicated Facilities and continues to use it although other than the change in its name, it has not been revised since its 2000 release. Similarly, the 2008 PBNDS and 2011 PBNDS are still in use, as they were originally released. In mid-June 2021, there were 38 dedicated and 84 non-dedicated adult detention facilities in use. Not all dedicated facilities were assigned performance-based detention standards, 36 were and 2 were not. Not all non-dedicated facilities were assigned national detention standards, 63 were and 21 were not.

Table 2. Adult Detention Facilities by Type and Assigned Detention Standards (ICE 2021b).

Type ICE Adult Facility	NDS 2000	NDS 2019	PBNDS 2008	PBNDS 2011	PBNDS 2011 (rev. 2016)	Totals
Dedicated (ICE only) Detention Facilities						
CDF				3	11	14
SPC					5	5
DIGSA		2		2	15	19
Subtotals		2		5	31	38
Non-dedicated (shared use) Detention Facilities						
IGSA	11	19	7	5	5	47
USMS CDF		1	1			2
USMS IGA	27	5	3			35
BOP						0
Subtotals	38	25	11	5	5	84
Totals	38	27	11	10	36	122

ICE occupied 122 facilities on 14 June 2021, of which 38 were dedicated and 84 were non-dedicated or shared use.

It is not unusual for an organization or professional association to promulgate more than one set of standards, when each set is tailored to a specific population to meet their unique needs. ICE understands this. ICE issued detention standards specifically for Family Residential Facilities in 2007 for that reason, and updated it in 2020, replacing one with other (ICE FRS 2020).

However, unlike the ACA and other professional organizations that replace older standards with newer ones when revised, ICE has kept the old and added each new set, assigning each facility one version or another. Now, ICE has five different sets, and all of them are still in use. More than confusing, it is unconscionable to detain the same population under appreciably different conditions, more so in order to qualify more facilities to house detainees, which is what ICE has done. Today, ICE assigns adult detainees to facilities operating under *five* different sets of expectations—2000 NDS, 2008 PBNDS, 2011 PBNDS, 2011 PBNDS (rev. 2016), *and* 2019 NDS—to maximize its bed capacity.

6. Government Oversight

Everyone is assured equal protection under the law. ICE's questionable use of detention standards, compounded by its inability to secure the facility operators' compliance with those standards, have been repeatedly scrutinized by the Government Accountability Office (GAO) and DHS Office of Inspector General (OIG), both of which are charged with oversight of federal agencies and focus on efficiency and integrity on behalf of the legislative and executive branches, respectively. To date, ICE appears to be neither deterred nor dissuaded.

In 2014, the GAO evaluated the three sets of detention standards that ICE had at that time and concluded employing more than one set of standards impeded ICE's ability to operate a uniformly effective and efficient system (GAO 2014). ICE disregarded its advice. In 2016, the GAO determined similar practices impeded IHSC's efforts to collect information about on-site and off-site health care services and assess utilization (GAO 2016a). Again, ICE disregarded its advice. Also in 2016, the GAO addressed ICE's inability to utilize the correct version of each set of detention standards—the abbreviated version for under "72-h" facilities or the complete version for "over 72-h" facilities (GAO 2016b). ICE disregarded its advice.

In 2018, the DHS OIG concluded ICE's methods for monitoring facilities' compliance with their respective detention standards had failed and many of the deficiencies that it had identified were longstanding (OIG 2018). In 2019, the OIG probed further and found just 28 of the 106 contracts that it reviewed, approximately half of ICE's 206 contracts for beds at that time, included the Quality Assurance Surveillance Plan (QASP), a provision enabling ICE to impose financial penalties to ensure facilities met performance standards. The OIG determined where there was a QASP in place, ICE had imposed financial penalties on only two occasions despite numerous documented instances of facilities' failures to comply with detention standards. Instead, ICE issued waivers, exempting facilities with deficient conditions from complying with certain standards. The OIG discovered ICE also failed to issue written instruction to govern the waiver process, thereby enabling staff to continue to grant waivers without clear authority to do so (OIG 2019).

6.1. ICE's Oversight

The GAO and DHS OIG reports illustrate another reason that ICE should have just one set of detention standards—one set comprised solely of evidence-based practices—and it is this. ICE is unable to get most of the facilities it uses to comply with one set of standards; it is at least five times as unlikely that it will ever achieve compliance when there are five different sets of expectations in the field. There are several reasons why this is the case.

First, ICE's standards for acceptable and unacceptable performance (ICE 2021a) do not adequately address conditions that detainees encounter. Both acceptable and unacceptable are highly subjective terms. Not all deficiencies are equal. Frequency and severity vary—and no objective benchmarks are provided.

Additionally, ICE monitors detention facilities by several means. It assigns on-site agency monitors to its largest facilities. Independent reviews and fairly thorough inspections are also conducted at some facilities every several years by the Office of Detention Oversight, an independent office within ICE but outside of ERO. ICE also contracts with the Nakamoto Group Inc. to inspect most facilities annually. Those inspections were suspended through much of 2020 due to the pandemic then resumed remotely. Both oversight agencies and Congressional committees have been critical of ICE's contract management including its continued use of Nakamoto, and its inability to achieve better results over time. Chief among their concerns, no matter how poorly facilities perform, both the on-site agency monitors and the Nakamoto Group report that they Meet Standards. The GAO and OIG have also issued reports about ICE's failed oversight of detention operators, the most recent of which were published by the DHS OIG in June 2018 (OIG 2018), and the GAO in August 2020 (GAO 2020).

6.2. ICE Detention Today

Mid FFY2021, ICE had agreements to house adult detainees in 131 facilities in 38 states of which, 122 were in use. They are 38 dedicated detention centers housing ICE detainees only, and include five Service Processing Centers (SPCs),[4] 19 dedicated Intergovernmental Service Agreement (DIGSA) facilities,[5] and 14 Contract Detention Facilities (CDF),[6] all of which are supposed to comply with ICE Performance-based National Detention Standards (PBNDS). The remaining 84 facilities are non-dedicated, housing detainees, inmates and other prisoners, and include 47 Intergovernmental Service Agreement (IGSAs),[7] 35 U.S. Marshals Service Intergovernmental Agreements (USMS IGAs),[8] and two U.S. Marshals Service Contract Detention Facilities (USMS CDFs).[9] No detainees were assigned to a DOJ Bureau of Prison (BOP) facility at that time.[10] Most of these facilities are supposed to comply with ICE's National Detention Standards. The USMS agreed to adopt the 2019 NDS at USMS CDF facilities but not at USMS IGA facilities; instead, ICE agreed to utilize the USMS contracts already in place with those providers. ICE also agreed to accept BOP standards when using its facilities.

Although dedicated detention facilities are supposed to comply with PBNDS detention standards and non-dedicated detention facilities, NDS detention standards, it does not always work out that way. Just these several detention practices—civilly held immigration detainees many of them comingled with criminally charged and convicted inmates, in over 100 correctional facilities, operating under five different sets of expectations, all of them based upon corrections policy and practice, in conditions more restrictive than many pre-trial prisoners are exposed—illustrate how insidious incarceration can be.

Currently, there is some discussion "on the Hill" about moving away from privately owned and operated correctional facilities altogether and using only those that are publicly owned and operated. Numerous studies by Congress and the White House have concluded most of the detention facilities that ICE uses are chronically deficient. Advocates point out, public or private, they are still correctional facilities, staffed with correctional personnel, operating pursuant to correctional detention standards, holding detainees in conditions as punitive as those in jails and prisons, perpetuating the belief that detainees are dangerous and should be punished. Some imagine readily available, non-secure settings appropriate for most civilly-held individuals, conveying the civil nature of their proceedings, the contributions they made already before their arrival, and their suitability to be our neighbors (Schriro 2009).

7. Detainee Healthcare: The Right to Receive Treatment

The case law is clear. Adequate healthcare is a fundamental right of the detained (Estelle v. Gamble 1976), and it cannot be conditioned upon the facility to which detainees are assigned (Cuoco v. Moritsugu 2000).[11] ICE must provide detainees with the actual care necessary to treat their medical conditions at every facility (Rosemarie M. v. Morton 2009). This can only occur when one clear set of expectations consistent with the corresponding case law is uniformly executed nationwide.

The overall responsibility for detainee healthcare rests with the Immigration Health Service Corps (IHSC) within Enforcement and Removal Operations (ERO). The IHSC serves as the medical authority for detainee healthcare issues, establishes the formulary, and oversees the financial authorization and payment for off-site specialty and emergency care services. The IHSC is also the healthcare provider at approximately half of 38 to 40 dedicated detention facilities and provides medical case management and oversight of the medical care administered by 84 non-IHSC providers at the other facilities (ICE IHSC 2021). Unlike correctional healthcare however, which is premised on the community standard of care, the IHSC deviates in its delivery, conditioning care on cost containment and anticipated time to removal or release, all too often delaying or denying care. Frequently occurring examples of IHSC's questionable decision-making include denials of corrective lenses and hearing aids to address vision and hearing impairments, dental cleanings within the first six months at a facility, and dental treatment for cavities—instead, detainees are redirected to the commissary to purchase "cheaters" regardless of their vision problem, and teeth requiring attention are extracted; cavities are not filled. Most physical ailments are treated with ibuprofen, and some mental health symptoms as well; there are no clinical services.

Although ICE's healthcare policy is established by IHSC, independently of ICE, IHSC is not responsible for healthcare outcomes. Instead, the delivery of detainee healthcare, and ultimately, detainees' health and safety, are the responsibility of each detention facility with which ICE contracts in accordance with that agreement which specifies in part, its assigned detention standards. This is an especially impactful provision at all the non-dedicated facilities where the state or local health department determines what is medically necessary.

7.1. Performance-Based National Detention Standards (PBNDS) for Dedicated Facilities

2008 PBNDS, 22 Medical Care, states, "All detainees shall have access to emergent, urgent, and non-emergent medical, dental, and mental health care within the scope of services provided by the Division of Immigration Health Services (ICE 2008c)".

2011 PBNDS, 4.3 Medical Care, states, "All detainees shall have access to appropriate and necessary medical, dental, and mental health care, including emergency services (ICE 2011c)".

2011 PBNDS (rev. 2016), 4.3 Medical Care, also provides, "All detainees shall have access to appropriate and necessary medical, dental, and mental health care, including emergency services (ICE 2016c)".

7.2. National Detention Standards for Non-Dedicated Facilities

2000 NDS, Medical Care, states, "All detainees shall have access to medical services that promote detainee health and general well-being (ICE 2002c)".

2019 NDS, 4.3 Medical Care, Policy, states, "All detainees shall have access to appropriate medical, dental, and mental health care, including emergency services (ICE 2019c)".

The inconsistencies in expectations and service delivery were especially apparent during the pandemic.

7.3. Pandemic Planning and Preparation

Pandemic planning and preparation are not new and there is no question as to its necessity. Over the course of DHS' 20-year history, the federal government has responded to the Severe Acute Respiratory Syndrome (SARS) between 2002 and 2004, H1N1 in 2009, Middle East Respiratory Syndrome (MERS) in 2012, Ebola between 2014 and 2016, Zika between 2015 and 2016, and the Coronavirus (COVID-19) since 2019 (Council on Foreign Relations 2021). Despite the continual threat each outbreak presents systemwide, ICE's Medical Care Detention Standards vary considerably in their responses to infectious disease and infection control.

7.4. Performance-Based National Detention Standards (PBNDS) for Dedicated Facilities

PBNDS 2008, PBNDS 2011, and PBNDS 2011 (rev. 2016) Detention Standard Medical Care considered Communicable Disease and Infection Control at length, and provide detailed instructions to identify and address tuberculosis, significant communicable diseases (the most commonly occurring, chicken pox, measles, mumps, whooping cough, and typhoid), and blood-borne pathogens (notably, hepatitis and HIV).

7.5. National Detention Standards for Non-Dedicated Facilities

NDS 2000 and 2019 NDS Detention Standards Medical Care are far narrower in their consideration of communicable diseases, contemplating just the identification of tuberculosis and only during the intake screening, although NDS 2019 is also the only Medical Care standard to reference CDC guidelines, including CDC Guidelines for Correctional Facilities, in its screening requirements for TB.

NDS 2000 also dedicated a section to HIV/AIDS, the only standard to address operational issues associated with HIV/AIDS when it was published. Although NDS 2000 is still in use, it has never been updated and this section is outdated and should be revised or removed.

Regarding the treatment all other Infectious and Communicable Diseases, both NDS 2000 and 2019 are quite terse. NDS 2000 states in its entirety, "[d]etainees diagnosed with a communicable disease shall be isolated according to local medical operating procedures". NDS 2019 directs, "[t]he facility will have written plans that address the management of infectious and communicable diseases, including testing, isolation, prevention, and education. This also includes reporting and collaboration with local or state health departments in accordance with state and local laws and recommendations". It is up to the state or local health department to determine what this is.

ICE's decision that non-dedicated facilities are governed by state or local law is consequential when trying to assess the impact of COVID-19 on detainees in those facilities: in keeping with NDS 2000 and NDS 2019, each facility shall report positive test results—and deaths attributed to the coronavirus—according to that jurisdiction's policy or practice. As of June 2021, ICE reported detention facilities had administered 219,547 COVID-19 tests to detainees of which, 18,797 tests were positive for the coronavirus (8.5%) including nine patients known to have died and 851 patients currently in ICE custody, (ICE 2021b), a considerable number at a time that the percent of infected people in the community was at its lowest value in over a year (CDC 2021b). Studies show the actual number of COVID-19 detainee deaths nationwide may be as much as 5.5 times greater than reported by ICE due to jurisdictional differences in testing and reporting practices (Dolovich 2021).

8. ICE's Adaptation of CDC Interim Guidance on Management of Coronavirus Disease 2019 in Correctional and Detention Facilities

IHSC issued ICE's initial instructions to the field (ICE IHSC 2020). Thereafter, ERO released an Action Plan (ICE ERO 2020f) and then, Pandemic Response Requirements (PRR) (ICE ERO 2020a), to implement the CDC Interim Guidance (CDC 2020). ICE's earliest releases are especially revealing as to the dichotomy that differing detention standards created.

Interim Reference Sheet on 2019-Novel Coronavirus (COVID-19), Version 6.0. The first Interim Reference Sheet to be made available to the public is Version 6.0, on 6 March 2020, concerning CDC's expanded testing to include a wider group of symptomatic detainees ICE. IHSC's Sheet directed facility providers use their judgement to determine whether patients should be tested. It also "strongly encouraged" them to test for other causes of respiratory illness such as influenza (ICE IHSC 2020).

Coronavirus Disease 2019 (COVID-19) Action Plan, Revision 1. The next publicly available document and ERO's first release is its COVID-19 Action Plan, Revision 1, dated 27 March 2020 (ICE ERO 2020f). It was ICE's most comprehensive effort to date to mitigate risk of infection and transmission among detainees and staff but applied *only* to IHSC-staffed and non-IHSC-staffed, ICE-dedicated facilities.

Intergovernmental partners and non-dedicated facilities were instructed to take their directions from their local, state, tribal, territorial, and federal public health authorities, although it recommended that they consider the dedicated facilities' instructions as "best practices". It was one of the earliest and clearest demarcations in ICE's expectations for the field's response to COVID-19: Dedicated facilities must comply, non-dedicated facilities may. In fact, few did.

COVID-19 Pandemic Response Requirements. ERO released COVID-19 Pandemic Response Requirements (PRR), Version 1, on 10 April 2010 (ICE ERO 2020a), the first of six, addressing an agency-wide healthcare crisis with some requirements for dedicated detention facilities, and others for non-dedicated facilities, and a statement of sorts for all facilities.

In June 2020, PRR Version 2 attempted to address the considerable confusion—and criticism—that its facility-specific approach to a nationwide threat had generated, now insisting ERO's PRR establishes mandatory requirements, as well as best practices, for *all* its detention facilities in response to COVID-19 (ICE ERO 2020b). The DHS Office of Inspector General (OIG) disagreed with ICE's assertion that it had issued universal expectations for all facilities in its in June 2020 report about detention facilities' early experiences with COVID-19), reiterating ICE had provided guidance regarding COVID-19, but only dedicated detention facilities must comply (OIG 2020).

PRR Version 2 brought to light another disparity in ICE's detention management. Not all its agreements with facility operators contained compliance measures, and where there were provisions, they varied by contract in their consequences, and others had no provisions for penalties. Specific to the pandemic, differences in the facilities' provisions to impose sanctions for non-compliance with the PRR varied considerably and none of the dedicated facilities without a certain mechanism, a quality-assurance surveillance plan (QASP), could be penalized (OIG 2020). In another report by the DHS OIG just the year before, and referenced above, it found only a few of the contracts it had reviewed included a QASP, and ICE had exercised this provision on only two occasions (OIG 2019).

PRR Version 3 issued in July 2020 (ICE ERO 2020c), PRR Version 4 issued in September 2020 (ICE ERO 2020d), PRR Version 5 issued in October 2020 (ICE ERO 2020e), and PRR Version 6 issued in March 2021 (ICE ERO 2021) continued to differentiate detention operators' responsibilities by facility type.

9. ICE's Pandemic Plan: Feedback from Federal Oversight Agencies

Both the GAO and the DHS OIG have released reports about ICE's readiness for and response to the pandemic.

Department of Homeland Security (DHS) Office of Inspector General. In April 2020, the DHS OIG surveyed 196 detention facilities in use at that time about their experiences and challenges managing COVID-19; 188 facility operators responded representing 31 dedicated and 157 non-dedicated facilities, of which only 18 dedicated facilities were IHSC-staffed. Overall, 93% (175) of the facilities reported they were prepared to handle COVID-19 (OIG 2020). Generally, respondents stated they had adequate supplies for detainees to mitigate the spread of COVID-19. Specifically, 89% (168) said they had enough masks for detainees who exhibited COVID-19 symptoms or tested positive for COVID-19. About 90% (170) of facilities reported having enough liquid soap for detainees but more than one-third (69) reported not having enough hand sanitizer for their use.

There were demonstrable differences however, in readiness by facility type. For example, 85% of dedicated facilities (26 of 31) had on-site testing capacity compared to 54% of non-dedicated facilities (84 of 157). The disparity and its impact are significant: The ability to test on-site frequently determines whether detainees are tested at all—77% (24 of 31) of dedicated facilities reported testing detainees for potential COVID-19, whereas only 20% (32 of 157) of non-dedicated facilities reported doing so (ICE 2020b).

Quite a few facilities also reported significant limitations due to their physical space, its configuration and size. Of note, 11% (21) did not have the capacity to quarantine or isolate detainees who exhibited suspected COVID-19 symptoms, 12% (23) could not quarantine or isolate a detainee who had tested positive for COVID-19; and 29% (55) did not have negative pressure ventilation rooms to isolate airborne infections. Another one-third (62) had only one or two negative pressure rooms in their facilities.

Again, survey results conveyed the disparity between dedicated and non-dedicated facilities. Every dedicated facility (31) reported being able to quarantine or isolate detainees with confirmed cases of COVID-19, whereas 15% (21 of 157) of non-dedicated facilities reported they could not, and all but one dedicated facility had negative pressure ventilation rooms while 34% (54 of 165) of non-dedicated facilities did not.

As mentioned in the previous section, the OIG also took note that ICE had provided guidance regarding COVID-19 to all the facilities, much of which was applicable only to dedicated facilities and facilities with IHSC staff, and non-dedicated facilities and those without IHSC staff—the majority—were not obligated to comply. The artificial line that ICE created as to facilities' accountability also affected its efforts to communicate effectively with the field. The OIG determined about 83% (156) of facilities had received COVID-19 guidance from ICE headquarters and 75% (141) had received guidance from IHSC. Responses regarding the receipt of guidance differed however, between dedicated and non-dedicated facilities. For example, every dedicated facility reported it had received guidance from ICE regarding COVID-19, whereas almost 20% (32) of non-dedicated facilities reported they had not. Similarly, all but one dedicated facility reported receiving IHSC guidance, while 27% (43) of non-dedicated facilities reported they did not. It is difficult for the non-dedicated facilities to consider information from ERO as best practices when they were not received.

In September 2021, the DHS OIG released its assessments of nine detention facilities' responses to COVID-19 (OIG 2021). The OIG conducted unannounced remote inspections in response to congressional requests for a more in-depth review than the year before to determine whether ICE effectively controlled COVID-19 and adequately safeguarded the health and safety of detainee and detention staff. The areas that the OIG considered included maintaining adequate supplies of personal protective equipment, enhanced cleaning, and proper screening for new detainees and staff. The OIG identified a number of areas where the facilities struggled to properly manage the health and safety of detainees. For example, they observed instances where staff and detainees did not consistently wear face masks or socially distance. They also noted that some facilities did not consistently manage sick calls and did not regularly communicate with detainees about their COVID-19 test results. Although the OIG found that ICE was able to decrease the detainee population to help mitigate the spread of COVID-19, information about their transfers was limited. Its staff also found that testing of both detainees and staff was insufficient, and that ICE headquarters generally did not provide effective oversight of the facilities during the pandemic. Overall, the OIG concluded, ICE must resolve these issues to ensure it can meet the challenges of the COVID-19 pandemic, as well as future pandemics.

The Government Accounting Office. In June 2021, the GAO released a report summarizing its examination of ICE's policies and procedures for responding to COVID-19 in the field and how they were implemented at six facilities; ICE's mechanisms for conducting oversight of COVID-19-related health and safety measures; and ICE's data on COVID-19 cases and identified high-risk health factors among detainees, between January 2020 and March 2021 (GAO 2021). The study had been requested by unspecified Congressional committees. GAO staff reviewed ICE documents and interviewed ICE officials at headquarters and select facility operators between May 2020 and June 2021 about initial ERO communication, interim guidance and policy documents, detainee intake screening and testing, the identification of high-risk detainees, quarantine and isolation, hygiene and PPE supplies, cleaning and disinfection, social distancing and education efforts, and visitation procedures. The report summarized the interviews and surveys upon which ERO relied to monitor facilities' COVID-19 activities remotely during the pandemic. The GAO staff did not consider detainee grievances, formulate opinions, or make any recommendations, as it often does.

10. Harm and Risk Mitigation

The purpose of a viable custody classification system is to ensure safety and security and contribute to orderly facility operations, by separating and managing detainees based on verifiable and documented data. A thorough screening by qualified personnel during the admissions process is also crucial for the identification of individuals for whom detention would be detrimental to their health and/or wellbeing therefore merit modification of the conditions of confinement, transfer to a suitable facility. Rarely are individuals considered for release, although policy does not prevent it.

In CY2020, ICE tested 80,200 of 137,749 detainees (58%) for COVID-19 and recorded 8622 positive cases (11%) at over 100 immigration detention facilities. Approximately, 30% (2566) of positive COVID-19 cases occurred at the 18 IHSC-staffed facilities whereas the remaining 70% (6056) of cases occurred at facilities operated by contract medical staff or the local health authority. Of the detainees who tested positive for COVID-19 in 2020, approximately 89% (7687) were exposed to the virus while in ICE custody, whereas 5% (435) were exposed before contact with ICE. Eight detainees died while in ICE custody as a result of COVID-19 (GAO-21-414). At least several more are believed to have died in 2020 shortly after their release or removal (Smart et al. 2021). The data strongly suggest adequate screening and testing for COVID-19, correct and consistent use of PPE, sufficient space for quarantine, and information and access to vaccination could have slowed the spread of COVID-19 and saved lives.

11. ICE Risk Assessment

The mission of the DOJ National Institute of Corrections (NIC) is to advance public safety by shaping and enhancing correctional policies and practices. The NIC created an objective classification system for the INS at its request to ensure every detainee is placed in the appropriate category of risk—low, medium–low, medium–high, or high—and physically separated from detainees in other custody levels in the least restrictive housing consistent with facility safety and security. To do so reduces lower custody detainees' exposure to any potential physical and psychological danger that higher custody detainees may pose (ICE 2002a). The risk assessment process in ICE's five Custody Classification detention standards is also used to ascertain detainees' suitability for release and the conditions, if any, that may be warranted to ensure their compliance with court appearances.

NDS 2000 Detention Standard Detainee Classification System (ICE 2002b) is the most comprehensive of the five standards. As written, custody staff *in consultation with* medical and mental health clinicians can consistently produce highly accurate assessments of risk and need for special housing.

PBNDS 2008 (ICE 2008b), PBNDS 2011 (ICE 2011b), and PBNDS 2011 (rev. 2016) (ICE 2016b) Detention Standard 2.2 Custody Classification lack some of its specificity however there is sufficient instruction that staff can accurately assess detainee risk. The primary difference between PBNDS 2008, 2011, and 2011 (rev. 2016) and NDS 2000 is that these three rely primarily on detention officers to assess the detainees thus there must be adequate training and continual oversight by healthcare personnel to achieve a good result.

Additionally, the NDS 2000, PBNDS 2008, PBNDS 2011, and PBNDS 2011 standards (rev. 2016) include a user's manual and assessment forms or worksheets to promote consistently reliable outcomes. NDS 2000 also includes a monitoring instrument, the Primary Assessment Form, to assess each facility's compliance with the policy.

NDS 2019 Standard Detainee Classification System (ICE 2019b) is by far the least likely to achieve a good result. It has few instructions and no worksheets or forms. Detention staff is expected to complete assessments without assistance or support. NDS 2000 with attachments is 33 pages whereas, NDS 2019 is just three pages. Sometimes size matters—this is one of those times. Since the advent of COVID-19, reliable risk assessments are more consequential than ever.

11.1. ICE Special Vulnerabilities and Management Concerns

The NIC recognized that some detainees have special vulnerabilities and/or management concerns and there also should be provision in the classification process for their identification to inform housing assignments and accommodate certain handicapping conditions.

NDS 2000 Detainee Classification System and PBNDS 2008 Classification System identified only several Special Management Concerns—psychological impairments, mental deficiency, substance abuse, and detainees with medical problems or physical impairments. PBNDS 2011 2.2 Custody Classification System, PBNDS 2011 (rev. 2016) Custody Classification System, and NDS 2019 Custody Classification recognized quite a few special vulnerabilities—the elderly, those who are pregnant or nursing; those with serious physical or mental illness, or other disabilities; those who would be susceptible to harm in general population related to their sexual orientation or gender identity; and victims of sexual assault, torture, trafficking, or abuse. Having reviewed hundreds of custody classification worksheets in numerous facilities over the past ten years however, I can attest most Intake Officers do not complete this section and I do not believe they have had the training to do so correctly if they were directed. That so few are completed, or completed correctly, also underscores the need for training and continual supervision.

11.2. Prosecutorial Discretion

As a matter of policy, ICE has always had prosecutorial discretion to release individuals with serious medical conditions and individuals who are vulnerable to medical harm. The release of individuals with special vulnerabilities from immigration detention is authorized under a range of statutory and regulatory provisions, notably INA §§ 212(d)(5), 235(b), 236, and 241, and 8 C.F.R. §§ 1.1(q), 212.5, 235.5, and 236.(b), and even individuals held under mandatory detention pursuant to INA §§ 236(c). As a matter of practice, ICE is usually unwilling to do so, even when ordered by the Court.

In 2000 when NDS 2000 was issued, there was no ATD program to which detainees with special vulnerabilities and certain management concerns could be referred. This is no longer the case. ICE has operated ATD programs since 2004 (ICE 2021d). In July 2021, ICE updated its policy on the arrest and detention of pregnant, postpartum, and nursing women (ICE 2021c). The new policy directs ICE and CBP to limit the arrest of pregnant and nursing women, and it establishes new guidelines on how to treat them if they are detained. It addresses only two of many at-risk categories of detainees identified by the CDC and the Court who are at risk of serious illness or death from the coronavirus unless released.

12. CDC Guidance, Underlying Medical Conditions Associated with High Risk for Severe COVID-19

The CDC identified a number of categories of people more likely to get severely ill from COVID-19 (CDC 2021a). With regard to adults, the CDC considered both at-risk adults of any age and older adults.

Adults of Any Age. Adults of any age with the following conditions can be more likely to get severely ill from COVID-19: cancer, chronic kidney disease, chronic lung diseases including COPD (chronic obstructive pulmonary disease), asthma (moderate-to-severe), interstitial lung disease, cystic fibrosis, and pulmonary hypertension, dementia or other neurological conditions, diabetes (type 1 or type 2), Down syndrome, heart conditions such as heart failure, coronary artery disease, cardiomyopathies or hypertension, HIV infection, immunocompromised state, liver disease, overweight and obesity, pregnancy, sickle cell disease or thalassemia, current and former smokers, recipients of a solid organ or blood stem cell transplant, stroke or cerebrovascular disease, and substance use disorders.

Older Adults. Older adults are more likely to get severely ill from COVID-19. More than 80% of COVID-19 deaths occur in people over age 65, and more than 95% of COVID-19 deaths occur in people older than 45. Additionally, people exposed to long-standing system health and social inequities including many racial and ethnic minority groups and people with disabilities are more likely to both get COVID-19 and have worse outcomes.

13. Fraihat Risk Factors

In March 2020, attorneys on behalf of Plaintiffs Fraihat et al., sought relief for detained people with certain risk factors including those who are older, pregnant, or who have underlying medical conditions and are at a heightened risk of serious illness, life-altering complications, and death from COVID-19 (Fraihat v. ICE 2020). Plaintiffs argued successfully that ICE's responses to COVID-19 and its inadequate healthcare system will not protect people with risk factors. In April 2020, the Court ordered ICE review for release every person in the class.

Since then, all immigration detention centers are required to evaluate every new admission within five days of admission, to identify the presence of factors that may place a detainee at higher risk for severe illness due to COVID-19-related risk factors or disabilities. Based on the *Fraihat* ruling and related CDC guidance, ERO's PRR now requires every facility identify all the detainees with these chronic health conditions—cancer, chronic kidney disease, chronic obstructive requires pulmonary disease, Down syndrome, weakened immune system, overweight and obesity, serious heart conditions, including heart failure, coronary artery disease and cardiomyopathies, sickle cell disease, type one and type two diabetes mellitus, asthma, cerebrovascular disease, cystic fibrosis, hypertension or high blood pressure, neurologic conditions, including dementia, liver disease, pulmonary fibrosis, smoking, and thalassemia (ICE ERO 2020b, 2020c, 2020d, 2020e, 2021).

According to ICE data, in CY2020 facility medical staff determined 14,728 detainees had one or more conditions that placed them at high risk for severe illness due to COVID-19 of which, ICE released 5801 detainees (39%) from custody, removed another 5432 high-risk detainees from the United States (37%), and continued to detain 3487 (24%) as of the end of CY2020 (GAO 2021).

ICE needs to do more, now. As of 30 March 2021, 528 high-risk detainees have tested positive for COVID-19 (GAO 2021). *Fraihat* demonstrates just how inadequate ICE's classification policy and practice are. Few, if any, of the detainees with conditions that placed them at high risk for severe illness due to COVID-19 were known to ICE, and it is unlikely that ICE would have exercised the discretion it already had to release any of them.

14. Is the Past Prologue? Summary, Conclusions, and Recommendations

ICE does not handle infectious and communicable diseases well. Every year, detention facilities encounter detainees with measles, mumps, and chicken pox, and the prospect of significant consequences for some. Nevertheless, with each outbreak, impacted facilities do the same things the same ways. They lock down entire housing units, and occasionally the entire building, even when a simple screening for prior infection and/or verification of inoculation is all that it needed to return many of those detainees to general population. Some lockdowns have been so large and lasted so long that court runs have been cancelled, attorney visits forfeited, and access to outdoor recreation, the legal orientation program, and the law library were suspended. These outbreaks, always addressed the same way, occur so often that what were once questionable practices are widely accepted now as best practices for handling infectious and communicable diseases. It should not come as a surprise then, when IHSC and ERO directed the field offices and detention facilities in early 2020 to review their communicable disease and infection control plans in anticipation of the pandemic, it only served to fortify bad practices already entrenched systemwide. They thought they knew everything that they would need to know: 'it will pass'.

Although all detainees are always in the custody of ICE, their access to personal protective equipment, sanitation and hygiene supplies, testing and vaccine, adequate conditions for quarantine, as well as routine and emergency healthcare is dependent upon the facilities to which ICE has assigned them; and, as was demonstrated with respect to access to test kits and kit processing—the ability to test increases the ability to identity and address infected detainees—facilities' access to essential supplies, staff and space also varies considerably, and to the detriment of the individuals for whom ICE is responsible.

ICE's failures to take measures to mitigate the harm to which detainees continue to be exposed, and the heightened danger to which ICE has exposed at-risk detainees throughout the pandemic, must be addressed.

These are several of the ways that measurable improvements can be realized.

One, ICE is a federal enforcement agency. ICE should ensure all its policies and practices comply with immigration case law, are uniform and uniformly enforced, and every person in its custody receives equal treatment.

Two, to that end, ICE should operate a unified system, a system with one set of standards expressing the highest expectations and a continuum of control ranging from no supervision to detention, the premise being most require little or no supervision.

Three, ICE should decriminalize its policies and procedures, its facilities and ATD programs. ICE should discontinue use of jails and prisons, especially non-dedicated facilities where detainees are collocated and comingled with correctional populations, as well as correctional supervision strategies and correctional policies and procedures to the greatest extent practicable, as quickly as practicable.

Four, decisions as to detainees' placement along the continuum of control should be based on objective assessments of risk and a thorough identification of vulnerabilities. ICE should retain expert assistance and revise its classification process and also, add instruments to identify vulnerable persons and accurately identify security risk groups and members.

Five, upon the revision of risks and needs assessments, all detainees should undergo reclassification and low risk and at-risk detainees reconsidered for release under the least restrictive means. Also, there always should be sufficient personnel qualified to assess risk and identify vulnerabilities and make timely referrals at all facilities.

Six, mandatory detention should reflect real risk, and "in the custody of" should be expanded to include alternatives-to-detention programs. ICE should conduct a review of detainees' custody classification files currently held under mandatory detention provisions to identify anyone who may be detained erroneously under its provisions and arrange for their release. Depending upon the outcome of the review, additional training of Intake staff, and revision of custody classification detention standard and/or the INA § 236(c) and § 235(b) may be required as well.

Seven, detainee healthcare should meet or exceed the community standard of care at every location. Detainees' access to healthcare should not be conditioned on county or state policy. Every facility that ICE uses to detain individual in its custody must also be capable of complying fully with CDC Guidance. It is essential that IHSC establishes a universal standard for detainee healthcare for all facilities.

Eight, IHSC should conduct an immediate review of every facility to determine what levels and kinds of healthcare and which handicapping conditions cannot be accommodated. ICE must ensure anyone who cannot be accommodated at their current location is relocated or released immediately.

Nine, ICE is better positioned to act in the event of a pandemic than any of the detention facilities with which it contracts or the communities in which those facilities are located. For planning purposes, ICE should assume responsibility for the nation's immigration detention system's pandemic preparedness and response. It must ensure all detainees have timely access to requisite supplies and equipment, space for medical treatment and isolation, medicine, medical personnel, all necessary components of routine and emergency medical services, all of the time and at every location.

Ten, every facility that ICE uses for detention should be capable of complying fully with ICE's current detention standards, and upon revision thereof, one set of detention standards that complies with the case law. When that occurs, ICE should discontinue the use of any facility or facility provider that cannot meet these requirements. Until then, ICE should not issue any variances but for temporary conditions that can be readily and timely resolved.

Funding: This research received no external funding.

Institutional Review Board Statement: Not applicable.

Informed Consent Statement: Not applicable.

Data Availability Statement: Data available in a publicly accessible repository that does not issue DOIs. Publicly available datasets were analyzed in this study. This data can be found at: https://www.ice.gov/doclib/detention/FY21-detentionstats.xlx, accessed on 21 September 2021.

Conflicts of Interest: The author declares no conflict of interest.

Notes

[1] Unless noted otherwise, all data is presented by U.S. Federal Fiscal Year (FFY), 1 October–30 September.
[2] ICE identified 28% more detainees subject to mandatory detention (70%) that it designated risk levels 1, 2, and 3 (42%).
[3] ICE determines the threat level by the criminality of a detainee, including the recency of the criminal behavior and its severity. A detainee may be graded on a scale of one to three with one being the highest severity. When a detainee has no criminal convictions, s/he shall be classified as "No ICE Threat Level".
[4] The average daily population (ADP) FFYTD on 14 June 2021, by ICE Threat Level.
[5] Typically, this population consists of pre-trial inmates and inmates sentenced in a state court to a year or less.
[6] The SPC (Service Processing Center) is a facility owned by the government and staffed by a combination of federal and contract employees.

7   The DIGSA (Dedicated Intergovernmental Service Agreement) is a publicly owned facility operated by state/local government(s), or private contractors, in which ICE contracts to use all bed space via a Dedicated Intergovernmental Service Agreement; or facilities used by ICE pursuant to Inter-governmental Service Agreements. Typically, the latter are operated by private contractors pursuant to their agreements with local governments.
8   The CDF (Contract Detention Facility) is owned and operated by a private company and contracts directly with ICE. A CDF houses only ICE detainees. Note: ICE no longer identifies the CDF on its website as one of the types of facilities it uses but lists 14 CDFs in its report.
9   The IGSA (Intergovernmental Service Agreement) is a publicly owned facility operated by state/local government(s), or private contractors, in which ICE contracts for bed space via an Intergovernmental Service Agreement; or local jails used by ICE pursuant to Inter-governmental Service Agreements, which house both ICE and non-ICE detainees, typically county prisoners awaiting trial or serving short sentences, but sometimes also USMS prisoners.
10 The USMS IGA (USMS Intergovernmental Agreement) is a facility where ICE agrees to utilize an already established US Marshals Service contract.
11 The USMS (United States Marshals Service) is a facility primarily contracted with the USMS for housing of USMS detainees, in which ICE contracts with the USMS for bed space.
12 The BOP (Federal Bureau of Prisons): a facility operated by the Federal Bureau of Prisons for federal inmates.
13 ICE must not disregard excessive risk to a detainee's health or safety at any facility.

References

Cases

Bell v. Wolfish, 441 U.S. 520, 535 (1979).
Biden, President of U.S.; et al. v. Texas; et al., 594 U.S. 21A21 (2021).
City of Revere v. Massachusetts General Hospital, 463 U.S. 239 (1983).
Cuoco v. Moritsugu, 222 F.3d. 99, 107 (2nd Cir., 2000).
Edwards v. Johnson, 209 F.3d 772, 778 (5th Cir. 2000).
Estelle v. Gamble, 429 U.S. 97, 104 (1976).
Fong Yue Ting v. United States, 149 U.S. 698, 728-30 (1893).
Fraihat et al. v. ICE et al., Case No. 19-cv-01546-JGB(SHKx), Mar. 24, 2020.
Helling v. McKinney, 509 U.S. 25, 31-32 (1993).
Jones v. Blanas, 393F. 3d. 918, 933-34, (9th Cir. 2004), cert denied, 546 U.S. 820 (2005).
Rosemarie M. v. Morton, 671 F. Supp. 2d 1311, 1313 (M.D. Fla. 2009).
United States v. Solano, 41 U.S. 739, 747 (1987).
Wilson v. Seiter, 501 U.S. 294, 303 (1991).
Wong Wing v. United States, 163 U.S. 228, 237-38 (1896).
Youngberg v. Romeo, 457 U.S. 307, 321-32, (1982).
Zadvydas v. Davis, 533 U.S. 678, 609 (2001).

Statutes

Immigration and Naturalization Act 8 CFR § 236(c) and § 235(b).
Public Health Service Act, 42 U.S.C. §§ 265 and 268.

American Correctional Association. 2004. *Performance-Based Standards for Adult Local Detention Facilities*, 4th ed. Alexandria: American Correctional Association. Available online: https://www.aca.org/ACA_Prod_IMIS/ACA_Member/Standards_and_Accreditation/StandardsInfo_Home.aspx?WebsiteKey=139f6b09-e150-4c56-9c66-284b92f21e51&hkey=7c1b31e5-95cf-4bde-b400-8b5bb32a2bad&New_ContentCollectionOrganizerCommon=2#New_ContentCollectionOrganizerCommon=2 (accessed on 1 July 2021).
American Correctional Association. 2016. Standards Supplement. Available online: https://www.aca.org/ACA_Prod_IMIS/ACA_Member/Standards_and_Accreditation/StandardsInfo_Home.aspx?WebsiteKey=139f6b09-e150-4c56-9c66-284b92f21e51&hkey=7c1b31e5-95cf-4bde-b400-8b5bb32a2bad&New_ContentCollectionOrganizerCommon=2#New_ContentCollectionOrganizerCommon=2 (accessed on 1 July 2021).
Anonymous. 2021. Chapter 4: Conditions of Confinement, COVID-19, and the CDC. *Harvard Law Review* 134: 2233–56. Available online: https://harvardlawreview.org/2021/04/conditions-of-confinement-covid-19-and-the-cdc/ (accessed on 12 April 2021).
Bowling, Ben, and Sophie Westenra. 2018. Theoretical Criminology, 'A really hostile environment', Adiaphorization, global policing and the crimmigration control system. *Sage Journal* 24: 163–83. [CrossRef]
Centers for Disease Control and Prevention. 2019. Mission. Available online: https://www.cdc.gov/about/organization/mission.htm (accessed on 13 May 2019).
Centers for Disease Control and Prevention. 2020. Interim Guidance on Management of Coronavirus Disease 2019 (COVID-19) in Correctional and Detention Facilities. Available online: https://www.cdc.gov/coronavirus/2019-ncov/community/correction-detention/guidance-correctional-detention.html (accessed on 23 March 2020).

Centers for Disease Control and Prevention. 2021a. COVID-19 Medical Conditions, Updated May 13. Available online: https://www.cdc.gov/coronavirus/2019-ncov/need-extra-precautions/people-with-medical-conditions.html (accessed on 13 May 2021).

Centers for Disease Control and Prevention. 2021b. COVID Data Tracker Weekly Review. July 23. Available online: https://www.cdc.gov/coronavirus/2019-ncov/covid-data/covidview/index.html (accessed on 23 July 2021).

Cole, David. 2014. *The Difference Prevention Makes: Regulating Preventive Justice*. Washington, DC: Georgetown University Law Center, Crim. L. & Phil. [CrossRef]

Council on Foreign Relations. 2021. Major Epidemics of the Modern Era, 1899–2021. Available online: https://www.cfr.org/timeline/major-epidemics-modern-era (accessed on 2 July 2021).

Dolovich, Sharon. 2021. COVID Behind Bars Data Project. UCLA COVID Behind Bars Data Project. Available online: https://uclacovidbehindbars.org (accessed on 8 July 2021).

Goffman, Erving. 1961. *On the Characteristics of Total Institutions in Asylums: Essays on the Social Situation of Mental Patients and other Inmates*. Garden City: Anchor Books.

Government Accountability Office. 2014. Immigration Detention, Additional Actions Needed to Strengthen Management and Oversight of Facility Costs and Standards. GAO-15-153. Available online: https://www.gao.gov/products/GAO-15-153 (accessed on 10 October 2014).

Government Accountability Office. 2016a. Immigration Detention, Additional Actions Needed to Strengthen Management and Oversight of Detainee Medical Care. GAO-16-231. Available online: https://www.gao.gov/assets/680/675484.pdf (accessed on 29 February 2016).

Government Accountability Office. 2016b. Immigration Detention, Additional Actions Needed to Strengthen DHS Management of Short-Term Holding Facilities. GAO-16-514. Available online: https://www.gao.gov/assets/680/677484.pdf (accessed on 26 May 2016).

Government Accountability Office. 2020. Immigration Detention: ICE Should Enhance Its Use of Facility Oversight Data and Management of Detainee Complaints. GAO-20-596. Available online: https://www.gao.gov/products/gao-20-596 (accessed on 19 August 2020).

Government Accountability Office. 2021. Immigration Detention, ICE Efforts to Address COVID-19 in Detention Facilities. GAO-21-414. Available online: https://www.gao.gov/assets/gao-21-414.pdf (accessed on 30 June 2021).

Immigration and Customs Enforcement. 2002a. 2000 National Detention Standards for Non-Dedicated Facilities. Available online: https://www.ice.gov/detain/detention-management/2000 (accessed on 11 February 2002).

Immigration and Customs Enforcement. 2002b. 2000 INS Detention Standard, Detainee Classification System. Available online: https://www.ice.gov/doclib/dro/detention-standards/pdf/classif.pdf (accessed on 11 February 2002).

Immigration and Customs Enforcement. 2002c. 2000 INS Detention Standard, Medical Care. Available online: https://www.ice.gov/doclib/dro/detention-standards/pdf/medical.pdf (accessed on 11 February 2002).

Immigration and Customs Enforcement. 2008a. 2008 Operations Manual ICE Performance-Based National Detention. Available online: https://www.ice.gov/detain/detention-management/2008 (accessed on 11 March 2021).

Immigration and Customs Enforcement. 2008b. 2008 Performance-Based National Detention Standard, ICE/DRO Detention Standard, Classification System. Available online: https://www.ice.gov/doclib/dro/detention-standards/pdf/classification_system.pdf (accessed on 11 March 2021).

Immigration and Customs Enforcement. 2008c. 2008 Performance-Based National Detention Standard, ICE/DRO Detention Standard, Medical Care. Available online: https://www.ice.gov/doclib/dro/detention-standards/pdf/medical_care.pdf (accessed on 11 March 2021).

Immigration and Customs Enforcement. 2011a. 2011 Operations Manual ICE Performance-Based National Detention Standards. Available online: https://www.ice.gov/detain/detention-management/2011 (accessed on 11 March 2021).

Immigration and Customs Enforcement. 2011b. 2011 Performance-Based National Detention Standard, 2.2 Custody Classification System. Available online: https://www.ice.gov/doclib/detention-standards/2011/2-2.pdf (accessed on 11 March 2021).

Immigration and Customs Enforcement. 2011c. 2011 Performance-Based National Detention Standard, 4.3 Medical Care. Available online: https://www.ice.gov/doclib/detention-standards/2011/4-3.pdf (accessed on 11 March 2021).

Immigration and Customs Enforcement. 2016a. 2011 Operations Manual ICE Performance-Based National Detention Standards (rev. 2016). Available online: https://www.ice.gov/detain/detention-management/2011 (accessed on 11 March 2021).

Immigration and Customs Enforcement. 2016b. 2011 Performance-Based National Detention Standard (rev. 2016), 2.2 Custody Classification System. Available online: https://www.ice.gov/doclib/detention-standards/2011/2-2.pdf (accessed on 11 March 2021).

Immigration and Customs Enforcement. 2016c. 2011 Performance-Based National Detention Standard (rev. 2016), 4.3 Medical Care. Available online: https://www.ice.gov/doclib/detention-standards/2011/4-3.pdf (accessed on 11 March 2021).

Immigration and Customs Enforcement. 2019a. 2019 National Detention Standards for Non-Dedicated Facilities. Available online: https://www.ice.gov/detain/detention-management/2019 (accessed on 11 March 2021).

Immigration and Customs Enforcement. 2019b. 2019 National Detention Standard, 2.2 Custody Classification System. Available online: https://www.ice.gov/doclib/detention-standards/2019/2_2.pdf (accessed on 11 March 2021).

Immigration and Customs Enforcement. 2019c. 2019 National Detention Standard, 4.3 Medical Care. Available online: https://www.ice.gov/doclib/detention-standards/2019/4_3.pdf (accessed on 11 March 2021).

Immigration and Customs Enforcement. 2019d. ICE Detention Statistics, Facilities Data, EOFY2019. Available online: https://www.ice.gov/doclib/detention/FY19-detentionstats.xlsx (accessed on 7 October 2019).

Immigration and Customs Enforcement. 2020a. ICE Detention Statistics, Facilities Data, EOFY2020. Available online: https://www.ice.gov/doclib/detention/FY20-detentionstats.xlsx (accessed on 30 September 2020).

Immigration and Customs Enforcement. 2020b. ICE ERO FY2020 Achievements. Available online: https://www.ice.gov/features/ERO-2020/feature (accessed on 1 March 2021).

Immigration and Customs Enforcement. 2021a. ICE Detention Statistics Facilities Data, FY21 YTD. Available online: https://www.ice.gov/doclib/detention/FY21-detentionstats.xlx (accessed on 24 June 2021).

Immigration and Customs Enforcement. 2021b. COVID-19 ICE Detainee Statistics by Facility as of June 30, 2021. Available online: https://www.ice.gov/coronavirus#detStat (accessed on 30 June 2021).

Immigration and Customs Enforcement. 2021c. ICE Directive 11032.4, Identification & Monitoring of Pregnant, Postpartum or Nursing Individuals. Available online: https://www.ice.gov/doclib/detention/11032.4_IdentificationMonitoringPregnantPostpartumNursingIndividuals.pdf (accessed on 1 July 2021).

Immigration and Customs Enforcement. 2021d. History of ICE. Available online: https://www.ice.gov/features/history (accessed on 26 January 2021).

Immigration and Customs Enforcement, Enforcement and Removal Operations. 2020a. COVID-19 Pandemic Response Requirements, Version 1. Available online: https://www.ice.gov/doclib/coronavirus/eroCOVID19responseReqsCleanFacilities-v1.pdf (accessed on 10 April 2020).

Immigration and Customs Enforcement, Enforcement and Removal Operations. 2020b. COVID-19 Pandemic Response Requirements, Version 2. Available online: https://www.ice.gov/doclib/coronavirus/eroCOVID19responseReqsCleanFacilities-v3.pdf (accessed on 22 June 2020).

Immigration and Customs Enforcement, Enforcement and Removal Operations. 2020c. COVID-19 Pandemic Response Requirements, Version 3. Available online: https://www.ice.gov/doclib/coronavirus/eroCOVID19responseReqsCleanFacilities-v4.pdf (accessed on 28 July 2020).

Immigration and Customs Enforcement, Enforcement and Removal Operations. 2020d. COVID-19 Pandemic Response, Version 4. Available online: https://www.ice.gov/doclib/coronavirus/eroCOVID19responseReqsCleanFacilities-v4.pdf (accessed on 4 September 2020).

Immigration and Customs Enforcement, Enforcement and Removal Operations. 2020e. COVID-19 Pandemic Response Requirements, Version 5. Available online: https://www.ice.gov/doclib/coronavirus/eroCOVID19responseReqsCleanFacilities-v5.pdf (accessed on 27 October 2020).

Immigration and Customs Enforcement, Enforcement and Removal Operations. 2020f. Memorandum on Coronavirus Disease Action Plan, Revision 1. Available online: https://www.ice.gov/doclib/coronavirus/attF.pdf (accessed on 27 March 2020).

Immigration and Customs Enforcement, Enforcement and Removal Operations. 2021. COVID-19 Pandemic Response Requirements, Version 6. Available online: https://www.ice.gov/doclib/coronavirus/eroCOVID19responseReqsCleanFacilities.pdf (accessed on 16 March 2021).

Immigrations and Customs Enforcement, Family Residential Centers. 2020. Family Residential Standards (rev. 2020). Available online: https://www.ice.gov/doclib/frs/2020/2020family-residential-standards.pdf (accessed on 28 July 2021).

Immigration and Customs Enforcement, Immigration Health Services Corp. 2020. Interim Reference Sheet on 2019-Novel Coronavirus, Version 6. Available online: https://www.aila.org/infonet/ice-interim-reference-sheet-coronavirus (accessed on 6 March 2020).

Immigration and Customs Enforcement, Immigration Health Service Corps. 2021. Available online: https://www.ice.gov/detain/ice-health-service-corps (accessed on 24 March 2021).

Kalhan, Anil. 2010. Rethinking Immigration Detention, Columbia Law Review. *Sidebar*. pp. 42–58. Available online: http://www.columbialawreview.org/sidebar/volume/110/42_Anil_Kalhan.pdf (accessed on 25 October 2011).

Koulish, Robert. 2016. Immigration Detention in the Risk Classification Assessment Era. *Connecticut Public Interest Law Journal* 16: 1. Available online: https://cpilj.law.uconn.edu/wp-content/uploads/sites/2515/2018/10/16.1-Immigration-Detention-in-the-Risk-Classification-Assessment-Era-by-Robert-Koulish.pdf (accessed on 10 November 2016).

Melugin, Bill. 2021. FOX News, REPORT: ICE Confirms '30% of Detainees' Refusing COVID-19 Vaccine While in Detention Centers, 2021. Available online: https://candaceowensfans.com/report-ice-confirms-30-of-detainees-refusing-covid-19-vaccine-while-in-detention-centers/ (accessed on 22 July 2021).

Miner, Horace. 1956. Body Ritual among the Nacirema. *American Anthropologist* 58: 503–7. [CrossRef]

Morrissey, Kate. 2021. San Diego Union-Tribune, Court Ordered Return of Remain in Mexico Worsens Nightmare for Asylum Advocates. Available online: https://www.sandiegouniontribune.com/news/immigration/story/2021-08-28/court-remain-in-mexico-asylum (accessed on 28 August 2021).

Rosenberg, Mica, and Reade Levinson. 2018. Trump's Catch-and-Detain Policy Snares Many Who Have Long Called U.S. Home. Reuters. Available online: https://www.reuters.com/investigates/special-report/usa-immigration-court/ (accessed on 20 June 2018).

Schriro, Dora. 2009. U.S. Department of Homeland Security, Immigration and Customs Enforcement. Immigration Detention Overview and Recommendations. Available online: https://www.ice.gov/doclib/about/offices/odpp/pdf/ice-detention-rpt.pdf (accessed on 6 October 2009).

Smart, Noelle, Adam Garcia, and Nina Siulc. 2021. One Year Later, We Still Don't Know How Many People in ICE Detention Have Been Exposed to COVID-19, VERA Institute of Justice. Available online: https://www.vera.org/blog/one-year-later-we-still-dont-know-how-many-people-in-ice-detention-have-been-exposed-to-covid-19 (accessed on 8 April 2021).

U.S. Department of Homeland Security, Office of Inspector General. 2018. ICE's Inspections and Monitoring of Detention Facilities Do Not Lead to Sustained Compliance or Systemic Improvements. OIG-18-67. Available online: https://www.oig.dhs.gov/sites/default/files/assets/2018-06/OIG-18-67-Jun18.pdf (accessed on 26 June 2018).

U.S. Department of Homeland Security, Office of Inspector General. 2019. ICE Does Not Fully USE Contracting Tools to Hold Detention Facility Contractors Accountable for Failing to Meet Performance Standards. OIG-19-18. Available online: https://www.oig.dhs.gov/sites/default/files/assets/2019-02/OIG-19-18-Jan19.pdf (accessed on 29 January 2019).

U.S. Department of Homeland Security, Office of Inspector General. 2020. Early Experiences with COVID-19 at ICE Detention Facilities. OIG-20-42. Available online: https://www.oig.dhs.gov/sites/default/files/assets/2020-06/OIG-20-42-Jun20.pdf (accessed on 18 June 2020).

U.S. Department of Homeland Security, Office of Inspector General. 2021. ICE's Management of COVID-19 in Its Detention Facilities. Provides Lessons Learned for Future Pandemic Responses. OIG-21-58. Available online: https://www.oig.dhs.gov/sites/default/files/assets/2021-09/OIG-21-58-Sep21.pdf (accessed on 7 September 2021).

U.S. Immigration and Customs Enforcement Fiscal Year 2020 Enforcement and Removal Operations Report. 2021. Available online: https://www.ice.gov/doclib/news/library/reports/annual-report/eroReportFY2020.pdf (accessed on 12 May 2021).

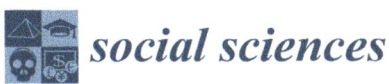

Article

Detained during a Pandemic: Human Rights behind Locked Doors

Justine N. Stefanelli

American Society of International Law, Washington, DC 20008, USA; jstefanelli@asil.org

Abstract: Every year, thousands of people are detained in United States immigration detention centers. Built to prison specifications and often run by private companies, these detention centers have long been criticized by academics and advocacy groups. Problems such as overcrowding and lack of access to basic healthcare and legal representation have plagued individuals in detention centers for years. These failings have been illuminated by the COVID-19 pandemic, which has disproportionately impacted detained migrants. Against a human rights backdrop, this article will examine how the U.S. immigration detention system has proven even more problematic in the context of the pandemic and offer insights to help avoid similar outcomes in the future.

Keywords: detention; immigration; human rights; healthcare; access to justice

Citation: Stefanelli, Justine N.. 2021. Detained during a Pandemic: Human Rights behind Locked Doors. *Social Sciences* 10: 276. https://doi.org/10.3390/socsci10070276

Academic Editor: Nigel Parton

Received: 23 June 2021
Accepted: 16 July 2021
Published: 20 July 2021

Publisher's Note: MDPI stays neutral with regard to jurisdictional claims in published maps and institutional affiliations.

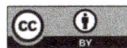

Copyright: © 2021 by the author. Licensee MDPI, Basel, Switzerland. This article is an open access article distributed under the terms and conditions of the Creative Commons Attribution (CC BY) license (https://creativecommons.org/licenses/by/4.0/).

1. Introduction

At the end of September 2020, the average daily population of detained immigrants in the United States (U.S.) was down to 19,068 because of COVID-19 mitigation efforts (U.S. Immigration and Customs Enforcement 2021; U.S. Immigration and Customs Enforcement). However, the 2019 average daily population was 50,165 (U.S. Immigration and Customs Enforcement 2020a). While there were fewer numbers of detainees in 2020, their length of stay in detention facilities went from an average of one month in 2019 to double that in 2020 (U.S. Immigration and Customs Enforcement 2020a, 2021), as it got harder to execute deportation orders and to apply for release from detention.

At the time of writing, U.S. ICE confirmed 15,056 COVID-19 cases among detainees since ICE began testing in February 2020.[1] Just over 10% of its detained population are positive for COVID-19 and are being actively monitored or are under isolation.[2] ICE has reported a total of nine deaths from COVID-19, but the accuracy of this number is disputed.[3] From the start, reports of insufficient sanitization supplies, staff without masks, and failures to facilitate social distancing hit the news. In response, angry and frightened detainees launched hunger strikes, and civil society organizations filed lawsuits advocating for the safety and human rights of detainees.

Described by one scholar as the "American Gulag" (Dow 2004), immigration detention centers have raised serious concerns for many years, particularly since the 1980s when the U.S. faced large numbers of migrants arriving from Cuba and Haiti. For the first time, U.S. detention capacity was stretched to its limits, and migrants were forced to reside in crude camps outdoors, particularly in Florida (Wilsher 2012). This period marked the start of the modern detention estate and the expansion of detention capacity in the United States (Wilsher 2012). The U.S. immigration detention system is now the largest in the world (Global Detention Project 2021). Though it began modestly, it has grown into a system that detains roughly 400,000 people annually (Jefferis 2020). This vast empire has unsurprisingly been the target of much criticism. Scholars and civil society organizations have raised concerns over every aspect of the detention framework, including the method by which a detention order is made;[4] the availability and quality of opportunities to be released from detention;[5] and the constitutional legitimacy of detaining noncitizens.[6] Beyond these, perhaps the greatest area of concern has been the conditions in detention centers[7] and the effect of such conditions on the mental and physical health of those detained.[8] These concerns only increased as the pandemic spread among immigration detention centers.

The pandemic hit immigration detention facilities hard. Pre-existing problems in detention centers, such as overcrowding, shared space, and lack of access to healthcare and legal representation were exacerbated by the pandemic and the slow and inadequate response of the U.S. Government to early concerns raised by human rights watchdogs. As two commentators put it in the early days of the pandemic, "Because the transmission of SARS-CoV-2 is predominantly from person to person through droplets, a pillar of infection prevention is social distancing and disinfection, which is antithetical to closed detention settings" (Meyer et al. 2020).

Although one year on the situation has improved, it is important to reflect on the U.S. Government's response to the pandemic's impact in detention centers in light of international and domestic law obligations concerning immigration detention and to identify some lessons learned to avoid a similar crisis in the future.

Following this introduction, Section 2 will introduce the nature and function of immigration detention in the United States and review the domestic and international standards applicable to the detention of noncitizens in the United States. It will also delve into criticisms of detention, particularly regarding healthcare, to more explicitly illustrate how the pandemic made a poor situation worse for immigration detainees.[9] Section 3 will review the response of ICE to the pandemic and demonstrate how detainees' access to healthcare was particularly compromised by ICE's insufficient reaction to the pandemic. Section 4 will look at the specific issue of access to justice and what happened in the immigration courts following the onset of the pandemic. Section 5 will identify what steps should and could have been taken to mitigate the impact of the COVID-19 pandemic and any similar situations that may arise in the future. Section 6 concludes that the U.S. immigration detention system must be reviewed using a human rights-based approach, to prevent what happened following the COVID-19 pandemic from happening again.

2. Detention and the Law

From its modest roots in the context of deporting Irish and French revolutionaries from the U.S., through its employment in the 1980s to address the sudden influx of Cubans and Haitians, immigration detention has grown to be an essential part of American immigration law enforcement (Wilsher 2012, pp. 1–118).[10] Although the procedures by which detention can be ordered are regulated by U.S. law, the manner in which detention is carried out is left largely unchecked. This section will briefly address the purpose of detention before moving on to the domestic and international standards that govern its implementation and an overview of criticisms of the U.S. detention regime that predated the pandemic.

2.1. The Detention Machine

The U.S. Department of Justice (DOJ) and the Department of Homeland Security (DHS) share jurisdiction over immigration detention. The DOJ essentially manages the operation of DHS, including the judicial review of immigration matters (excluding detention). Within the DOJ, the Executive Office for Immigration Review is responsible for immigration adjudication. It includes three units: (1) the Office of the Chief Immigration Judge (which comprises a number of immigration courts throughout the U.S.); (2) the Board of Immigration Appeals (BIA) (which hears appeals from the immigration courts); and (3) the Office of the Chief Administrative Hearing Officer (which deals exclusively with cases relating to the employment of migrants without the right to reside in the U.S.). Decisions of the BIA can be appealed to the federal courts, though their review powers are very limited (Stefanelli 2020, pp. 74–75). If a person wants to be released from detention, he or she must apply for habeas corpus at a federal district court.[11]

Within DHS, there are two immigration departments: Customs and Border Protection (CBP) to enforce immigration law at the borders of the country, and Immigration and

Customs Enforcement (ICE), which enforces immigration law within the United States and manages immigration detention. DHS has the power to detain noncitizens in a number of circumstances, including (1) detention pending a decision on removal from the U.S., (2) detention pending removal after it has been ordered, (3) detention pending a decision on entry at the borders, and (4) detention pending a decision on asylum.[12] Whether someone is detained largely depends on whether the immigration authorities believe that the person's release would pose a risk of harm to the United States or the public, or a risk of flight (i.e., to avoid prosecution by immigration authorities for violations of the law). Noncitizens who have committed certain qualifying crimes while in the U.S., or those who are deportable on grounds of terrorism, must be detained pending a decision on removal.[13] For most other noncitizens, risk is determined on a case-by-case basis using an automated risk assessment tool that assigns a public safety and flight risk score based on DHS enforcement priorities. However, the algorithm has been criticized as being unduly weighted in favor of detention (Noferi and Koulish 2014; Koulish 2016).

If a person is detained, he or she will be housed in one of ICE's 134 detention facilities, primarily located in major cities across the U.S.[14] These facilities come in many shapes and sizes, and they house adults and children—sometimes together in special family residential centers.[15] Some are run by state or federal authorities, while others are privately owned and/or operated by for-profit companies such as the GEO Group or CoreCivic (Ryo and Peacock 2018; Kennedy 2020).[16] Some are wholly dedicated to housing immigration detainees, while others (typically prisons that house both those convicted under criminal law and those detained under immigration powers) will include people convicted of criminal activity. In 2009, Congress issued what has become known as the "bed mandate" for detention centers. Under that mandate, ICE is required to maintain 34,000 beds in detention centers on a daily basis. In other words, immigration detention is subject to a statutory quota (Sinha 2016).

2.2. Domestic Detention Standards

Regardless of the type of detention facility, standards for operation apply. Immigration-detainee-only facilities must abide by certain standards.

The Performance-Based National Detention Standards (PBNDS). This 455-page set of standards was created in 2011 in an "ongoing effort to tailor the conditions of immigration detention to its unique purpose . . . [and] to improve medical and mental health services [and] increase access to legal services" (U.S. Immigration and Customs Enforcement 2011, p. I; Papst 2009). In the words of one scholar, "the PBNDS standards are relatively high and would make immigration detention centers habitable" (Kennedy 2020). The PBNDS cover seven main subjects, some of which provide basic human rights, such as a grievance system and medical screening (Noferi 2014, pp. 555–56), and they include a number of "expected outcomes", which are specific implementation targets for each aspect of the PBNDS. However, the PBNDS do not indicate whether, and to what extent, there are consequences for a failure to reach an expected outcome, nor are there any legal means for ICE to ensure that privately-run detention centers adhere to the standards (Sthanki 2013, p. 465).

Non-immigration-exclusive detention facilities (such as prisons) are expected to comply with the 2019 National Detention Standards for Non-Dedicated Facilities (NDSNDF). According to ICE, these are "facilities used by ICE . . . with an Average Daily Population of less than 10" (U.S. Immigration and Customs Enforcement 2019). NDSNDF standard 4.3 notes that it is policy for "All detainees [to] have access to appropriate medical, dental, and mental health care, including emergency services" (U.S. Immigration and Customs Enforcement 2019, p. 112). The NDSNDF also calls for each facility to have "written plans" to address infectious and communicable diseases (U.S. Immigration and Customs Enforcement 2019, p. 114). Unlike the PBNDS, the NDSNDF does not include subject-specific expected outcomes.

Finally, family detention centers must abide by the Family Residential Standards 2020 (U.S. Immigration and Customs Enforcement 2020b). Like the PBNDS, these standards include expected outcomes and include provisions governing healthcare. For example, section 4.3 requires that residents "have access to a continuum of health care services including screening, prevention, health education, diagnoses, and treatment".

The way that ICE manages its detention facilities has long been criticized. For a start, the use of three sets of standards has been called confusing, making "it difficult for entities to hold facilities accountable" and collect accurate data concerning the healthcare of detainees (Bowen 2020, p. 299). More substantively, it has been highlighted that "'[n]o checks and balances currently exist within ICE. ICE investigates itself", and that detention center abuses are conducted "with impunity, and without recourse" (Sthanki 2013, pp. 448–49; United Nations Working Group on Arbitrary Detention 2010, para. 35).[17] Moreover, because the standards are not legally binding, they are effectively unenforceable (Sthanki 2013, p. 464; Global Detention Project 2010, p. 13). Though both the PBNDS and the NDSNDF include an internal grievance mechanism whereby detainees can file a complaint with a designated facility representative or committee, detainees rarely make recourse to this option, for fear of retribution by facility staff (Sthanki 2013, p. 466). Prior to the adoption of the PBNDS, Amnesty International commented that "conditions of detention in many facilities do not meet either international human rights standards or ICE guidelines" (Amnesty International 2009, p. 7). In 2017, the DHS Office of Inspector General conducted unannounced inspections of five immigration detention facilities to evaluate their compliance with ICE standards (U.S. Department of Homeland Security Office of Inspector General, "About Us" 2017).[18] It found a number of violations, including "unsafe and unhealthy detention conditions", but noted that ICE had begun to take "corrective action" in response to the report (U.S. Department of Homeland Security Office of Inspector General, "About Us" 2017, p. 1). Despite such action, violations continue. For example, A 2020 report by the House Committee on Homeland Security found that ICE facilities fail to meet basic standards of care for migrants (U.S. House of Representatives Committee on Homeland Security 2020). In particular, the report condemned ICE's failure to properly oversee detention facilities and to provide sufficient medical care, including for COVID-19 (U.S. House of Representatives Committee on Homeland Security 2020, pp. 7–10, 13–19).

Beyond this, there is no U.S. law that governs the way that detention centers are managed.[19] Thus, it is necessary to turn to international law for guidance.

2.3. International Detention Standards

Although various international human rights law instruments govern immigration detention, they are not all legally binding on the United States. This article will therefore focus on the two main binding legal instruments that address the rights of migrants in detention: the International Covenant on Civil and Political Rights (ICCPR)[20] and the United Nations Convention Against Torture and Cruel, Inhuman or Degrading Treatment (UNCAT).[21] These standards apply to all government entities and agencies, as well as private contractors that carry out government functions, such as running immigration detention centers.

The U.S. ratified the ICCPR in 1992. It applies to government entities and agents, but it provides no enforceable rights for individuals in U.S. courts. However, the U.S. must report to the United Nations (UN) Human Rights Committee to demonstrate its compliance with the Convention. The U.S. is therefore obligated to ensure that all government officials are complying with the Convention's obligations with respect to detained persons (Skinner 2008, p. 292). Article 6 ICCPR guarantees the right to life to "every human being". The UN Human Rights Committee has explained that this requires states to "take special measures of protection towards persons in situation [sic] of vulnerability", including refugees and asylum seekers, and that a "heightened duty of care" applies to those "deprived of their liberty by the State" (United Nations Human Rights Committee 2018, para. 23). Article 7 of the ICCPR provides that, "No one shall be subjected to torture or to cruel, inhuman or degrading treatment or punishment". This means that governments are required to provide "adequate medical care during detention", (United Nations Human Rights Committee 1990, p. 69) including "prompt and regular access be given to doctors and lawyers" to prevent "physical and mental suffering".[22]

The U.S. ratified the UNCAT in 1994 and has enacted a number of domestic laws to implement its provisions (Garcia 2009).[23] As with the ICCPR, the U.S. must report periodically on its compliance with the UNCAT to the Committee Against Torture. UNCAT includes a general prohibition on torture and other inhuman and degrading treatment. Together, Articles 10 and 11 make clear that parties to the Convention must comply with its provisions with respect to individuals held in custody (Skinner 2008, p. 292). The Committee has found that the UNCAT may be violated if a state fails to provide adequate medical care (Amon 2020).

Although this article focuses on the two legal instruments just described, it is worth highlighting the UN Standard Rules for the Treatment of Prisoners (also known as the Nelson Mandela Rules). Although not legally binding, the Nelson Mandela Rules go beyond the standards set forth in the two instruments above (United Nations General Assembly 2016). For example, they provide detailed standards regarding accommodation, hygiene, clothing and bedding, food, and healthcare services, including the rule that detainees "should enjoy the same standards of health care that are available in the community, and should have access to necessary health-care services free of charge without discrimination on the grounds of their legal status" (United Nations General Assembly 2016, Rule 24).

2.4. Criticisms

Despite the existence of the above standards, conditions in detention centers regarding healthcare have long been a subject of criticism from scholars, civil society organizations, and the UN.[24] For example, Detention Watch Network has referred to "ICE's shameful record of medical negligence . . . poor sanitation, and demonstrated inability to properly respond to past infectious disease outbreaks" (Detention Watch Network 2020a, p. 1), and the medical care provided in immigration detention centers has been called "dangerously substandard" (Human Rights Watch 2018).

The UN Human Rights Committee last issued its observations on the U.S. in 2014, mandating that the U.S. ensure compliance with Articles 7 and 10 (United Nations Human Rights Committee 2014a, para. 20). The Committee is currently awaiting another report from the U.S. and, in particular, an update on "the conditions within immigrant detention facilities, both publicly and privately owned, including access to healthcare" (United Nations Human Rights Committee 2019, para. 21). The UN Committee Against Torture expressed concern about "reports of substandard conditions of detention in immigration facilities" (United Nations Committee against Torture and Other Cruel, Inhuman or Degrading Treatment or Punishment 2014, para. 19) and has specifically asked the U.S. to respond to such reports (United Nations Committee against Torture and Other Cruel, Inhuman or Degrading Treatment or Punishment 2017, para. 28). Moreover, the UN Working Group on Arbitrary Detention noted in a 2017 report on a visit to the U.S. that detainees in private facilities "expressed concern about . . . the poor quality of food and drinking water . . . and access to medical services" (United Nations Working Group on Arbitrary Detention 2017, para. 34).

When COVID-19 reached the U.S., the immigration detention system was therefore already struggling to meet the healthcare needs of detainees. Detention facilities were overcrowded, despite then-President Donald Trump's increasing the number of detention facilities (American Civil Liberties Union 2020, p. 14 (American Civil Liberties Union)). ICE was already under fire for its poor monitoring and prevention of disease in its facilities.[25] As the first few months of the pandemic demonstrated, immigration detainees were particularly vulnerable to the pandemic and did not have adequate resources to avoid its impact.

3. The Pandemic Strikes

It is important to emphasize that closed environments, such as detention centers, are particularly vulnerable to the spread of disease. In addition to overcrowding, the communal nature of detention centers means that people are unable to socially distance—bathrooms and sinks are shared, as are mealtimes, and staff come and go from the outside world (Amon 2020). In fact, it was reported in November 2020 that COVID-19 infection rates in detention centers were 13 times higher than the national infection rate (Driesbach 2020).[26]

As indicated in Section 1 above, ICE issues statistics regarding the impact of COVID-19 on detention centers. To supplement reports from a system that has sometimes been called a "black box", a number of other organizations also began tracking the effect of COVID-19 in detention centers from the start of the pandemic (Cho 2020). In April 2020, the organization Freedom for Immigrants (FFI) began issuing regular analyses and updates on the impact of COVID-19 on those in ICE custody. In its first update, just over a month after the World Health Organization declared COVID-19 a pandemic (World Health Organization 2020), FFI reported on the dire circumstances in detention facilities, including "crowded and unsanitary conditions, continued transfers of people between facilities with known or suspected outbreaks, and a lack of or insufficient quantities of soap and personal protective equipment (PPE), for the people in custody as well as staff and guards" (Freedom for Immigrants 2020, p. 1). The update also included detainees' concerns "that ICE was either failing to provide or deliberately blocking information about the spread of COVID-19 inside detention" (Freedom for Immigrants 2020, p. 1). The FFI updates continued in this vein, noting that the observations in their reports "remained consistent—at every stage of the pandemic, ICE failed to implement even basic public health protocols to mitigate against the spread of COVID-19" (Freedom for Immigrants 2021, p. 1). Reports surfaced of detainees' lack of access to soap and hand sanitizer, or in some instances, being required to purchase these items in detention center commissaries (Zwick 2020).

In recognition of the vulnerability of detainees, the Centers for Disease Control issued "Interim Guidance on Management of COVID-19 in Correctional and Detention Facilities" in March 2020.[27] ICE detention facilities are required to comply with CDC guidelines on environmental health (U.S. Immigration and Customs Enforcement 2011, sct. V.A). The CDC recommended that ICE "provide a no-cost supply of soap" to detained persons, in quantities sufficient to allow for multiple hand washings; provide alcohol-based sanitizer with at least 50% alcohol; implement social distancing strategies; and provide clear information about the existence of COVID-19 cases within detention centers and the need to maintain good hygiene and distance from other detainees. Despite this, ICE continued to operate its detention centers largely unchanged.

Although ICE announced in March 2020 that it would be focusing its immigration enforcement efforts on "public-safety risks and individuals subject to mandatory detention based on criminal grounds",[28] ICE continued to transfer detainees between ICE facilities, and between ICE facilities and prisons, even when ICE facilities were dealing with known outbreaks (American Civil Liberties Union 2021, p. 6). In April, ICE ordered its officers to reassess the need to detain those over 60 years of age and anyone with immune-system-compromising illnesses (Hsu 2020). This led to the release of approximately 700 people (Flynn 2020). That same month (and for several more thereafter), judges around the U.S. were ordering detention centers to reduce their populations (Brennan Center for Justice 2021). Staff at some facilities were told not to wear masks to prevent the spread of panic among detainees and, reportedly, some centers offered masks to detainees who were willing to sign a waiver releasing one of the private detention centers from liability, should they become ill (Detention Watch Network 2020b). Some facilities began using quarantines to isolate and stop the spread of infection, but it appears that their use was not uniform and sometimes included quarantines of groups of people (Zwick 2020). ICE also continued deporting detainees, sometimes without testing them for COVID-19 (ibid). Later, when travel bans were imposed, an inability to remove even those who tested negative for COVID-19 only served to worsen the problem of overcrowding in centers (Chishti and

Pierce 2020). Detainees at a privately-run detention center in Georgia reported that they were routinely denied COVID-19-related medical care and punished harshly for asking for such treatment (Del Valle and Olivares 2020; Olivares 2020). In late 2020, it became evident that communities with ICE facilities were experiencing more serious outbreaks and a faster rate of infection than communities without detention centers (Detention Watch Network 2020b, p. 26).

A related problem was ICE's failure to halt *all* enforcement operations at the start of the pandemic. As indicated above, ICE refocused its enforcement operations on safety risks, but because it did not stop completely, new people were detained, thus exacerbating conditions in detention centers. As the Brennan Center recommended, "ICE and CBP should release all individuals who are not a 'credible threat' to public safety on parole/bond, including all people without a criminal record or with only a minor violation as their most serious criminal conviction. This would encompass most of the detained population" (Brennan Center for Justice 2021).

In addition to an ICE-led decision to release, ICE has the discretion to grant parole to noncitizens in certain circumstances. In particular, the governing statute gives ICE the discretion to temporarily parole individuals "on a case-by-case basis for urgent humanitarian reasons or significant public benefit".[29] It must be requested by the detainee. Guidance on humanitarian parole provides examples of the types of people in detention that should be considered for release, including people who have "serious medical conditions" and people "whose continued detention is not in the public interest".[30] In addition, it must normally be demonstrated that the immigrant applicant for parole does not pose a flight or security risk.[31] Several organizations called on attorneys to apply for humanitarian parole, especially for high-risk detainees (Meyer et al. 2020; Immigration Justice Campaign 2020). However, because most detainees have no legal representation (discussed below), this option remained largely unknown to them.[32]

In response to these circumstances, a number of detainees launched hunger strikes, and several civil society organizations filed lawsuits on behalf of detainees to secure their release, many of which are ongoing at the time of writing.[33]

4. Access to Justice

Section 2.3 above indicated that the Human Rights Committee has interpreted Article 7 to require access to lawyers. In addition, Article 9(4) provides a right to judicial review for those deprived of their liberty that has also been interpreted by the Committee as including "prompt and regular access" to lawyers (United Nations Human Rights Committee 2014b, para. 58). Once it became evident that the pandemic could have a devastating effect in the United States, the Executive Office for Immigration Review (EOIR), the office that manages the immigration court system, began grappling with how to respond to COVID-19. On 15 March 2020, the EOIR announced that hearings scheduled for people not in detention would be postponed, but that the courts would remain open for other matters. It later began to close immigration courts and announced rules requiring visitors (including attorneys) to courts operated by DHS and located in detention centers to wear PPE—some even specified that visitors must provide their own (Adelstein and Keith 2020).

While it may seem a positive development that the EOIR did not suspend hearings for detainees, given the poor quality of protection measures implemented in ICE facilities, continuing in-person hearings for detained immigrants posed an unnecessary risk of contamination for all people present in the immigration courts, including the immigrants themselves. Speaking to the Texas Tribune, Judge Ashley Tabaddor, president of the National Association of Immigration Judges, commented that "[f]ailing to close all of the nation's Immigration Courts, both non-detained and detained settings, now will exacerbate a once-in-a-century public health crisis and lead to a greater loss of life" (Aguilar 2020). In addition, the requirement to wear PPE at a time when there was a shortage of PPE, meant that some lawyers were unable to go to the courts and detention centers to see clients whose cases were progressing (Aguilar 2020).

These specific circumstances must be viewed in the larger context of access to justice for immigrants. In particular, unlike criminal defendants, immigrants do not have the right to a court-appointed lawyer. This leaves most immigrants without representation when it comes to contesting their detention and deportation orders (Eagly and Shafer 2015).[34] Without legal representation, it is often extremely difficult to obtain release. In fact, represented immigrants are "three times more likely to be released and 10.5 times more likely to establish their right to remain in the United States" than unrepresented immigrants (Vera Institute of Justice 2020, p. 1). Not being able to obtain release from detention because of a lack of access to a lawyer means that many immigrants are unnecessarily detained for prolonged periods of time in facilities that were already struggling to meet human rights minimums before the pandemic.

Each of these issues together created a perfect storm in immigration detention facilities. Although pandemics on the scale of COVID-19 are infrequent, it is not smart to assume that they will continue to be so rare. It is also not wise to presume that the low number of detainees reported by ICE at the end of 2020 is a sign of a change in detention practice. Indeed, as of 4 June 2021, ICE reported 24,100 people in detention.[35] That is a 26% increase from the 19,068 people detained at the end of 2020. It seems that ICE is returning to its pre-pandemic level of detaining immigrants. It is therefore of the utmost importance to consider what can and should be done to safeguard the fundamental rights of detainees in future outbreaks.

5. Lessons Learned

From the start of the pandemic, people and organizations working in immigration and human rights law identified a number of ways to prevent or mitigate the spread of COVID-19 (or any other virus on this scale) in immigration detention facilities, including the immediate release of all detainees (Detention Watch Network 2020a, p. 5; Vera Institute of Justice 2020; García Hernández and Moctezuma García 2020). While it may not be feasible to empty all of the detention centers, releasing detainees who do not pose a risk of harm or flight is reasonable and effective. Fewer detainees in facilities means that those who remain detained can more easily socially distance themselves from one another. Some even called for a commitment from DHS not to re-detain those who were released because of COVID-19 "absent a compelling, individualized reason to do so" (American Civil Liberties Union 2020, p. 8). ICE should have temporarily stopped all enforcement operations so that new people were not detained and added to the facilities' populations (Detention Watch Network 2020a, pp. 4–5; Vera Institute of Justice 2020, p. 4). To stop the spread of disease between facilities and the community, ICE should have also halted all detainee transfers. Within detention centers and immigration courts, clear and honest information about the virus should have been provided to detainees in a language they could understand, and hygiene products should have been made freely and widely available. Steps should also have been taken to ensure that detainees have access to vaccines under the same conditions as the general public, taking into account detainees who pose a higher risk for contracting the virus (American Civil Liberties Union 2020, p. 8). Finally, the immigration courts should have suspended all types of proceedings, not just those for non-detained immigrants, and ICE should have immediately halted the execution of all deportation orders.

ICE's inadequate and delayed response to the pandemic worsened its impact in detention centers. The fallout made it clear that there is work to be done beyond the need to respond quickly and intelligently when a pandemic strikes. Several systemic issues must be addressed so that if and when another pandemic strikes, an already-strained system is not put under further pressure.

First, detention should be used as a last resort, imposed only after an individual assessment has concluded that the person poses a risk of harm or flight. Those who do not pose such risks should be released, and an alternative to detention should be applied. The UN Working Group on Arbitrary Detention has explained that "[a]lternatives to detention can take various forms: reporting at regular intervals to the authorities; release on bail;

or stay in open centers or at a designated place. Such measures are already successfully applied in a number of countries. They must however not become alternatives to release" (United Nations Working Group on Arbitrary Detention 2010, para. 65). To that end, the ACLU has recommended that the DHS "[e]stablish a nationwide program of community-based alternatives to detention run by nonprofit organizations providing case management services" (American Civil Liberties Union 2020, p. 8). Second, where people are detained, it is essential for them to have effective access to legal representation. Although immigrants do not have the right to court-appointed lawyers like criminal defendants do, communities should "continue to invest in and grow publicly funded legal representation programs" (Vera Institute of Justice 2020, p. 3). Although some programs currently exist, they are by no means sufficient to provide resources for the thousands of people detained without legal representation.[36] Third, while in detention, access to healthcare should be improved. In particular, it makes sense to ensure that immigration detention healthcare systems are connected with general healthcare and emergency planning systems and that there is information sharing between the health and justice departments (Kinner et al. 2020). Fourth, in recognition that under normal circumstances ICE violates its own standards without consequence (Hamilton YEAR, p. 120), it is vital that independent oversight mechanisms with enforcement power are put in place to ensure that any breaches of the rules are corrected and punished and that detainees can effectively report wrongdoing to an independent body or agency. This is especially important considering that more than two-thirds of detainees are housed in private detention centers (Amnesty International 2020, p. 29). Relatedly, the U.S. should take seriously its commitments to the ICCPR and the UNCAT, for example by implementing recommendations from the Human Rights Committee and the Committee Against Torture and ensuring that detainees can enforce the standards in U.S. courts. A review of the ICE detentions standards should be conducted against the international legal framework, including the superior standards set forth in the Nelson Mandela Rules, and the rules should be consolidated insofar as possible to avoid inconsistent implementation. Fifth, immigration detention facilities should engage in pandemic response strategy development. To assist in this process, ICE should be factored into the broader public health response planning so that it is not left to develop strategies in isolation (Kinner et al. 2020). On a more granular level, each facility should have protocols in place for screening visitors, supplying PPE, social distancing, cleaning and disinfection, and restricting movement—including limiting staff and visitors to essential personnel (Kinner et al. 2020). Sixth, the U.S. Government should put an end to the use of private immigration detention facilities. In January 2021, the Biden Administration ordered the U.S. Department of Justice to take steps to end its reliance on private prisons for federal prisoners,[37] and human rights experts have since called for an extension of that mandate to immigration detention facilities (Scaffidi 2021). Bringing all immigration detention centers under the direct control of ICE, combined with revamping the standards applicable in those centers, are essential steps on the journey toward achieving a human rights-compliant immigration detention system.

Beyond policy, it may be possible to achieve binding legislative change for detention centers. There are currently two bills before Congress that seek to improve the immigration detention framework. The New Way Forward Act was introduced to Congress in January 2021 and aims to reform the enforcement of U.S. immigration law (U.S. Congress 2021a). In particular, it seeks to end the use of mandatory detention of those who have committed certain crimes considered "aggravated felonies",[38] thereby extensively reducing the number of immigrants placed in detention. It also provides for automatic review by the Secretary of Homeland Security of the decision to detain an immigrant within 48 h of the person being taken into custody Noferi (2016). That same provision also imposes a rebuttable presumption that the immigrant should be released. Essentially, if enacted, the Act would reduce the use of detention and improve the quality of detention, where it is imposed.

The Dignity for Detained Immigrants Act was introduced to Congress in April 2021 and sets minimum standards for the protection of immigrants in DHS custody (U.S.

Congress 2021b). The bill includes provisions on oversight and transparency for detention facilities, including a process to deal with a failure to comply with the standards set forth in the bill; it provides a cause of action for detainees in facilities out of compliance with the standards; and it addresses broader concerns such as the pervasive use of private detention facilities and procedures for detaining noncitizens.

Though it may be difficult to achieve consensus on the sort of legislative change described above, it should not be difficult to put in place plans and procedures to ensure that detainees are taken care of both within and outside the context of a pandemic. At a bare minimum, detention centers should meet detainees' basic human rights requirements. Detainees should have been informed accurately about the virus and provided with free PPE and hygienic supplies, and all detention facility staff should have been wearing masks. DHS's failure to act quickly and intelligently and the U.S.'s failure to meet its international human rights obligations meant that detainees were without the information and resources necessary to avoid contracting COVID-19.

6. Conclusions

To avoid repeating the events of 2020, the U.S. must take more control over its detention estate. It should ensure that it meets its international obligations, and that ICE adheres to its own standards at all times. If the U.S. remains committed to detention as a primary means of immigration law enforcement, decisions to detain should be made more carefully and detention centers should be managed more strictly. Detention should be used sparingly so that facilities are not overcrowded and are able to provide the resources needed to combat the spread of infection. A more effective response also requires a detailed review of the operation of ICE facilities. ICE should not operate in a vacuum. It must be involved in pandemic and emergency response planning, and it should not be the judge of its own actions. It is important that we learn from this pandemic to avoid making the same mistakes in the future. Ultimately, a holistic and human rights-based approach to reforming immigration detention is a necessary part of accomplishing this goal.

Funding: This research received no external funding.

Institutional Review Board Statement: Not applicable.

Informed Consent Statement: Not applicable.

Data Availability Statement: Not applicable.

Conflicts of Interest: The author declares no conflict of interest.

Notes

[1] ICE maintains a website that includes COVID-19 ICE Detainee Statistics, available online https://www.ice.gov/coronavirus#detStat (accessed on 16 June 2021). The website is updated frequently.

[2] ICE Detainee Statistics, available online https://www.ice.gov/coronavirus#detStat (accessed on 16 June 2021).

[3] There have been conflicting reports of the numbers of death. For example, the Brennan Center for Justice reports that there were 21 deaths in ICE custody in fiscal year 2020, most of which were due to Covid-19 (see Brennan Center for Justice 2021). Moreover, ICE number do not include those who died in the hospital after being released from detention (American Civil Liberties Union 2021, p. 6).

[4] See, e.g., Noferi and Koulish (2014); Koulish (2016).

[5] See, e.g., Legomsky (1999); Kimball (2009); Stefanelli (2020).

[6] See, e.g., Caloz-Tschopp (1997); Chelgren (2011); Wilsher (2012).

[7] See, e.g., Dow (2004); Bosworth and Kaufman (2011).

[8] See, e.g., American Civil Liberties Union (2020); Hing (2010); Mukhopadhyay (2009); Pyntikova (2010); Saadi (2020).

[9] The author wishes to emphasize that this article is in no way intended to infer that similar problems are not occurring on a similar, if not worse, level in the context of the detention of convicted persons in prisons. The discussion of the impact of COVID-19 on people in prison is beyond the scope of this article. However, the Equal Justice Initiative provides up-to-date information on the impact of the pandemic on prisons, and may be a good starting point for the reader who may not be familiar with that

10 The history and purpose of immigration detention in the U.S. is the subject of much scholarship and beyond the scope of this article. See, e.g., Stefanelli (2020), pp. 24–28 and notes therein).
11 The origin and functioning of habeas corpus is beyond the scope of this article, but see Stefanelli (2020), pp. 73–75 and related citations for more information).
12 The Immigration and Nationality Act 1952 provides DHS with the power to detain. See INA, Pub. L. 82–414, 66 Stat. 163 (enacted 27 June 1952) [hereinafter INA], §§ 235(b)(1)(B)(iii)(IV); 235(b)(2)(A); 236; 241.
13 INA § 236(c).
14 U.S. Immigration and Customs Enforcement, Detention Facilities, https://www.ice.gov/detention-facilities (accessed on 18 May 2021).
15 See Detention Watch Network, "Family Detention," available online at: https://www.detentionwatchnetwork.org/issues/family-detention (accessed on 7 July 2021).
16 In fact, roughly two-thirds of immigration detention is managed by private companies such as these (Ryo and Peacock 2018).
17 The situation is compounded when it comes to privately-managed facilities, whose liability for detention center harms has been limited by the U.S. Supreme Court (Global Detention Project 2010, p. 13). See also Sthanki (2013, p. 450), discussing *Minneci v. Pollard*, 565 U.S. 118 (2012) and *Corr. Servs. Corp. v. Malesko*, 534 U.S. 61 (2001).
18 The Office of Inspector General was established in 2002 and its mission is "to provide independent oversight and promote excellence, integrity, and accountability within DHS".
19 The U.S. Supreme Court has held that if the conditions in a detention facility amount to cruel and unusual punishment under the Eighth Amendment of the U.S. Constitution, the Due Process Clause of the Fifth Amendment may be violated. Skinner discusses two relevant cases on this issue and points out that the UN Human Rights Committee has criticized the U.S. approach as not being in line with the object and purpose of the ICCPR (Skinner 2008, p. 284).
20 G.A. res. 2200A (XXI), 21 U.N. GAOR Supp. (No. 16) at 52, U.N. Doc. A/6316 (1966), 999 U.N.T.S. 171 (entered into force 23 March 1976, ratified by U.S. 8 September 1992).
21 Convention Against Torture and Other Cruel, Inhuman or Degrading Treatment or Punishment, 10 December 1984, 1465 U.N.T.S. 113, 116 (entered into force June signed by U.S 18 April 1988, ratified by U.S. 21 October 1994). The Convention was implemented by provisions in the Foreign Affairs Reform and Restructuring Act of 1998, Pub. L. 105–277, div. G, 21 October 1998, 112 Stat. 2681–761.
22 The UN Human Rights Committee has indicated that Article 10 ICCPR complements Article 7 so that together, they stand for the notion that "not only may persons deprived of their liberty not be subjected to treatment that is contrary to article 7 ... but neither may they be subjected to any hardship or constraint other than that resulting from the deprivation of liberty; respect for the dignity of such persons must be guaranteed under the same conditions as for that of free persons" (United Nations Human Rights Committee 1992, para. 3).
23 See, in particular, the Detainee Treatment Act of 2005, Pub. L. No. 109–148, §§ 1001–1006, 119 Stat. 2680, 2739 (2005) (codified at 42 U.S.C. § 200dd(a)). As Zivec writes, the Alien Tort Claims Act (28 U.S.C. § 1350 (2006)) "grants federal courts 'original jurisdiction of any civil action by an alien for a tort ... committed in violation of the law of nations or a treaty of the United States.' Therefore, in theory a detainee could bring suit under the [Act] for violations of [UNCAT] and the Detainee Treatment Act of 2005. However, the Supreme Court has not yet addressed whether gross medical negligence can amount to cruel, inhuman, or degrading treatment or punishment" (Zivec 2011).
24 See, e.g., Zivec (2011), Tovino (2016a, 2016b), Bowen (2020), Morehouse (2010).
25 See Amnesty International (2020, p. 7), citing in note 13 the U.S. Congress's 2019 instruction to DHS to examine "how the Department delivers healthcare to individuals in its custody and to departmental personnel," including "outbreak response".
26 The vulnerability of detainees has previously been identified and examined in the context of HIV and AIDS. See Burris and Lipscombe (Sowder 1992; Burris 1992; Lipscombe 2013).
27 CDC, "Interim Guidance on Management of Coronavirus Disease 2019 (COVID-19) in Correctional and Detention Facilities" (23 March 2020), available online at: https://www.cdc.gov/coronavirus/2019-ncov/community/correction-detention/guidance-correctional-detention.html. Updates are continually added to the Guidance, the most recent being from 6 May 2021.
28 ICE website, supra note 1.
29 INA, supra note 9, § 212(d)(5) (8 U.S.C. § 1182(d)(5)).
30 8 C.F.R. § 212.5(b).
31 8 C.F.R. § 212.5(d).
32 The Southern Poverty Law Center, for example, created a webinar for unrepresented detainees teaching them about humanitarian parole in English and Spanish. See https://www.splcenter.org/webinar-ice-humanitarian-parole-time-covid-19 (accessed on

33 See, e.g., American Civil Liberties Union (2021); Langona (2020). In addition, the American Immigration Council has filed a number of suits against ICE in the context of the pandemic. See https://www.americanimmigrationcouncil.org/what-we-do/litigation for more information (accessed on 16 June 2021).

34 Detainees applying for release from detention via an application for habeas corpus can apply for appointed counsel, but the likelihood of a court granting the application is low. See Stefanelli (2020, p. 78).

35 ICE website, supra note 1.

36 Major cities, such as New York, Los Angeles, and Washington D.C. tend to have pro bono immigrant legal services to assist in litigation, including habeas corpus applications. For example, in Washington, D.C., the CAIR Coalition serves this function, as well as local general legal aid societies. More broadly, the American Bar Association has run projects that provide legal services to migrants detained in South Texas. However, these programs and organizations are severely understaffed and under-resourced.

37 President Biden's Executive Order to that effect is available online https://www.federalregister.gov/documents/2021/01/29/2021-02070/reforming-our-incarceration-system-to-eliminate-the-use-of-privately-operated-criminal-detention (accessed on 16 June 2021).

38 For a discussion of mandatory detention, see, e.g., Noferi (2016).

Also at the top:
16 June 2021). See also Innovation Law Lab, "Instructions for Completing the Pro Se COVID-19 Parole Request," https://www.ilcm.org/wp-content/uploads/2020/04/Pro-Se-HPR-Packet-COVID-19.pdf (accessed on 16 June 2021).

References

Adelstein, Janna, and Douglas Keith. 2020. Initial Court Responses to Covid-19 Leave a Patchwork of Policies. *Brennan Center for Justice*. April 14. Available online: https://www.brennancenter.org/our-work/analysis-opinion/initial-court-responses-covid-19-leave-patchwork-policies (accessed on 16 June 2021).

Aguilar, Julián. 2020. Immigration attorneys worry ICE rules will take away needed medical supplies. *The Texas Tribune*. March 22. Available online: https://www.texastribune.org/2020/03/22/immigration-attorneys-worry-ices-new-ppe-rule-take-away-needed-supplie/ (accessed on 16 June 2021).

American Civil Liberties Union. 2020. Justice-Free Zones: U.S. Immigration Detention under the Trump Administration. Available online: https://www.aclu.org/report/justice-free-zones-us-immigration-detention-under-trump-administration?redirect=justicefreezones (accessed on 16 June 2021).

American Civil Liberties Union. 2021. The Survivors: Stories of People Released from ICE Detention during the COVID-19 Pandemic. Available online: https://www.aclu.org/report/survivors (accessed on 16 June 2021).

Amnesty International. 2009. Jailed Without Justice: Immigration Detention in the USA. Available online: https://www.amnestyusa.org/pdfs/JailedWithoutJustice.pdf (accessed on 7 July 2021).

Amnesty International. 2020. USA: 'We are Adrift, about to Sink': The Looming COVID-19 Disaster in United States Immigration Detention Facilities. Available online: https://www.amnesty.org/en/documents/amr51/2095/2020/en/ (accessed on 16 June 2021).

Amon, Joseph J. 2020. COVID-19 and Detention: Respecting Human Rights. *Health and Human Rights Journal*. Available online: https://www.hhrjournal.org/2020/03/covid-19-and-detention-respecting-human-rights/ (accessed on 16 June 2021).

Bosworth, Mary, and Emma Kaufman. 2011. Foreigners in a Carceral Age: Immigration and Imprisonment in the United States. *Stanford Law & Policy Review* 22: 429–54.

Bowen, Allison Michelle. 2020. The Importance of Standardized Data Collection and Reporting in Improving Medical Care for Immigration Detainees. *Saint Louis University Journal of Health Law & Policy* 13: 291–316.

Brennan Center for Justice. 2021. Immigration Detention and Covid-19. Available online: https://www.brennancenter.org/our-work/research-reports/immigration-detention-and-covid-19 (accessed on 16 June 2021).

Burris, Scott. 1992. Prisons, Law and Public Health: The Case for a Coordinated Response to Epidemic Disease behind Bars. *University of Miami Law Review* 47: 291–336. [PubMed]

Caloz-Tschopp, Marie-Claire. 1997. On the Detention of Aliens: The Impact on Democratic Rights. *Journal of Refugee Studies* 10: 165–80. [CrossRef]

Chelgren, Whitney. 2011. Preventive Detention Distorted: Why it is Unconstitutional to Detain Immigrants Without Procedural Protections. *Loyola of Los Angeles Law Review* 44: 1477–528.

Chishti, Muzaffar, and Sarah Pierce. 2020. Crisis within a Crisis: Immigration in the United States in a Time of COVID-19. *Migration Policy Institute*. March 26. Available online: https://www.migrationpolicy.org/article/crisis-within-crisis-immigration-time-covid-19 (accessed on 16 June 2021).

Cho, Eunice. 2020. Immigration Detention Was a Black Box Before COVID-19. Now, it's a Death Trap. *ACLU*. April 30. Available online: https://www.aclu.org/news/immigrants-rights/immigration-detention-was-a-black-box-before-covid-19-now-its-a-death-trap/ (accessed on 16 June 2021).

Del Valle, Gaby, and José Olivares. 2020. Immigrants at Privately Run ICE Detention Center were Thrown Out of Wheelchairs when they Asked for Medical Help. *The Intercept*. July 23. Available online: https://theintercept.com/2020/07/23/ice-guards-excessive-force-sick-immigrants/ (accessed on 16 June 2021).

Detention Watch Network. 2020a. Courting Catastrophe: How ICE is Gambling with Immigrant Lives Amid a Global Pandemic. Available online: https://www.detentionwatchnetwork.org/pressroom/reports/2020/courting-catastrophe-how-ice-gambling-immigrant-lives-amid-global-pandemic (accessed on 16 June 2021).

Detention Watch Network. 2020b. Hotbeds of Infection: How ICE Detention Contributed to the Spread of COVID-19 in the United States. Available online: https://www.detentionwatchnetwork.org/pressroom/releases/2020/hotbeds-infection-new-report-details-contribution-ice-s-failed-pandemic (accessed on 16 June 2021).

Dow, Mark. 2004. *American Gulag: Inside Immigration Prisons*. Berkeley and Los Angeles: University of California Press.

Driesbach, Eamon N. 2020. COVID-19 case rates among ICE detainees 13 times higher than US average. *Healio News*. November 4. Available online: https://www.healio.com/news/infectious-disease/20201104/covid19-case-rates-among-ice-detainees-13-times-higher-than-us-average (accessed on 16 June 2021).

Eagly, Ingrid V., and Steven Shafer. 2015. A National Study of Access to Counsel in Immigration Court. *University of Pennsylvania Law Review* 164: 1–91.

Flynn, Meagan. 2020. ICE delayed its pandemic response, putting detainees at 'substantial' risk of harm, judge finds. *The Washington Post*. April 21. Available online: https://www.washingtonpost.com/nation/2020/04/21/ice-coronavirus-detention-ruling/ (accessed on 16 June 2021).

Freedom for Immigrants. 2020. COVID-19 in ICE Custody Biweekly Analysis & Update, April 14. Available online: https://www.freedomforimmigrants.org/s/FFI-April-14-COVID-19-FINAL.pdf (accessed on 16 June 2021).

Freedom for Immigrants. 2021. COVID-19 in ICE Custody Biweekly Analysis & Update, March 26. Available online: https://www.freedomforimmigrants.org/s/March-Conditions-Report-_FINAL.pdf (accessed on 16 June 2021).

Garcia, Michael John. 2009. The U.N. Convention Against Torture: Overview of U.S. Implementation Policy Concerning the Removal. Available online: https://www.hsdl.org/?abstract&did=38823 (accessed on 16 June 2021).

García Hernández, César Cuauhtémoc, and Carlos Moctezuma García. 2020. Close Immigration Prisons Now. *The New York Times*. March 19. Available online: https://www.nytimes.com/2020/03/19/opinion/coronavirus-immigration-prisons.html (accessed on 16 June 2021).

Global Detention Project. 2010. Immigration Detention and the Law: U.S. Policy and Legal Framework. Available online: https://www.globaldetentionproject.org/immigration-detention-and-the-law-us-policy-and-legal-framework (accessed on 16 June 2021).

Global Detention Project. 2021. United States Overview. Available online: https://www.globaldetentionproject.org/countries/americas/united-states (accessed on 16 June 2021).

Hing, Bill Ong. 2010. Systemic Failure: Mental Illness, Detention, and Deportation. *U.C. Davis Journal of International Law & Policy* 16: 341–82.

Hsu, Spencer S. 2020. U.S. judge orders ICE to say how many detained migrants are being released under expanded coronavirus medical reviews. *The Washington Post*. April 9. Available online: https://www.washingtonpost.com/local/legal-issues/us-judge-orders-ice-to-say-how-many-detained-migrants-are-being-released-under-expanded-coronavirus-medical-reviews/2020/04/09/aaecf0b0-79b6-11ea-9bee-c5bf9d2e3288_story.html (accessed on 16 June 2021).

Human Rights Watch. 2018. Code Red: The Fatal Consequences of Dangerously Substandard Medical Care in Immigration Detention. Available online: https://www.hrw.org/report/2018/06/20/code-red/fatal-consequences-dangerously-substandard-medical-care-immigration# (accessed on 16 June 2021).

Immigration Justice Campaign. 2020. Parole from ICE Detention: An Overview of the Law. On File with Author. Available online: https://immigrationjustice.us/get-trained/covid-19-updates/ (accessed on 16 June 2021).

Jefferis, Danielle C. 2020. Constitutionally Unaccountable: Privatized Immigration Detention. *Indiana Law Journal* 95: 145–82.

Kennedy, Patrick. 2020. ICE Detention Contracts, Third-Party Beneficiary Suits, and Private Contractors in Immigration Detention. *Marquette Law Review* 104: 465–510.

Kimball, Kimere Jane. 2009. A Right to be Heard: Non-Citizens' Due Process Right to In-Person Hearings to Justify Their Detentions Pursuant to Removal. *Stanford Journal of Civil Rights & Civil Liberties* 5: 159–90.

Kinner, Stuart A., Jesse T. Young, Kathryn Snow, Louse Southalan, Daniel Lopez-Acuña, Carina Ferreira-Borges, and Éamonn O'Moore. 2020. Prisons and custodial settings are part of a comprehensive response to COVID-19. *The Lancet*. March 17. Available online: https://www.thelancet.com/journals/lanpub/article/PIIS2468-2667(20)30058-X/fulltext (accessed on 16 June 2021).

Koulish, Robert. 2016. Immigration Detention in the Risk Classification Assessment Era. *Connecticut Public Interest Law Journal* 16: 1–37.

Langona, Kim. 2020. Ongoing Litigation Over Migrants' Release Amid COVID-19. *Crimmigration*. April 3. Available online: http://crimmigration.com/2020/04/03/ongoing-litigation-over-migrants-release-amid-covid-19/ (accessed on 16 June 2021).

Legomsky, Stephen H. 1999. The Detention of Aliens: Theories, Rules, and Discretion. *The University of Miami Inter-American Law Review* 30: 531–49.

Lipscombe, Carl Kenneth. 2013. Tylenol and an Ice Pack: An Inadequate Prescription for HIV/AIDS in Immigration Detention Centers. *Cardozo Public Law, Policy & Ethics Journal* 11: 529–62.

Meyer, Jaimie P., Carlos Franco-Paredes, Parveen Parmar, Faiza Yasin, and Matthew Gartland. 2020. COVID-19 and the coming epidemic in US immigration detention centers. *The Lancet*. April 15. Available online: https://www.thelancet.com/journals/laninf/article/PIIS1473-3099%2820%2930295-4/fulltext (accessed on 16 June 2021).

Morehouse, Angela. 2010. Changes in the Wind: How Increased Detention Rates, New Medical Care Standards, and ICE Policy Shifts Alter the Debate on Immigrant Detainee Healthcare. *Intercultural Human Rights Law Review* 5: 187–240.

Mukhopadhyay, Riddhi. 2009. Death in Detention: Medical and Mental Health Consequences of Indefinite Detention of Immigrants in the United States. *Seattle Journal for Social Justice* 7: 693–736.

Noferi, Mark. 2014. Making Civil Immigration Detention Civil, and Examining the Emerging U.S. Civil Detention Program. *Journal of Civil Rights and Economic Development* 27: 533–87.

Noferi, Mark. 2016. Mandatory Immigration Detention for U.S. Crimes: The Noncitizen Presumption of Dangerousness. In *Immigration Detention, Risk and Human Rights*. Edited by Maria João Guia, Robert Koulish and Valsamis Mitsilegas. Cham: Springer, ISBN 978-3-319-79660-4.

Noferi, Mark, and Robert Koulish. 2014. The Immigration Detention Risk Assessment. *Georgetown Immigration Law Journal* 29: 45–93.

Olivares, José. 2020. ICE's Immigration Detainees Protested Lack of Coronavirus Precautions—And Swat-Like Private-Prison Guards Pepper-Sprayed Them. *The Intercept*. May 5. Available online: https://theintercept.com/2020/05/05/ice-stewart-immigration-detention-coronavirus-protest-pepper-spray/ (accessed on 16 June 2021).

Papst, Kelsey E. 2009. Protecting the Voiceless: Ensuring ICE's Compliance with Standards That Protect Immigration Detainees. *McGeorge Law Review* 40: 261–290.

Pyntikova, Eugenia. 2010. Mental Illness in Immigration Detention Facilities: Searching for the Rights to Receive & Refuse Treatment. *Georgetown Immigration Law Journal* 25: 151–76.

Ryo, Emily, and Ian Peacock. 2018. The Landscape of Immigration Detention in the United States. American Immigration Council Special Report. Available online: https://www.americanimmigrationcouncil.org/research/landscape-immigration-detention-united-states (accessed on 15 June 2021).

Saadi, Altaf. 2020. Understanding U.S. Immigration Detention: Reaffirming Rights and Addressing Social-Structural Determinants of Health. *Health and Human Rights Journal* 22: 187–98.

Scaffidi, Elizabeth. 2021. US should end use of private 'for profit' detention centres, urge human rights experts. *United Nations News*. February 4. Available online: https://news.un.org/en/story/2021/02/1083862 (accessed on 16 June 2021).

Sinha, Anita. 2016. Arbitrary Detention: The Immigration Detention Bed Quota. *Duke Journal of Constitutional Law and Policy* 12: 77.

Skinner, Gwynne. 2008. Bringing International Law to Bear on the Detention of Refugees in the United States. *Willamette Journal of International Law and Dispute Resolution* 16: 270–99.

Sowder, D. Stuart. 1992. AIDS in Prison: Judicial Indifference to the AIDS Epidemic in Correctional Facilities Threatens the Constitutionality of Incarceration. *New York Law School Law Review* 37: 663–88.

Stefanelli, Justine N. 2020. *Judicial Review of Immigration Detention in the UK, US and EU: From Principles to Practice*. Oxford and New York: Hart Publishing.

Sthanki, Maunica. 2013. Deconstructing Detention: Structural Impunity and the Need for an Intervention. *Rutgers Law Review* 56: 447–504.

Tovino, Stacey A. 2016a. Of Mice and Men: On the Seclusion of Immigration Detainees and Hospital Patients. *Minnesota Law Review* 100: 2381–432.

Tovino, Stacy A. 2016b. The Grapes of Wrath: On the Health of Immigration Detainees. *Boston College Law Review* 57: 167–227.

U.S. Congress. 2021a. New Way Forward Act, H.R. 536, 117th Cong. Available online: https://www.congress.gov/bill/117th-congress/house-bill/536/text?q=%7B%22search%22%3A%5B%22new+way+forward%22%5D%7D&r=1&s=6 (accessed on 19 July 2021).

U.S. Congress. 2021b. Dignity for Detained Immigrants Act, S. 1186, 117th Cong. Available online: https://www.congress.gov/bill/117th-congress/house-bill/2222/all-info (accessed on 19 July 2021).

U.S. Department of Homeland Security Office of Inspector General, "About Us". 2017. Available online: https://www.oig.dhs.gov/about (accessed on 7 July 2021).

U.S. House of Representatives Committee on Homeland Security. 2020. Ice Detention Facilities: Failing to Meet Basic Standards of Care. Available online: https://homeland.house.gov/download/staff-report-ice-detention-facilities (accessed on 16 June 2021).

U.S. Immigration and Customs Enforcement. 2011. Performance-Based National Detention Standards. Available online: https://www.ice.gov/detain/detention-management/2011 (accessed on 16 June 2021).

U.S. Immigration and Customs Enforcement. 2019. National Detention Standards for Non-Dedicated Facilities. Available online: https://www.ice.gov/detain/detention-management/2019 (accessed on 16 June 2021).

U.S. Immigration and Customs Enforcement. 2020a. *Fiscal Year 2019 Enforcement and Removal Operations Report*. Available online: https://www.ice.gov/sites/default/files/documents/Document/2019/eroReportFY2019.pdf (accessed on 19 July 2021).

U.S. Immigration and Customs Enforcement. 2020b. Family Residential Standards. Available online: https://www.ice.gov/doclib/frs/2020/2020familyresidentialstandards.pdf (accessed on 7 July 2021).

U.S. Immigration and Customs Enforcement. 2021. *Fiscal Year 2020 Enforcement and Removal Operations Report*. Available online: https://www.ice.gov/doclib/news/library/reports/annual-report/eroReportFY2020.pdf (accessed on 19 July 2021).

United Nations Committee against Torture and Other Cruel, Inhuman or Degrading Treatment or Punishment. 2014. Concluding Observations on the Combined Third to Fifth Periodic Reports of the United States of America. CAT/C/USA/CO/3-5. Available online: https://digitallibrary.un.org/record/790513?ln=en (accessed on 16 June 2021).

United Nations Committee against Torture and Other Cruel, Inhuman or Degrading Treatment or Punishment. 2017. List of Issues Prior to Submission of the Sixth Periodic Report of the United States of America. UN Doc. CAT/C/USA/QPR/6. Available online: https://digitallibrary.un.org/record/1306808?ln=en (accessed on 16 June 2021).

United Nations General Assembly. 2016. Resolution Adopted by the General Assembly on 17 December 2016: United Nations Standard Minimum Rules for the Treatment of Prisoners (the Nelson Mandela Rules). U.N. Doc. No. A/RES/70/175, Adopted at the General Assembly's Seventieth Session. Available online: https://undocs.org/A/RES/70/175 (accessed on 7 July 2021).

United Nations Human Rights Committee. 1990. *Pinto v. Trinidad and Tobago* (Communication no. 232/1987), Report of the Human Rights Committee, vol. 2, UN Doc. A/45/40. Available online: http://www.worldcourts.com/hrc/eng/decisions/1990.07.20_Pinto_v_Trinidad_and_Tobago.htm (accessed on 16 June 2021).

United Nations Human Rights Committee. 1992. General Comment No. 21: Article 10 (Humane Treatment of Persons Deprived of Their Liberty). Available online: https://www.refworld.org/docid/453883fb11.html (accessed on 16 June 2021).

United Nations Human Rights Committee. 2014a. Concluding Observations on the Fourth Periodic Report of the United States of America. UN Doc. CCPR/C/USA/CO/4. Available online: https://digitallibrary.un.org/record/771176?ln=en (accessed on 16 June 2021).

United Nations Human Rights Committee. 2014b. General Comment No. 35: Article 9 (Liberty and Security of Person). UN Doc. CCPR/C/GC/35. Available online: https://tbinternet.ohchr.org/_layouts/15/treatybodyexternal/Download.aspx?symbolno=CCPR%2fC%2fGC%2f35&Lang=en (accessed on 16 June 2021).

United Nations Human Rights Committee. 2018. General Comment No. 36 on Article 6 of the International Covenant on Civil and Political Rights, on the Right to Life. UN Doc. CCPR/C/GC/36. Available online: https://tbinternet.ohchr.org/Treaties/CCPR/Shared%20Documents/1_Global/CCPR_C_GC_36_8785_E.pdf (accessed on 16 June 2021).

United Nations Human Rights Committee. 2019. List of Issues Prior to Submission of the Fifth Periodic Report of the United States of America. UN Doc. CCPR/C/USA/QPR/5. Available online: https://undocs.org/pdf?symbol=en/CCPR/C/USA/QPR/5 (accessed on 16 June 2021).

United Nations Working Group on Arbitrary Detention. 2010. Promotion and Protection of All Human Rights, Civil, Political, Economic, Social and Cultural Rights, Including the Right to Development. UN Doc. A/HRC/13/30. Available online: https://www2.ohchr.org/english/bodies/hrcouncil/docs/13session/A.HRC.13.30_AEV.pdf (accessed on 16 June 2021).

United Nations Working Group on Arbitrary Detention. 2017. Report of the Working Group on Arbitrary Detention on Its Visit to the United States of America. UN Doc. A/HRC/36/37/Add.2. Available online: https://digitallibrary.un.org/record/1655103?ln=en (accessed on 16 June 2021).

Vera Institute of Justice. 2020. How Local Leaders Can Ensure Immigrant Justice During COVID-19. Available online: https://www.vera.org/downloads/publications/coronavirus-guidance-local-leaders-immigrant-justice.pdf (accessed on 16 June 2021).

Wilsher, Daniel Wilsher. 2012. *Immigration Detention: Law, History, Politics*. Cambridge: Cambridge University Press.

World Health Organization. 2020. Director General's Opening Remarks at the Media Briefing on COVID-19. *WHO*. March 11. Available online: https://www.who.int/director-general/speeches/detail/who-director-general-s-opening-remarks-at-the-media-briefing-on-covid-19---11-march-2020 (accessed on 16 June 2021).

Zivec, Allyson. 2011. Don't Give Us Your Sick: Inadequate Medical Care in Immigration Detention Centers and How it Violates International Human Rights Law. *Phoenix Law Review* 5: 229–58.

Zwick, Keren. 2020. ICE Detention in the Time of COVID-19: Accounts from NIJC's Detained Clients. Available online: https://immigrantjustice.org/staff/blog/ice-detention-time-covid-19-accounts-nijcs-detained-clients (accessed on 16 June 2021).

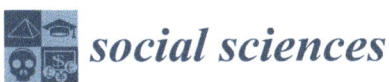

Article

The House Is on Fire but We Kept the Burglars Out: Racial Apathy and White Ignorance in Pandemic-Era Immigration Detention

Wenjie Liao [1], Kim Ebert [2,*], Joshua R. Hummel [2] and Emily P. Estrada [3]

[1] Department of Sociology and Anthropology, Rochester Institute of Technology, Rochester, NY 14623, USA; wxlgss@rit.edu
[2] Department of Sociology and Anthropology, North Carolina State University, Raleigh, NC 27607, USA; jrhummel@ncsu.edu
[3] Department of Sociology, SUNY Oswego, Oswego, NY 13126, USA; emily.estrada@oswego.edu
* Correspondence: klebert@ncsu.edu

Abstract: Past research shows that crises reveal the sensitive spots of established ideologies and practices, thereby providing opportunities for social change. We investigated immigration control amid the pandemic crisis, focusing on potential openings for both challengers and proponents of immigration detention. We asked: How have these groups responded to the pandemic crisis? Have they called for transformative change? We analyzed an original data set of primary content derived from immigrant advocates and stakeholders of the immigration detention industry. We found as the pandemic ravaged the world, it did not appear to result in significant cracks in the industry, as evidenced by the consistency of narratives dating back to pre-pandemic times. The American Civil Liberties Union's (ACLU) criticisms of inhumane conditions in immigration detention resembled those from its pre-pandemic advocacy. Private prison companies, including CoreCivic and GEO Group, emphasized their roles as ordinary businesses rather than detention managers during the pandemic, just as they had before the crisis. U.S. Immigration and Customs Enforcement (ICE), however, manufactured an alternative storyline, emphasizing "COVID fraud" as the real threat to the "Homeland." Although it did not call for radical change, it radically shifted its rhetoric in response to the pandemic. We discuss how these organizations' indifference towards structural racism contributes to racial apathy and how the obliviousness and irresponsibility of industry stakeholders resembles white ignorance.

Keywords: COVID; immigration detention; racial apathy; white ignorance; crimmigration; institutional legitimacy

Citation: Liao, Wenjie, Kim Ebert, Joshua R. Hummel, and Emily P. Estrada. 2021. The House Is on Fire but We Kept the Burglars Out: Racial Apathy and White Ignorance in Pandemic-Era Immigration Detention. *Social Sciences* 10: 358. https://doi.org/10.3390/socsci10100358

Academic Editor: Robert E. Koulish

Received: 28 July 2021
Accepted: 18 September 2021
Published: 27 September 2021

Publisher's Note: MDPI stays neutral with regard to jurisdictional claims in published maps and institutional affiliations.

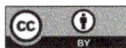

Copyright: © 2021 by the authors. Licensee MDPI, Basel, Switzerland. This article is an open access article distributed under the terms and conditions of the Creative Commons Attribution (CC BY) license (https://creativecommons.org/licenses/by/4.0/).

1. Introduction

The pandemic has been a time of crisis, a crisis of greater magnitude than most of us have ever experienced. In such times, people tend to seek stability and order to escape the chaos brought on by crises, turning to institutions of social control for a sense of normalcy and security, which can strengthen such institutions (Berger 2009; Olmo 1990). In the era of COVID-19, however, the precariousness and vulnerability brought on by the pandemic and people's reactions to it potentially destabilized institutions of social control. Indeed, conditions within places where people live and work together indoors, such as detention facilities,[1] accelerate the spread of the virus (Hooks and Libal 2020). Although immigration detention has long been the subject of scholarly and activist criticism (e.g., see Golash-Boza 2016; Kirkham 2012; Sullivan 2010), the devastating effects of the pandemic have prompted new and more urgent condemnations of the immigration detention industry and its practices. Meanwhile, the Movement for Black Lives (M4BL) has challenged the foundation of the criminal justice system, calling for transformative cultural and community changes that would involve the disbanding of police and defunding of prisons (Bell 2016; Carruthers 2018; M4BL 2019). Accordingly, the legitimacy of the immigration detention industry, which is embedded in the criminal justice system, has likely deteriorated further.

The pandemic and the corresponding condemnation of the industry, in addition to M4BL's compelling criticisms of the criminal justice system, have created an opportunity for immigrant advocates to call for radical, transformative change. We might expect the current environment to inspire the ACLU, for example, to advocate for changes such as "abolishing ICE" and ending immigration detention. We also might expect this context to prompt industry stakeholders to utilize explicitly racist and nativist narratives that pathologize migrant bodies, characterizing them as diseased, in order to rationalize enforcement, detention, and deportation. After all, migrants have historically been a convenient target for such discourse (Li and Nicholson 2021; Markel and Stern 1999). However, we know relatively little about the effects of the pandemic on not only immigrant advocacy but also the reactions of the immigration detention industry. Specifically, a dearth of research examines the apparent decline in the industry's legitimacy, the challenges from advocacy groups, and the responses of industry stakeholders. This gap is significant because the legitimacy or lack thereof of immigration detention has implications for the institution's future and the fates of thousands of migrants. Additionally, the discursive politics of immigration control, including immigration detention, is embedded in the broader immigration politics that inform ideologies and practices that affect all migrants and their communities far beyond the walls of detention facilities.

To address this gap, we qualitatively analyzed an original data set of primary content of over 700 public documents released in 2020 by the American Civil Liberties Union (ACLU), the private prison industry, including CoreCivic and the GEO Group, Inc. (hereafter, GEO), and the U.S. Immigration and Customs Enforcement (ICE). Using a critical race theory lens (Bracey 2015; Watkins Liu 2018), we examined what these groups say and what they do not say, considering that omissions and oversights could be equally as important as what is said. Given the white supremacist history of immigration policy (Glenn 2015; Golash-Boza et al. 2019), continued racist practices at every stage and level of immigration control and the criminal justice system more broadly (Alexander 2012; Aranda and Vaquera 2015; Armenta 2017; Arriaga et al. 2020), and overrepresentation of Black and Brown men in lockup[2] and deportation numbers (Golash-Boza 2016; Golash-Boza and Hondagneu-Sotelo 2013; Zarrugh 2020), it is telling if these groups fail to mention race in the immigration detention industry.

We found that the ACLU continues to criticize practices within immigration detention during the pandemic, but it does so within the confines of its pre-pandemic criticisms. Industry stakeholders also relied on pre-pandemic narratives. They are outwardly indifferent towards the pandemic crisis and relatively silent about their role in exacerbating the spread of the virus within detention facilities and the surrounding communities. Private prison companies continued to characterize themselves as ordinary service-providing businesses, bemoaning the financial losses due to the pandemic, thus demonstrating not only apathy but also insensitivity and recklessness towards individuals in detention facilities and to all adversely affected by the pandemic. Moreover, ICE not only appears unconcerned about the plight of at-risk and infected individuals in detention, but it has also manufactured an alternative storyline with a new enemy: "COVID fraud." In directing its efforts towards "Operation Stolen Promise," ICE overlooks its actions in enforcement, detainment, and deportation that amplified the deadly effects of the pandemic and emphasizes its role as protector of law and order of the "Homeland," demonstrating a remarkably irresponsible and cruel position. ICE ignores the pandemic spreading across the country like a wildfire and instead chooses to focus on those "stealing our promises."

These findings further our understanding of the discursive environment of U.S. immigration politics and offer critical insights into the processes of maintaining and challenging the status quo in the context of crises. They inform existing work on the racialization of migrants within immigration control in two meaningful respects. First, the seemingly contradictory narratives presented by the critics and enforcers of immigration detention during the pandemic did not effectively loosen the foundation of the institution. Altogether, this collection of claims contributes to *racial apathy* (Forman and Lewis 2006). The conversation remains largely disengaged with the interlocking systems of exclusion and exploitation underlying migrant suffering, thus minimizing the racism faced by migrants and reinforcing color blindness. Second, the storylines of the immigration detention industry contribute not only to racial apathy but to *white ignorance* as well (Mills 2007; Mueller 2020). This is evident in aspects of their accounts, including how they aggressively disregard the effects of the pandemic in detention and unmistakably overlook their role in spreading the virus. In the context of not only the pandemic but also Black movements that are effectively centering racial oppression on the global stage and promoting the dissolution and defunding of multiple aspects of the criminal justice system, ICE and private prison companies are so divorced from reality their obliviousness appears willful, aggressive, and militant.

2. Background: Immigration Detention in the Pandemic

COVID-19, caused by the novel, severe, acute respiratory syndrome coronavirus 2 (SARS-CoV-2), was first reported in December 2019 in Hubei Province, China. Since then, the World Health Organization has declared it a pandemic (WHO 2021). As of September 2021, over 200 million people globally have contracted the disease that led to more than 4.5 million deaths. The U.S. alone has totaled more than 40 million cases and over 500,000 deaths (Johns Hopkins Coronavirus Resource Center 2021).

As an industrialized country with unparalleled clinical and research capacity, the exceptionally high rates of COVID-19 in the U.S. are largely due to the federal government's failure in forming and executing effective policies in response to the pandemic (Carter and May 2020; Haffajee and Mello 2020). Among other things, the poor response to COVID-19 was a symptom of a medical system that prioritizes profits and reinforces health inequity (Carter and May 2020; Okonkwo et al. 2020).

For a multitude of reasons, migrants in detention are among the groups disproportionately impacted by the virus. Above all, institutionalized populations, such as those living in orphanages, nursing homes, and custodial settings, constitute some of the most vulnerable groups to infectious diseases as they live in close quarters with limited mobility (Barnett and Grabowski 2020; Marouf 2021; Wang et al. 2020). Their frequent interaction with staff members also increases the chance of cross-infection (Barnett and Grabowski 2020). Meanwhile, overcrowding, poor ventilation, rudimentary healthcare, lack of basic hygiene, and insufficient testing in prisons, jails, and immigration detention centers further exacerbate the danger of contagious diseases (Arriaga et al. 2020; Franco-Paredes et al. 2020; Keller and Wagner 2020). Such damning conditions, combined with the already elevated risk for a variety of diseases among migrant detainees due to existing health disparities (Meyer et al. 2020), have led to exceptionally high rates of COVID-19 in immigration detention centers (UCLA Law n.d.). The pandemic persists as we write. On one hand, the introduction of effective vaccines encourages cautious optimism. On the other hand, unequal access to vaccines and treatments both globally and domestically is accompanied by reports of outbreaks among the hardest hit and least protected populations, including migrants in detention. As of early September 2021, ICE reported that 27,149 detainees have tested positive for COVID-19 since the start of the pandemic and that nine people have died while in ICE custody (ICE Staff 2020c). However, researchers criticize these numbers, arguing ICE is severely underreporting the spread of the pandemic in its facilities. They estimate that the number of people in lockup who have contracted the virus is up to 15 times higher than what ICE has reported (Smart et al. 2021). Predictive models suggest that the vast majority of detainees will contract the disease even under the most optimistic scenario (Irvine et al. 2020).

Furthermore, immigrant detention in the pandemic presents a threat not only to migrant detainees but also to public health in general. Research indicates that prison staff also experience substantially higher COVID-19 case prevalence than the U.S. population overall (Ward et al. 2021) as they share "an environment known to amplify, accelerate, and act as a reservoir for outbreaks of respiratory diseases" with the prison inmates (Montoya-Barthelemy et al. 2020, p. 888). As staff members commute between work and home, carrying the virus into the communities where they live (Keller and Wagner 2020; Kinner et al. 2020), the local healthcare systems could have been or may still be overwhelmed as new variants spread, as most ICE detention facilities are often located in small, isolated towns (Eason 2017) with limited medical resources (Keller and Wagner 2020). Additionally, the frequent transfer of detainees among facilities risks transmitting the disease across different communities (Keller and Wagner 2020; Meyer et al. 2020).

Alerted by the rapid spread of COVID-19 among ICE detainees and detention facility staff, public health experts called for the release of most if not all ICE detainees to minimize the risk of exacerbating the pandemic (Lopez et al. 2021). While claiming to heed these suggestions, ICE continued its enforcement efforts throughout the pandemic and failed to adhere to COVID-19 safety guidelines (Dyer 2021; Miller et al. 2020). Given the record level of immigration detention under the Trump administration (Cho et al. 2020), ICE's (in)action during COVID-19 poses a tremendous risk to both the detainees and public health. Meanwhile, ICE also continued to deport migrants (e.g., ICE Staff 2020a), many from COVID-infested facilities and some diagnosed with the disease, demonstrating that the U.S. and its agencies are actively and knowingly spreading the virus globally (Miller et al. 2020; Montes 2020).

ICE's failure in addressing the COVID-19 crisis has not gone unnoticed. In addition to criticism from immigrant rights advocates such as the ACLU (e.g., see Cho 2020a), mainstream media have also covered the disastrous impacts of ICE's insufficient response to the pandemic both domestically (e.g., Hackman 2020; La Gorce 2020) and globally (e.g., Keller and Wagner 2020; Montes 2020). For instance, in April 2021, the *New York Times* (Niu et al. 2021) published a thorough account of ICE's mishandling of COVID-19 that ended with a call to release more detainees. Although immigration detention has long been the subject of scholarly and activist criticism (see Ebert et al. 2020 and references therein), the current pandemic appears to have provided a new entry point to expose the cruelty of the industry and to challenge its legitimacy. We therefore ask: Have critics of immigration detention taken advantage of this opening to expose and further delegitimize this practice? How has the immigration detention industry responded to its critics and the crisis?

3. Materials and Methods

3.1. Research Design

To answer these questions, we analyzed an original data set of primary content of over 700 documents released in 2020 by ACLU, the private prison industry (including CoreCivic and GEO Group), and ICE.[3] We selected these groups because they represent a diverse network of organizations with varying connections to and interests in immigration control, allowing us to examine criticisms and responses to those criticisms in relation to one another. We selected ACLU based on our investigation of news media coverage of immigration detention between 1995 and 2018 (see Ebert et al. 2020; Estrada et al. 2020). Among all of the quotes from representatives of advocacy organizations, ACLU was the most frequently quoted. The ACLU is a well-known civil rights organization with a long history of advocacy related to immigration detention. Because of this history, the ACLU holds a political "insider" status and maintains a degree of institutional authority on par with ICE and private prison companies. The ACLU is opposed to immigration detention that violates the rights of immigrants. Even though it has not historically been opposed to immigration detention, per se, we included the ACLU in this study because we were curious if the pandemic prompted it to fundamentally shift its position regarding immigration detention.

Because private prison companies have physical custody of over 70% of immigrants detained in the U.S. (Freedom for Immigrants 2018), which generates a substantial portion of their revenue (Gilman and Romero 2018), they also have a vested interest in maintaining the legitimacy of immigration detention. Thus, the way they frame immigrant detention during the pandemic is central to addressing our research questions. We selected CoreCivic and GEO Group[4] specifically because they are the two largest publicly traded prison companies and constitute more than 50% of the market share in private immigration detention (Juárez et al. 2018; Oliver 2018). Finally, ICE is the federal agency empowered to enforce and regulate immigration policies, and, as such, holds a degree of power, status, and resources beyond what is available to other groups. ICE has a vested interest in promoting dominant ideologies that legitimate immigration control, a system from which it benefits (Jackman 1994; Lamont et al. 2014). Thus, the way ICE frames immigration detention in the midst of the pandemic provides insight into how powerful groups legitimate and reproduce inequality in the context of a crisis.

We based our analysis on documents available to the public because they provide insight into the "front stage" image a group is trying to project (Goffman 1959). Press releases, in particular, represent an official view on a topic, designed to project a carefully crafted and negotiated public image or argument. In order to maintain legitimacy, organizations will often engage in " ... elaborate displays of confidence, satisfaction, and good faith ... " (Meyer and Rowan 1977, p. 358) to demonstrate to the public that their goals have merit and their methods in achieving these goals are reputable. Furthermore, press releases serve as a source of other media, such as the news media (Majstorović 2007), and are important for the dissemination of seemingly convincing messages (Bail 2012). Thus, discussions of the pandemic within these documents provide a measure of how groups used the "opportunity" of the crisis to reframe their positions in relation to the immigrant detention industry.

3.2. Data Collection

To collect data from the ACLU, we searched all press releases and blog posts in 2020 that the ACLU released under the topic "Immigrants' Rights and Detention." This search returned 32 press releases and 23 blog posts. Most of these—28 and 13, respectively—covered COVID-19 in immigration detention, primarily pertaining to the increased risks of the virus among migrants in lockup. The majority of those that did not discuss the pandemic (eight of 14) were published prior to 12 March 2020,[5] in the weeks before the pandemic became widespread in the U.S., and the remaining six covered topics ranging from abortion access to unlawful detainment of migrants. We searched the websites of CoreCivic and GEO Group to gather their press releases. We also searched Wayback Machine and GlobeNewswire after discovering that the companies do not include all of their past press releases on their websites. Altogether, these searches returned 38 CoreCivic press releases and 16 GEO Group press releases from 2020, of which 22 and four, respectively, mentioned the pandemic in some capacity. Eleven of the remaining 28 were released prior to 12 March 2020, and the other 17 discussed such topics as financial reports, new policies and programs (such as reentry-focused legislation), and facility contract information. To collect data from ICE, we examined 631 news releases from 2020. In the heading of each news release, ICE included a label that identified the topic of the news release, such as "Enforcement and Removal," "Narcotics," and "Operational." Of its 631 news releases, 170 were released prior to 12 March and of the remaining 461, ICE labeled 49 of these "COVID-19."

3.3. Data Analysis

We began data analysis in summer 2020 with the intent of examining how narratives changed during the early months of the pandemic, specifically with documents from January through April 2020. We began by conducting a pilot analysis of approximately 10% of the data, taking notes on patterns that emerged from the text. This preliminary analysis served as the foundation of a codebook that the four-person research team developed across multiple meetings and rounds of testing. After reaching an intercoder reliability score of 90%, we divided the remaining data between authors for systematic coding. We used NVivo, a qualitative software program that facilitates the coding process and provides a systematic way of analyzing data, for paragraph-level coding of documents that mentioned COVID-19 (or a variation of the term).

During this phase of coding, we continued to meet regularly to discuss concerns and periodically conduct further intercoder reliability checks. Through these conversations, we realized that, to fully address our research question on how groups have responded to the pandemic crisis, we needed to expand data analysis to include documents from the entirety of 2020. We also realized the importance of including documents that did not specifically address COVID-19 but were nonetheless published during this period, which allowed us to consider what these organizations were talking about when their conversations did not center on the pandemic. Thus, we expanded our initial data collection and analysis efforts to include all documents published in the year 2020. In addition, we supplemented our primary data with a sample of news media coverage[6] on both the pandemic and the immigration detention industry in order to contextualize the emergent patterns.

4. Results

4.1. The Continuing Attack on Inhumane Conditions in Immigration Detention: ACLU

The ACLU responds to the COVID-19 pandemic by taking a critical stance on the conditions within detention—not on detention itself. Of the 32 press releases and 23 blog posts regarding immigration detention from 2020, the majority (28 and 13, respectively) focused on COVID-19 in immigration detention. Given the current social context of the pandemic, ACLU relied more heavily on narratives related to the health risks of imprisoned migrants rather than other factors. Often, this narrative involved ACLU presenting living conditions within detention facilities as a public health issue that creates unnecessary health risks for detained immigrants. In the following, Andre Segura, legal director for the ACLU of Texas, described these risks, arguing that immigration detention is a "clear violation of their constitutional rights":

> Detention centers like the Montgomery Processing Center cannot adequately protect the lives of those like our clients: There is no way to practice social distancing in a detention center, and they do not have access to face masks or even regular access to basic hygiene. Limiting the number of people held in jails is critical to prevent a COVID-19 outbreak at MPC and the surrounding community. (ACLU Staff 2020b)

The ACLU's critical stance towards aspects of immigrant detention, however, was not limited to the context of the pandemic alone. In some cases, the ACLU used the pandemic and the increased health risks that it poses as evidence to support the ACLU's position on immigrant detention that predated the pandemic. The following quote from Bobby Hodgson, a staff attorney for the NYCLU, continued calls for ICE to end its "No-Release Policy" that began well before the COVID-19 pandemic (e.g., see Kang 2018):

> ICE improperly manipulated the detention process to imprison almost everyone they arrest, and right now that decision is putting many people in harm's way as COVID-19 spreads. (ACLU Staff 2020c)

Hodgson emphasized the vulnerability of immigrants as a result of the pandemic and used this victimization as a reason for ICE to act "right now." However, the pandemic itself is not what made ICE's "No-Release Policy" a problem. Other passages about immigration detention operations more generally displayed a similar pattern. The one below, for example, connected problems with immigration detention during the pandemic to a larger pattern of conduct associated with the Trump administration:

> The rapid spread of COVID-19 in immigration detention facilities is a prime example of everything that has gone wrong with immigration detention ... It is little coincidence that a disproportionate number of detention centers that now

have confirmed cases of COVID-19 came online under the Trump administration. (Cho 2020b)

In the passage, Cho used the pandemic as "a prime example" of problems related to immigration detention under the Trump administration. Rather than depicting COVID-19 as a qualitatively new problem and challenge for immigration detention, Cho employed the pandemic as the latest opportunity to criticize the Trump administration's overall handling of immigration detention without calling for radical change.

While COVID-19 is a prominent part of the passages above, the narratives mirror those that ACLU has used to discuss a number of pre-pandemic topics, such as detention conditions and family separation. Typically, these narratives present immigrants as victims of poor physical and legal conditions at the hands of federal government entities. To provide one pre-pandemic example from January 2020, the following quote from Alanah Odoms Herber, ACLU of Louisiana executive director, explained how the Trump administration and immigration agencies victimized asylum seekers by failing to release them from detention on parole in Louisiana:

> Seeking asylum is a legal right, but the Trump administration has continued to subject asylum seekers . . . to unconscionable and unlawful cruelty . . . We will not stand by while ICE uses private contractors to detain and abuse vulnerable people exercising their right to seek asylum at our borders. (ACLU Staff 2020a)

As in passages from the pandemic, Herber's statement expressed how detained immigrants suffered "unconscionable and unlawful cruelty" at the hands of the Trump administration and other federal government branches. ACLU, then, did not entirely change its messaging to focus solely on the COVID-19 pandemic. Rather, it adapted many previous campaigns to fit within the altered context of immigrant detention in the pandemic era.

4.2. Business as Usual: Private Prison Companies

Private prison companies never discussed the increased risk of infection and spread of the virus in detention facilities, nor did they acknowledge their role in exacerbating the spread of the virus. Of its 16 press releases in 2020, GEO Group referenced the pandemic in four, but the virus was not the focal point of any of them. CoreCivic was more responsive; 22 of its 38 press releases in 2020 discussed COVID-19. However, of these 22, only 11 focused on the pandemic, including announcements regarding testing, deaths, and CoreCivic's Coronavirus Medical Action Plan. The other 11 mentioned the pandemic, but centered on other topics such as financial reports, contract information, and changes in corporate structure. Regardless of CoreCivic's increased acknowledgment of the virus, neither company actually responded to public criticisms of detention in the pandemic era.

When referencing their operations in the context of the pandemic, private prison companies often characterized COVID-19 as a threat to business, and they presented their response to the crisis in a favorable light. They discussed their handling of the pandemic in ways similar to how other businesses might respond to any other challenge. The following quote from Damon Hininger, president and CEO of CoreCivic, illustrates this:

> This pandemic is creating unprecedented challenges for businesses and industries... But I believe it can also be an opportunity for organizations to support current employees and help those who may be looking for a new career following a job loss. We are proud to step forward to help in both of these ways. (CoreCivic Staff 2020a)

Here, Hininger distanced CoreCivic from the negative consequences of ongoing immigration detention amid a pandemic to present the company as a positive opportunity for prospective employees in a time when jobs were scarce. Although certainly insensitive to the people who suffered serious health consequences of COVID-19, this tactic of discussing the pandemic in economic terms was common. The passage below from a GEO Group press release, for example, used the pandemic to explain decreases in the number of people it detained and resultant "lower full-year 2020 revenues":

> Our ICE Processing Centers and U.S. Marshals Service facilities began experiencing lower overall occupancy in late March 2020 as a result of declines in crossings and apprehensions along the U.S. Southwest border, as well as, a decrease in court and sentencing activity at the federal level in the United States due to the COVID-19 pandemic. (GEO Group Staff 2020a)

Beyond perpetuating the abstraction of detained people as a profit-generating capacity (Doty and Wheatley 2013; Douglas and Sáenz 2013; Golash-Boza 2016), this passage enabled GEO Group to identify the pandemic as a force defined by its loss of corporate dollars rather than human lives.

When private prison companies acknowledged the effect of the pandemic on individuals, this discussion tended to happen in economic terms with a focus on their employees—not on the individuals they imprison. For example, after discussing the financial impact of the pandemic on GEO Group, the chairperson and CEO, George Zoley, thanked employees:

> During the second quarter, we experienced some favorable cost trends that resulted in better than expected financial performance. While we are encouraged by these favorable trends, our company continues to face challenges associated with the COVID-19 pandemic, which has had a negative operational and financial impact across several segments of our company. In the face of these challenges, our frontline employees have shown incredible commitment and perseverance, helping our company manage through these difficult times, and we are thankful for their dedication and daily sacrifice. (GEO Group Staff 2020b)

Rather than discussing how the pandemic affected the people that GEO Group detains, Zoley described the economic challenges and thanked the employees for sacrificing themselves. The CEO of CoreCivic went so far as to highlight the company's beneficent approach towards its employees by rewarding them a $500 Hero bonus for "steadfastly answering the call to serve and protect our communities and those in our care." Hininger explained, "The bonus program is one way we can show our appreciation for their focus and dedication during this challenging time" (CoreCivic Staff 2020a). Once again, any discussion of the companies' commitment to ensure the safety of the individuals they imprison was conspicuously absent.

Despite attempts to focus on their role as an ordinary service-providing business in the midst of the pandemic, private prison companies could not completely escape acknowledging the actual service they provide: prison management. When discussing this aspect of their business, private prison companies described the need for more cautious operations posed by the pandemic and their fulfillment of necessary changes without addressing the increased risk of infection and spread of the virus in detention facilities or acknowledging their role in accelerating the spread of COVID-19. This message appeared as an affirmation that private prison companies prepared and implemented plans to protect those in detention facilities. For example,

> CoreCivic is working hard to protect our employees, those entrusted to our care, and our communities during the COVID-19 pandemic. We have a Coronavirus Medical Action Plan in place at each of our facilities, which we've been working on since January. (CoreCivic Staff 2020c)

In this passage, CoreCivic framed itself as a good steward that developed widespread policies to protect its employees, wards, and communities. As it related to detained immigrants, "those entrusted to our care" is a vague and palatable phrase that reinforces CoreCivic's paternalistic authority over a vulnerable and dependent population. When evidence suggested that detention during the COVID-19 pandemic poses a high risk of transmission, private prison companies reaffirmed their implementation of sufficient safety practices and used descriptions of cases as "asymptomatic" to minimize the perceived harm caused by COVID-19 (e.g., see CoreCivic Staff 2020b). These descriptions of COVID-19 cases within facilities framed private prison companies as beneficent caregivers, which, in turn, deflected attention away from the dangers faced by immigrant detainees related to confinement in a pandemic.

4.3. Silence and the "Stolen Promise": ICE

Instead of applying a generous spin to its role in immigration detention that resembled those used by private prison companies, ICE generally avoided discussing the effects of the pandemic within detention altogether. As an alternative, ICE turned to the "customs" side of its operations to present itself as the solution to a so-called COVID-19 contraband crisis.

ICE's unique presentation of the pandemic became apparent when comparing it both to other organizations' pandemic coverage and to its own pre-pandemic news releases. In 2020, ICE produced 631 news releases, 49 (8%) of which mentioned COVID-19 in some capacity. Notably, 8% is a much smaller relative share of documents compared to those produced by the ACLU (41 of 55, or 75%) or GEO Group and CoreCivic (26 of 55, or 48%) during the same time. While this is not entirely surprising given that each are different groups with distinct (but overlapping) foci, the magnitude of the difference in coverage is still striking, particularly when we examined the content of the material. Prior to the pandemic, ICE typically presented itself as an "immigration" agency that handled enforcement through practices such as detention and deportation. When discussing the pandemic in its 2020 coverage, however, ICE appeared much less consistent in its emphasis on immigration enforcement.

Of the 49 news releases, only six discussed ICE's response to the pandemic within detention facilities, such as reports of people in detention testing positive for the virus and announcements of testing in facilities. For example, Henry Lucero, executive associate director for ICE's Enforcement and Removal Operations (ERO), talked about ICE's plans to prioritize testing for families in detention:

> We take the responsibility to care for the families in our custody very seriously and we are working with all of our partners to determine how to reduce the spread of COVID-19, not only at our FRCs, but at all locations housing ICE detainees. (ICE Staff 2020b)

Here, ICE directly addressed the effects of the virus within its facilities and described its "caring" response, a notable rarity in its news releases given its insistent silence on the prevalence of the virus within its facilities. One possible reason for the small number of news releases directly describing ICE's response to the pandemic in detention facilities might be that ICE developed a webpage devoted to COVID-19 guidance, which was initially posted on 14 March 2020 (ICE Staff 2020c). However, there was a meaningful, qualitative difference between the two forms of communication. A webpage devoted to COVID-19 in detention is not as publicly visible and proactive as press releases and, accordingly, is likely something that would only be discovered by parties actively seeking it out. On the other hand, press releases are documents meant for more widespread public consumption. Given these differences, it is telling that ICE did not actively release many public statements about its response to the virus and instead, relegated this coverage to a single webpage.

Instead of publicly addressing the risks of detention during the COVID-19 pandemic, ICE diverted attention elsewhere in the vast majority of its public content. Oftentimes, ICE focused on other operations and policies that were in place pre-pandemic. Out of the 49 press releases that mentioned COVID-19, 10 addressed policy updates, such as increases in flexibility in workplace compliance and updates to the Student and Exchange Visitor Program (SEVP), and nine discussed additional operations in place, including "removal flights." For example, a news release reported on the return of 209 U.S. citizens "on the return leg of two removal flights via ICE Air Operations":

> ICE will continue to work with the State Department to facilitate the safe return of U.S. citizens on future removal flight returns from Guatemala, Honduras and

El Salvador throughout the duration of the COVID-19 pandemic. (ICE Staff 2020a)

In such announcements, ICE emphasized its benevolent role in providing the safe return of U.S. citizens, and, in turn, downplayed its unpleasant role in deportations. ICE did not refer to these as "deportations" but instead used the term "removals," further masking its distasteful practice of continuing deportations amid a global pandemic, which served to spread the virus globally (Kassie and Marcolini 2020). Again, instead of addressing the risks of enforcement, detention, and deportation during the COVID-19 pandemic and its role in amplifying the risks, ICE continued its pre-pandemic narratives of focusing on policies and procedures that existed before the crisis.

ICE not only minimized the seriousness of deportations and detention in its news releases but also diverted attention away from the severity of the pandemic within detention facilities and from its own failures and transgressions. ICE's creation of an alternate reality, in which it functioned primarily as a customs agency that protects Americans from the alleged threat of "COVID fraud", is especially illustrative of this pattern. While ICE discussed the customs side of its operations in a handful of pre-pandemic news releases from 2020, it primarily did so in its limited coverage of counterfeit merchandise (five out of the 175 news releases prior to 12 March 2020[7]). Of the 49 news releases that mentioned the virus, however, approximately half (n = 24) covered COVID-related criminal activity, including news releases on "COVID fraud."

For example, ICE announced the launch of Operation Stolen Promise in April 2020 "to protect the Homeland from the increasing and evolving threat posed by COVID-19-related fraud and criminal activity" (ICE Staff 2020e). On 30 November, it announced Operation Stolen Promise 2.0 "with the specific goal of countering the threat of counterfeit vaccines, treatments and supplies" (ICE Staff 2020g). ICE framed the fraud as a major problem amid the pandemic that required ICE's attention: "Surging criminal activity surrounding the COVID-19 pandemic requires an equally robust investigative response to protect the American public" (ICE Staff 2020e). In announcing its efforts to combat "COVID fraud," ICE relied on nationalist and racist language to celebrate its role as protector of "the Homeland," ensuring the "health and safety of the American public" (ICE Staff 2020f). It also publicized that NBC's Today Show and ABC's Good Morning America featured its "efforts to combat COVID-19 fraud" (ICE Staff 2020d), creating the image that mainstream media (and, hence, likely the public) approve of its work.

For ICE, then, immigration control during the pandemic was more about touting its valiant efforts protecting Americans from potential foreign contraband and criminals than about protecting detained immigrants from an actual deadly pandemic within its detention facilities. It is not surprising that ICE failed to acknowledge its role in spreading the virus in communities throughout the U.S. and across the globe, but it is remarkable how little attention ICE paid to the effects of the pandemic on people it imprisons and deports.

5. Discussion: Racial Apathy and White Ignorance

Berger (2009, p. 493) argued that "[c]rises present ruptures, breaks in the norm that provide opportunities to exacerbate or overturn existing ideologies and practices." Given this and the well-documented threat immigration detention poses to public health during a pandemic, we might have expected ACLU to adopt new and more subversive arguments against the institution. In the context of the global racial justice movement, we might have expected these new arguments to target structural racism as the root cause of the violations of immigrant rights and to call for radical change, such as ending detention entirely and abolishing ICE. We might also have expected the current context of the pandemic to inspire industry stakeholders to use historical narratives that pathologize migrant bodies, characterizing them as diseased, in order to rationalize enforcement, detention, and deportation (Li and Nicholson 2021; Markel and Stern 1999).

Our results suggested that, although each organization adapted its narratives about immigration detention to various degrees, the pandemic did not lead to significant cracks in the system. We argue that the collection of varying and dialogic frames contributes to *racial apathy*, as they remain largely indifferent to the interlocking systems of exclusion and exploitation underlying migrant suffering, thus minimizing the racism migrants experience and reinforcing color blindness. In 2020, private prison companies, ICE, and ACLU, failed to mention anything about how the immigration system in the U.S. was built to maintain a certain racial order, i.e., white supremacy (Sáenz and Douglas 2015). In other words, they assumed the immigration system's racial innocence (Murakawa and Beckett 2010). Under such assumption, it is extremely difficult, if not impossible, to challenge the system itself and propose transformative change: If the system is innocent, one can only critique the practices. Meanwhile, the system, through the frames presented by ICE and private prison companies and even ACLU, continues to depict migrants as "exotic others," i.e., criminals, profitable bodies, victims to be saved and cared for, etc. As such, while the frames from ACLU appeared to contradict those from ICE and private prison companies, the narratives presented by the three parties formed a dialogue that naturalizes "immigrant" as a degraded category and immigration detention as a legitimate institution, despite its sometimes questionable practices.

Furthermore, we argue that, in the context of not only the pandemic but also Black movements that are effectively placing racial oppression on the global stage and promoting the dissolution and defunding of multiple aspects of the criminal justice system, the frameworks of industry stakeholders, including ICE and private prison companies, contribute to racial apathy as well as the epistemology of *white ignorance*. Mills (2007, p. 13) introduced it as follows:

> Imagine an ignorance militant, aggressive, not to be intimidated, an ignorance that is active, dynamic, that refuses to go quietly—not at all confined to the illiterate and uneducated but propagated at the highest levels of the land, indeed presenting itself unblushingly as knowledge.

This militant unawareness denies the racial reality that defines the structure of American society. In doing so, it reinforces the racial order of white supremacy. Aspects of white ignorance are evident in accounts by ICE and private prison companies, including the ways in which they aggressively disregarded the effects of the pandemic in detention and unmistakably overlooked their role in spreading the virus. In the current context, they appear so divorced from reality that their obliviousness appears proactive. In the following, we further discuss how the groups contribute to the process of racial apathy and the epistemology of white ignorance.

5.1. Comfortable and Convenient Criticism: ACLU

In 2020, ACLU did not call for transformative change in response to the pandemic. Much of ACLU's coverage of COVID-19 within immigrant detention aligned with critical framing against immigration detention prior to the pandemic, where news media coverage focused on human rights violations within these facilities and bad management practices (Ebert et al. 2020). Although the content of its press releases and blogs may have contained strongly worded language (e.g., referring to immigration detention as a "death trap," calling for Congress to "reduce funding to ICE for detention operations and shift to community-based alternatives to immigration detention that are not driven by profit" (Cho 2020b)), the targets of this criticism were specific individuals, practices, and organizations, not the existence of immigration detention. As such, ACLU failed to question the legal system that categorizes certain migrants as "illegal."

ACLU's criticisms of immigration detention represented racial apathy in that its relatively superficial critiques resemble the "minimization of racism" frame of color-blind racism (Bonilla-Silva 2017). Though critiques related to human rights violations and bad management are clearly intended to advocate for the rights of migrants, ACLU avoids any discussions of how the racialization and criminalization of migrants serves to rationalize their expropriation. In this way, its rhetoric plays a role in minimizing systematic inequality and does little to question how "illegality" is socially constructed and rooted in global power dynamics (Armenta 2017; De Genova 2004; Golash-Boza 2016; Gómez Cervantes 2021; Menjívar 2021).

5.2. Profiting from Crises: Private Prison Companies

Private prison companies prioritized the concerns of their shareholders, their employees, and even themselves as businesses over the oppression and suffering of migrants. Despite acknowledging base concerns about the pandemic in their detention facilities, private prison companies failed to engage meaningfully with critiques from ACLU or other public health experts. Instead, CoreCivic and GEO Group framed the pandemic as threatening to business and employees. They continued to present themselves as ordinary businesses rather than prison operators, much in the same way as they did before the pandemic (Ebert et al. 2020). However, the companies also took advantage of the opportunity of this crisis to present themselves as solutions to the hardships created by the pandemic.

Given the pivotal role the industry played in spreading COVID-19 and in reinforcing a carceral state that deprives poor communities of color access to resources needed to respond to major disasters effectively, this form of self-presentation represents a distortion of reality that reinforces the epistemology of white ignorance. Such narratives resemble those emerging from the aftermath of many other crises: The most dispossessed groups (in this case, migrant detainees, poor communities, and communities of color with little access to medical resources or space for quarantine) suffer disproportionately as a direct consequence of neoliberal reforms (in this case, privatized mass incarceration), yet these groups are relegated back to the same oppressive private market that is thought to be the most "efficient" place to fulfill their needs after the disaster (Silva 2016). Naomi Klein (2010) described this phenomenon as disaster capitalism, wherein beneficiaries of neoliberal marketization exploit the fear and disorientation generated by unexpected crises to further advocate for their agenda. These strategies are not surprising given the private prison companies' financial interests and pre-COVID narratives, but they nonetheless provide insight into how, without directly vilifying or criminalizing migrants, the companies implicate immigrant detainees as the "Other," whose well-being is of little concern.

5.3. Smoke and Mirrors and Moral Panics: ICE

In contrast to both the ACLU and the private prison industry, ICE attempted to take advantage of the pandemic by creating an alternative reality that not only excused itself from its responsibilities in worsening the pandemic through immigration detention but also reinforced its role as enforcer and protector of law and order. Although it maintained its self-characterization as a law-and-order agency, the agency manufactured a moral panic (Cohen 2011; Flores-Yeffal et al. 2019) to change its, and thus America's, enemy from "illegal" immigrant to foreign contraband. Nonetheless, this new focus continued to criminalize and dehumanize immigrants as threats, classifying them as invisible criminal others who do not matter and racializing them without resorting to explicit racial language. Indeed, in the pandemic era, ICE characterized itself less as an "immigration" agency that manages enforcement and more as a "customs" agency that protects Americans from COVID-related fraud. By making this change, ICE deflected attention away from the increased risk of the virus among detained individuals and surrounding communities. This narrative instantiated white ignorance, expressed apathy towards immigrants, and demonstrated remarkable irresponsibility and cruelty towards those negatively impacted by the pandemic.

Instead of rationalizing immigration detention through characterizing migrants as diseased, ICE practically ceased discussion of immigration detention altogether. It is not surprising that ICE failed to acknowledge its role in spreading the virus, but what is surprising is how little attention ICE paid to the effects of the pandemic on people affected by its practices. Differences in uses of the pandemic aside, industry stakeholders, including private prison companies and ICE, stand together in their rare responses to criticisms of their practices and their silence about their role in exacerbating the negative effects of the pandemic. Again, these patterns reinforce white ignorance, in that they were indifferent towards migrants in detention and seemingly oblivious about the effects of the virus in detention and their role in spreading the virus within detention facilities and beyond. In its news releases, ICE seldom talked about the virus in detention facilities, as was the case with GEO Group and to a lesser extent CoreCivic. This silence is conspicuous.

The quietness of the industry is particularly evident when we examined calls from public health experts and news media coverage of the pandemic in these months. Our supplementary sample of *New York Times* (*NYT*) coverage of COVID-19 and the industry (see page 11) illustrated the peculiarity of ICE's and private prison companies' inaction and lack of attention paid to the pandemic within their facilities. In articles published from 12 March to 30 April 2020 that mentioned the industry and COVID-19, nearly all (30 out of 32) reported on problems and criticisms of (mostly) ICE's actions/efforts in heightening the negative effects of the pandemic in terms of detainment, enforcement, and deportation. For example, an 18 March article on the pandemic reported problems with ICE's inactions:

> Many ICE detainees say they feel like sitting ducks who will inevitably be infected. "The officials here have not said anything to us about what is happening outside, or any extra precautions that we should take," said a 40-year-old man from the Congo who is detained in a Karnes City, Texas, facility. (NYT Staff 2020b)

Another article reported on ICE's practice of continuing arrests in places with growing numbers of COVID-19 cases, noting that:

> One agency whose operations did not appear to have been affected by the outbreak was the U.S. Immigration and Customs Enforcement, or ICE, whose agents have continued to arrest immigrants around New York City over the past 10 days ... alarming advocates and lawyers who believe they could endanger vulnerable people who are already in custody. (NYT Staff 2020a)

The *NYT* articles discussed the role of the industry in amplifying the pandemic, the increased risk of the virus in detention, and the increased risk of spreading the virus in deportation efforts. In the face of similar messages, some governments, such as that of Spain, decided to close down immigration detention (Brandariz and Fernández-Bessa 2021). ICE, on the other hand, carried on and discussed contraband.

6. Conclusions

We argue that the narratives concerning immigration detention in the U.S. during the pandemic crisis represent a form of racial apathy in that they play upon deeply embedded broader discourses that racialize migrants as either threatening or vulnerable, all the while assuming the legal and economic systems through which they are racial and exploited as racially innocent (Murakawa and Beckett 2010). In the context of the pandemic and of the broader movements that have effectively highlighted racial oppression and challenged the foundation of the criminal justice system, the doggedness of industry stakeholders in remaining apathetic and their resistance against acknowledging reality also reinforces white ignorance.

The implications and significance of our findings should be understood within the history of the U.S. immigration system and its deep connections to racial formation in this country. Prior studies have established that race and racism are both the basis and products of immigration management in the U.S., an institution initially designed with the explicit goal to maintain white supremacy, which it continues to do so albeit more subtly (for a review, see Sáenz and Douglas 2015). As such, it not only constitutes the ideological boundaries of racial categories but also has material implications for which races can be physically present on U.S. soil and the consequences of this presence (Lopez 2006). Therefore, the complete absence of a racial perspective from all three groups is curious and significant in understanding the contemporary ideological terrain of immigration politics. This absence or amnesia needs to be situated in the context of post-Civil Rights color blindness. Since the Civil Rights movement, as explicit racism became publicly less acceptable, "crime" and "law and order" emerged as racially coded language, adopted by many politicians in order to appeal to white voters (Campbell and Schoenfeld 2013). White racial backlash against civil disobedience during the Civil Rights movement and the war on drugs are prime examples of this tactic (Beckett 1997; Weaver 2007). The consequence of this shift is the expansion of racialized social control in the form of hyper-policing and mass incarceration of people of color, which increasingly includes migrants, and the contraction of language we can use to talk about racism (Murakawa and Beckett 2010). Critical race theorists and sociologists have named this contradiction "racism without racists" or color-blind racism (Bonilla-Silva 2017; Lopez 2006).

ICE's story surrounding its "Operation Stolen Promise" appears to be an extension of the racist "law and order" tactic wherein Latinx migrants are increasingly criminalized (e.g., see Armenta 2017). In contrast, the frames used by the private companies reveal another key aspect of immigration control in contemporary U.S.—its neoliberal transformation (Silva 2016). The "racial neutrality" in their story appears to stem not from the legal system but from the market. The divergence between ICE and the private prison companies in their presentation of the pandemic might lead one to think that their logics are parallel alternatives. Yet, considering how closely they must work with one another to enable immigration detention, we should see these stories as complementary and as a clear illustration of how, under a neoliberal paradigm, governmentality becomes infused with market logic (Peters 2006). Therefore, the campaign for "law and order" is not only a racial project but also a capitalist enterprise, constituting the contemporary chapter of the long history of interdependence between capitalism and racism (Alexander 2012). In short, through examining how racial apathy and white ignorance manifest in frames around immigration detention during a pandemic, our research threaded together the two pillars of racialized immigration enforcement—white supremacy and capitalism—and exemplified how violence against migrants is tolerated, justified, and normalized in these intersecting systems of oppression.

Although our results imply that the pandemic did not lead to significant cracks in the system, the cracks may yet arrive and cracks may exist in other arenas. The ACLU did not meaningfully change in response to the pandemic in terms of its arguments concerning immigration detention, at least during our study's time frame. Although the organization has not yet recommended (that we are aware of) abolishing ICE, ending immigration detention, or closing the more than 200 ICE facilities nationwide, in an April 2021 press release, it recommended the closure of 39 ICE detention facilities (ACLU Staff 2021a). ACLU reiterated and expanded upon this press release in a May 2021 report, recommending that the DHS "close detention facilities located in remote areas, opened without clear justification, and those with established records of abuse" and replace them with "community-based case management," run by nonprofit organizations (ACLU Staff 2021b). Additionally, in 2021, ACLU called for transformative change in other arenas, and it linked racism and immigration detention. Through avenues outside of press releases and blogs, the ACLU publicized its support for reparations and for abolishing the police (ACLU Staff 2021c; Fernandez 2021), and it connected ICE and law enforcement in documents other than press releases (Mukpo 2020). Future research could analyze if ACLU continues to recommend more radical change and to target structural racism as the root cause of the violations of immigrant rights.

We chose to focus on the ACLU as a major critic of immigration detention practices due to the organization's large scale of coverage of such practices and the frequency with which media outlets reference the organization. Yet ACLU's politics are also limited by these characteristics: It is outwardly opposed to detention practices that violate immigrants' rights, not the practice of immigration detention itself. While this might be a strategic choice not fully reflective of the intentions of the actors within the organization, it is nonetheless the outward facade of the organization and it contributes to public discourses about migrants and immigration control. Other organizations and movements grounded in intellectual traditions that are more explicit in their systemic critique of the root causes of migration and migrant suffering exist. For example, the Detention Watch Network has published several reports explicitly calling for the abolishment of the U.S. immigrant detention system, many of which have recently connected this call for action to the pandemic by pointing to the inhumane and unsafe treatment migrants have experienced in detention during the pandemic. Likewise, the Occupy ICE protest movement, which began in Portland, Oregon, in 2018, placed the dissolution of ICE at the forefront of their demands. The initial protest in Portland generated similar "occupations" of immigrant detention centers across the nation. A systematic, longitudinal examination of more radical organizations and collective action was beyond the scope of the current investigation, but it is, nonetheless, important and worthy of study. As we have witnessed in recent years, at least some ideas from radical movements are being introduced to mainstream audiences. A glimpse of this change can indeed be found in the ACLU's response to policing and reparations. A study of this process could very well demonstrate that the pandemic and additional contextual factors loosened the foundation of immigration control as well.

Author Contributions: Conceptualization, K.E., W.L., J.R.H. and E.P.E.; Methodology, K.E., W.L., J.R.H. and E.P.E.; Software, K.E., W.L., J.R.H. and E.P.E.; Validation, J.R.H.; Formal Analysis, K.E., W.L., J.R.H. and E.P.E.; Investigation K.E., W.L., J.R.H. and E.P.E.; Data Curation, J.R.H.; Writing—Original Draft Preparation, K.E., W.L., J.R.H. and E.P.E.; Writing—Review & Editing, K.E., W.L., J.R.H. and E.P.E.; Supervision, K.E.; Project Administration, J.R.H.; Funding Acquisition, K.E., W.L. and E.P.E. All authors have read and agreed to the published version of the manuscript.

Funding: This research was funded by the National Science Foundation grant number #SES-1850712, 2019–2021.

Institutional Review Board Statement: The study was approved by the Institutional Review Board of North Carolina State University (protocol code 15450 and date of approval 20 July 2020).

Informed Consent Statement: Not Applicable.

Data Availability Statement: The data presented in this study are available on request from the corresponding author. The data are not publicly available through a repository because all sources are publicly available directly from the data sources.

Conflicts of Interest: The authors declare no conflict of interest.

Notes

[1] We periodically use the term "facility" to describe places migrants and non-migrants are imprisoned. We understand that this term conceals the severity of these places where people are held against their will, but we use it because it is commonly used in our data.

[2] An examination of the immigrant population in the U.S. reveals that immigrant detention is highly racialized and gendered (which is also reflective of the classed, racialized, and gendered processes of border crossing, legality, and authorization, to name a few). Although ICE does not report racial and ethnic characteristics of the people it detains, we can see from these numbers that foreign-born individuals who are most likely racialized as white (i.e., people born in Europe and living in the U.S.) are vastly underrepresented in immigration lockup. Of the 41,268 individuals in immigration detention in March 2018, 85.2% were reported as men and 28.5% were born in Mexico, 41% in Central America, and approximately 1% in Europe (TRAC Immigration 2019). However, of the 44,760,622 foreign-born individuals in the U.S. in 2018, 48.2% were reported as men, and 25% were born in Mexico, 8% in Central America, and 10.8% in Europe (Budiman et al. 2020).

[3] Available upon request.

[4] We did not include Management and Training Corporation (MTC) in our study because it is a privately held prison contractor and, consequently, does not publicize much of its business operations.

[5] 12 March 2020 emerged from our data as the start date for the recognition of the pandemic, as the first reference to COVID-19 from ACLU and CoreCivic appeared on this date. ICE initially issued COVID-19 guidance on 14 March and GEO Group released its first press release about the virus on 30 April.

[6] Using Nexus Uni to search for *New York Times* articles released between 12 March 2020 and 30 April 2020 with the keywords ("COVID" OR "coronavirus") and ("Immigration and Customs Enforcement" OR "CoreCivic" OR "GEO Group"), we found 32 eligible articles (35 total returns, with three repeat articles). See the previous footnote for the rationale of the 12 March start date. The end date of 30 April 2020 was somewhat arbitrary; in order to contextualize the emergent patterns, we wanted a snapshot of data to compare coverage and, therefore, we did not need to examine the remainder of the year.

7   Here, we discuss a few irregularities and discrepancies in these data. Although these five news releases were comparable to the pandemic-era discussion of COVID-19 contraband, a total of 28 out of the 175 news releases were customs-related in that they discussed some form of contraband, but they primarily discussed drug-related offenses of groups or individuals. Furthermore, we initially collected these 175 news releases in October 2020; in May 2021, however, ICE's website included only 170 news releases in this same time period.

References

ACLU Staff. 2020a. ACLU of Louisiana Demands Humanitarian Parole for Asylum Seeker with Severe Disabilities. Available online: https://www.aclu.org/press-releases/aclu-louisiana-demands-humanitarian-parole-asylum-seeker-severe-disabilities (accessed on 22 June 2021).

ACLU Staff. 2020b. ACLU of Texas Files Lawsuit against ICE to Release Medically Vulnerable People from Texas Detention Facility. Available online: https://www.aclu.org/press-releases/aclu-texas-files-lawsuit-against-ice-release-medically-vulnerable-people-texas (accessed on 14 June 2021).

ACLU Staff. 2020c. NYCLU and Bronx Defenders Seek Emergency Relief for People in ICE Detention. Available online: https://www.aclu.org/press-releases/nyclu-and-bronx-defenders-seek-emergency-relief-people-ice-detention (accessed on 22 June 2021).

ACLU Staff. 2021a. ACLU Calls on Biden Administration to Shut Down ICE Detention Facilities. Available online: https://www.aclu.org/press-releases/aclu-calls-biden-administration-shut-down-ice-detention-facilities (accessed on 1 September 2021).

ACLU Staff. 2021b. The Survivors: Stories of People Released from ICE Detention during the COVID-19 Pandemic. Available online: https://www.aclu.org/report/survivors (accessed on 1 September 2021).

ACLU Staff. 2021c. Reparation, H.R. 40 and the Path Forward. Available online: https://www.aclu.org/news/topic/reparations-h-r-40-and-the-path-forward/ (accessed on 14 June 2021).

Alexander, Michelle. 2012. *The New Jim Crow: Mass Incarceration in the Age of Colorblindness*. New York: The New Press.

Aranda, Elizabeth, and Elizabeth Vaquera. 2015. Racism, the immigration enforcement regime, and the implications for racial inequality in the lives of undocumented young adults. *Sociology of Race and Ethnicity* 1: 88–104. [CrossRef]

Armenta, Amada. 2017. Racializing Crimmigration: Structural Racism, Colorblindness, and the Institutional Production of Immigrant Criminality. *Sociology of Race and Ethnicity* 3: 82–95. [CrossRef]

Arriaga, Felicia, Jasmine Heiss, and Max Rose. 2020. Incarceration during covid-19: Jail shouldn't be a death sentence. In *Social Problems in the Age of COVID-19, Volume 1: US Perspectives*. Bristol: Bristol University Press, pp. 25–34.

Bail, Christopher. 2012. The Fringe Effect: Civil Society Organizations and the Evolution of Media Discourse about Islam since the September 11th Attacks. *American Sociological Review* 77: 855–79. [CrossRef]

Barnett, Michael, and David Grabowski. 2020. Nursing Homes Are Ground Zero for COVID-19 Pandemic. *JAMA Health Forum* 1: e200369. [CrossRef]

Beckett, Katherine. 1997. *Making Crime Pay: Law and Order in Contemporary American Politics*. Oxford: Oxford University Press.

Bell, Joyce. 2016. Introduction to the special issue on Black movements. *Sociological Focus* 49: 1–10. [CrossRef]

Berger, Dan. 2009. Constructing Crime, Framing Disaster: Routines of Criminalization and Crisis in Hurricane Katrina. *Punishment and Society* 11: 491–510. [CrossRef]

Bonilla-Silva, Eduardo. 2017. *Racism without Racists: Color-Blind Racism and the Persistence of Racial Inequality in America*, 5th ed. Lanham: Rowman and Littlefield Publishers.

Bracey, Glenn. 2015. Towards a Critical Race Theory of the State. *Critical Sociology* 41: 553–72. [CrossRef]

Brandariz, José, and Cristina Fernández-Bessa. 2021. Coronavirus and Immigration Detention in Europe: The Short Summer of Abolitionism? *Social Sciences* 10: 226. [CrossRef]

Budiman, Abby, Christine Tamir, Lauren Mora, and Luis Noe-Bustamante. 2020. Facts on U.S. immigrants, 2018. *Pew Research Center*. Available online: https://www.pewresearch.org/hispanic/2020/08/20/facts-on-u-s-immigrants-current-data/ (accessed on 3 September 2021).

Campbell, Michael, and Heather Schoenfeld. 2013. The Transformation of America's Penal Order: A Historicized Political Sociology of Punishment. *American Journal of Sociology* 118: 1375–423. [CrossRef]

Carruthers, Charlene. 2018. *Unapologetic: A Black, Queer, and Feminist Mandate for Radical Movements*. Boston: Beacon Press.

Carter, David, and Peter May. 2020. Making Sense of the U.S. COVID-19 Pandemic Response: A Policy Regime Perspective. *Administrative Theory and Praxis* 42: 265–77. [CrossRef]

Cho, Eunice Hyunhye, Tara Tidwell Cullen, and Clara Long. 2020. Justice-free zones: U.S. immigration detention under the Trump administration. *ACLU*. Available online: https://www.aclu.org/report/justice-free-zones-us-immigration-detention-under-trump-administration (accessed on 19 July 2021).

Cho, Eunice. 2020a. DHS Watchdog Confirms: ICE Is Failing to Protect Detained People from COVID. *ACLU*. Available online: https://www.aclu.org/news/immigrants-rights/dhs-watchdog-confirms-ice-is-failing-to-protect-detained-people-from-covid/ (accessed on 12 June 2021).

Cho, Eunice. 2020b. Immigration Detention Was a Black Box Before COVID-19. Now, It's a Death Trap. *ACLU*. Available online: https://www.aclu.org/news/immigrants-rights/immigration-detention-was-a-black-box-before-covid-19-now-its-a-death-trap/ (accessed on 14 June 2021).

Cohen, Stanley. 2011. *Folk Devils and Moral Panics*. London: Routledge.

CoreCivic Staff. 2020a. CoreCivic Announces Hiring Commitment, Employee Hero Bonus Program Amid COVID-19. Available online: https://www.corecivic.com/corecivic-announces-hiring-commitment-employee-hero-bonus-program-amid-covid-19 (accessed on 14 June 2021).
CoreCivic Staff. 2020b. CoreCivic Expands COVID-19 Testing at Trousdale Turner Correctional Center. Available online: https://www.corecivic.com/corecivic-expands-covid-19-testing-at-trousdale-turner-correctional-center (accessed on 14 June 2021).
CoreCivic Staff. 2020c. CoreCivic Statement on COVID-19 Prevention. *CoreCivic*. Available online: https://www.corecivic.com/en/corecivic-statement-on-covid-19-prevention (accessed on 14 June 2021).
De Genova, Nicholas. 2004. The Legal Production of Mexican/Migrant 'Illegality'. *Latino Studies* 2: 160–85. [CrossRef]
Doty, Roxanne Lynne, and Elizabeth Shannon Wheatley. 2013. Private Detention and the Immigration Industrial Complex. *International Political Sociology* 7: 426–43. [CrossRef]
Douglas, Karen Manges, and Rogelio Sáenz. 2013. The Criminalization of Immigrants & the Immigration-Industrial Complex. *Daedalus* 142: 199–227.
Dyer, Owen. 2021. COVID-19: US Immigration Enforcement Flouts Safety Guidelines, Report Claims. *British Medical Journal* 372: 1–3.
Eason, John. 2017. Prisons as Panacea or Pariah? The Countervailing Consequences of the Prison Boom on the Political Economy of Rural Towns. *Social Sciences* 6: 7. [CrossRef]
Ebert, Kim, Wenjie Liao, and Emily Pate Estrada. 2020. Apathy and Color-Blindness in Privatized Immigration Control. *Sociology of Race and Ethnicity* 6: 533–47. [CrossRef]
Estrada, Emily P., Kim Ebert, and Wenjie Liao. 2020. Polarized Toward Apathy: An Analysis of the Privatized Immigration-Control Debate in the Trump Era. *PS: Political Science & Politics* 53: 679–684.
Fernandez, Paige. 2021. This system cannot be reformed. *ACLU*. Available online: https://milled.com/aclu/this-system-cannot-be-reformed-WvPK2-U1SY2vEjKq (accessed on 14 June 2021).
Flores-Yeffal, Nadia, Guadalupe Vidales, and Girsea Martinez. 2019. #WakeUpAmerica,#IllegalsAreCriminals: The role of the cyber public sphere in the perpetuation of the Latino cyber-moral panic in the US. *Information, Communication & Society* 22: 402–19.
Forman, Tyrone, and Amanda Lewis. 2006. Racial Apathy and Hurricane Katrina: The Social Anatomy of Prejudice in the Post-Civil Rights Era. *Du Bois Review* 3: 175–202. [CrossRef]
Franco-Paredes, Carlos, Katherine Jankousky, Jonathan Schultz, Jessica Bernfeld, Kimberly Cullen, Nicolas G. Quan, Shelley Kon, Peter Hotez, Andrés Henao-Martínez, and Martin Krsak. 2020. COVID-19 in Jails and Prisons: A Neglected Infection in a Marginalized Population. *PLoS Neglected Tropical Diseases* 14: e0008409. [CrossRef]
Freedom for Immigrants. 2018. Detention by the Numbers. Available online: https://www.freedomforimmigrants.org/detention-statistics# (accessed on 23 July 2021).
GEO Group Staff. 2020a. The GEO Group Reports First Quarter 2020 Results. Available online: https://investors.geogroup.com/news-events-and-reports/investor-news/news-details/2020/The-GEO-Group-Reports-First-Quarter-2020-Results/default.aspx (accessed on 14 June 2021).
GEO Group Staff. 2020b. The GEO Group Reports Second Quarter 2020 Results and Issues Updated Financial and Dividend Guidance. Available online: https://investors.geogroup.com/news-events-and-reports/investor-news/news-details/2020/The-GEO-Group-Reports-Second-Quarter-2020-Results-and-Issues-Updated-Financial-and-Dividend-Guidance/default.aspx (accessed on 14 June 2021).
Gilman, Denise, and Luis Romero. 2018. Immigration Detention, Inc. *Journal on Migration and Human Security* 6: 145–60. [CrossRef]
Glenn, Evelyn Nakano. 2015. Settler colonialism as structure: A framework for comparative studies of US race and gender formation. *Sociology of Race and Ethnicity* 1: 52–72. [CrossRef]
Goffman, Erving. 1959. *The Presentation of Self in Everyday Life*. New York: Doubleday.
Golash-Boza, Tanya, and Pierrette Hondagneu-Sotelo. 2013. Latino immigrant men and the deportation crisis: A gendered and racial removal program. *Latino Studies* 11: 271–92. [CrossRef]
Golash-Boza, Tanya, Maria D. Duenas, and Chia Xiong. 2019. White supremacy, patriarchy, and global capitalism in migration studies. *American Behavioral Scientist* 63: 1741–59. [CrossRef]
Golash-Boza, Tanya. 2016. The Parallels between Mass Incarceration and Mass Deportation: An Intersectional Analysis of State Repression. *Journal of World-Systems Research* 22: 484–509. [CrossRef]
Gómez Cervantes, Andrea. 2021. "Looking Mexican": Indigenous and non-indigenous Latina/o immigrants and the racialization of illegality in the Midwest. *Social Problems* 68: 100–17. [CrossRef]
Hackman, Michelle. 2020. Immigrant detainee becomes first covid-19 casualty in ICE facility. *Wall Street Journal*, May 7.
Haffajee, Rebecca L., and Michelle M. Mello. 2020. Thinking Globally, Acting Locally: The U.S. Response to COVID-19. *New England Journal of Medicine* 382: e75. [CrossRef]
Hooks, Gregory, and Bob Libal. 2020. Hotbeds of Infection: How ICE Detention Contributed to the Spread of COVID-19 in the United States. Available online: https://www.detentionwatchnetwork.org/sites/default/files/reports/DWN_Hotbeds%20of%20Infection_2020_FOR%20WEB.pdf (accessed on 12 June 2021).
ICE Staff. 2020a. ICE Air Flying Home US Citizens from Central America during COVID-19 Outbreak. Available online: https://www.ice.gov/news/releases/ice-air-flying-home-us-citizens-central-america-during-covid-19-outbreak (accessed on 12 June 2021).
ICE Staff. 2020b. ICE Expands Voluntary COVID-19 Testing to All at Family Residential Centers. Available online: https://www.ice.gov/news/releases/ice-expands-voluntary-covid-19-testing-all-family-residential-centers (accessed on 14 June 2021).

ICE Staff. 2020c. ICE Guidance on COVID-19. Available online: https://web.archive.org/web/20200314113345/https://www.ice.gov/covid19 (accessed on 14 June 2021).
ICE Staff. 2020d. ICE HSI Efforts to Combat COVID-19 Fraud Featured on NBC Today Show, ABC Good Morning America. Available online: https://www.ice.gov/news/releases/ice-hsi-efforts-combat-covid-fraud-featured-nbc-today-show-abc-good-morning-america (accessed on 14 June 2021).
ICE Staff. 2020e. ICE HSI Launches Operation Stolen Promise. Available online: https://www.ice.gov/news/releases/ice-hsi-launches-operation-stolen-promise (accessed on 14 June 2021).
ICE Staff. 2020f. ICE HSI Warns Public to Remain Vigilant about COVID Fraud. Available online: https://www.ice.gov/news/releases/ice-hsi-warns-public-remain-vigilant-about-covid-fraud (accessed on 14 June 2021).
ICE Staff. 2020g. ICE pivots to combat COVID-19 vaccine fraud with launch of Operation Stolen Promise 2.0. Available online: https://www.ice.gov/news/releases/ice-pivots-combat-covid-19-vaccine-fraud-launch-operation-stolen-promise-20 (accessed on 19 June 2021).
Irvine, Michael, Daniel Coombs, Julianne Skarha, Brandon del Pozo, Josiah Rich, Faye Taxman, and Traci C. Green. 2020. Modeling COVID-19 and Its Impacts on U.S. Immigration and Customs Enforcement (ICE) Detention Facilities, 2020. *Journal of Urban Health* 97: 439–47. [CrossRef]
Jackman, Mary. 1994. *The Velvet Glove: Paternalism and Conflict in Gender, Class, and Race Relations*. Berkeley: University of California Press.
Johns Hopkins Coronavirus Resource Center. 2021. COVID-19 dashboard by the Center for Systems Science and Engineering (CSSE) at Johns Hopkins University (JHU). *Johns Hopkins University*. Available online: https://coronavirus.jhu.edu/map.html (accessed on 11 September 2021).
Juárez, Melina, Bárbara Gómez-Aguiñaga, and Sonia Bettez. 2018. Twenty Years after IIRIRA: The Rise of Immigrant Detention and its Effects on Latinx Communities across the Nation. *Journal on Migration and Human Security* 6: 74–96. [CrossRef]
Kang, Stephen. 2018. Judge Blocks Blanket Detention of Asylum Seekers. Available online: https://www.aclu.org/blog/immigrants-rights/immigrants-rights-and-detention/judge-blocks-blanket-detention-asylum-seekers (accessed on 6 July 2021).
Kassie, Emily, and Barbara Marcolini. 2020. How ICE Exported the Coronavirus. Available online: https://www.themarshallproject.org/2020/07/10/how-ice-exported-the-coronavirus (accessed on 28 July 2021).
Keller, Allen, and Benjamin Wagner. 2020. COVID-19 and Immigration Detention in the USA: Time to Act. *The Lancet Public Health* 5: E245–E246. [CrossRef]
Kinner, Stuart, Jesse Young, Kathryn Snow, Louise Southalan, Daniel Lopez-Acuña, Carina Ferreira-Borges, and Éamonn O'Moore. 2020. Prisons and Custodial Settings Are Part of a Comprehensive Response to COVID-19. *The Lancet Public Health* 5: e188–e189. [CrossRef]
Kirkham, Chris. 2012. Private Prisons Profit from Immigration Crackdown, Federal and Local Law Enforcement Partnerships. *Huffington Post*. Available online: https://www.huffingtonpost.com/2012/06/07/private-prisons-immigration-federal-law-enforcement_n_1569219.html (accessed on 4 May 2018).
Klein, Naomi. 2010. *The Shock Doctrine: The Rise of Disaster Capitalism*. New York: Henry Holt and Company.
La Gorce, Tammy. 2020. 'Everybody Was Sick': Inside an ICE Detention Center. *The New York Times*. Available online: https://www.nytimes.com/2020/05/15/nyregion/coronavirus-ice-detainees-immigrants.html (accessed on 14 June 2021).
Lamont, Michèle, Stefan Beljean, and Matthew Clair. 2014. What is Missing? Cultural Processes and Causal Pathways to Inequality. *Socio-Economic Review* 12: 573–608. [CrossRef]
Li, Yao, and Harvey Nicholson Jr. 2021. When "model minorities" become "yellow peril"—Othering and the racialization of Asian Americans in the COVID-19 pandemic. *Sociology Compass* 15. [CrossRef]
Lopez, Ian Haney. 2006. *White by Law: The Legal Construction of Race*. New York: NYU Press.
Lopez, William, Nolan Kline, Alana Lebrón, Nicole Novak, Maria-Elena De Trinidad Young, Gregg Gonsalves, Ranit Mishori, Basil Safi, and Ian Kysel. 2021. Preventing the Spread of COVID-19 in Immigration Detention Centers Requires the Release of Detainees. *American Journal of Public Health* 111: 110–15. [CrossRef] [PubMed]
M4BL. 2019. Vision for Black Lives. Available online: m4bl.org/policy-platforms/ (accessed on 6 July 2019).
Majstorović, Danijela. 2007. Construction of Europeanization in the High Representative's discourse in Bosnia and Herzegovina. *Discourse and Society* 18: 627–51. [CrossRef]
Markel, Howard, and Alexandra Minna Stern. 1999. Which Face? Whose Nation? Immigration, Public Health, and the Construction of Disease at America's Ports and Borders, 1891–928. *American Behavioral Scientist* 42: 1314–31. [CrossRef]
Marouf, Fatma E. 2021. The Impact of COVID-19 on Immigration Detention. *Frontiers in Human Dynamics* 2: 1–12. [CrossRef]
Menjívar, Cecilia. 2021. The Racialization of "Illegality". *Daedalus* 150: 91–105. [CrossRef]
Meyer, Jaimie, Carlos Franco-Paredes, Parveen Parmar, Faiza Yasin, and Matthew Gartland. 2020. COVID-19 and the Coming Epidemic in US Immigration Detention Centres. *The Lancet Infectious Diseases* 20: 646–48. [CrossRef]
Meyer, John, and Brian Rowan. 1977. Institutionalized Organizations: Formal Structure as Myth and Ceremony. *American Journal of Sociology* 83: 340–63. [CrossRef]
Miller, Holly Ventura, Melissa Ripepi, Amy Ernstes, and Anthony Peguero. 2020. Immigration Policy and Justice in the Era of COVID-19. *American Journal of Criminal Justice* 45: 793–809. [CrossRef] [PubMed]

Mills, Charles. 2007. White ignorance. In *Race and Epistemologies of Ignorance*. Edited by Shannon Sullivan and Nancy Tuana. Albany: State University of New York Press, pp. 13–38.

Montes, Juan. 2020. U.S. fails to prevent deportation of migrants infected with covid-19, Guatemalan officials say. *Wall Street Journal*, June 25.

Montoya-Barthelemy, Andre, Charles Lee, Dave Cundiff, and Eric Smith. 2020. COVID-19 and the Correctional Environment: The American Prison as a Focal Point for Public Health. *American Journal of Preventive Medicine* 58: 888–91. [CrossRef] [PubMed]

Mueller, Jennifer. 2020. Racial ideology or racial ignorance? An alternative theory of racial cognition. *Sociological Theory* 38: 142–69. [CrossRef]

Mukpo, Ashoka. 2020. For Black Immigrants, Police and ICE Are Two Sides of the Same Coin. *ACLU*. Available online: https://www.aclu.org/news/criminal-law-reform/for-black-immigrants-police-and-ice-are-two-sides-of-the-same-coin/ (accessed on 1 September 2021).

Murakawa, Naomi, and Katherine Beckett. 2010. The Penology of Racial Innocence: The Erasure of Racism in the Study and Practice of Punishment. *Law and Society Review* 44: 695–730. [CrossRef]

Niu, Isabelle, Emily Rhyne, and Aaron Byrd. 2021. How ICE's Mishandling of COVID-19 Fueled Outbreaks around the Country. *The New York Times*. Available online: https://www.nytimes.com/video/us/100000007707896/immigration-detention-covid.html (accessed on 12 June 2021).

NYT Staff. 2020a. Rush for Jobless Benefits Crashes New York State Website. *The New York Times*. Available online: https://www.nytimes.com/2020/03/16/nyregion/coronavirus-new-york-update.html (accessed on 10 July 2021).

NYT Staff. 2020b. Trump signs relief package; China reports zero new local infections. *The New York Times*. March 18. Available online: https://www.nytimes.com/2020/03/18/world/coronavirus-news.html (accessed on 24 September 2021).

Okonkwo, Ijeoma, Alder Howie, C. Parry, C. L. Shelton, S. Cobley, R. Craig, N. Permall, S. H. El-Sheikha, N. Herbert, and P. Arnold. 2020. The Safety of Paediatric Surgery between COVID-19 Surges: An Observational Study. *Anaesthesia* 75: 1605–33. [CrossRef]

Oliver, Kelsey. 2018. Correctional Facilities in the US. Available online: https://clients1.ibisworld.com/reports/us/industry/default.aspx?entid=1461 (accessed on 8 November 2018).

Olmo, Rosa del. 1990. The Economic Crisis and the Criminalization of Latin American Women. *Social Justice* 17: 40–53.

Peters, Michael. 2006. Neoliberal governmentality: Foucault on the birth of biopolitics. In *Gouvernementalität und Erziehungswissenschaft: Wissen—Macht—Transformation*. Edited by Susanne Weber and Susanne Maurer. Wiesbaden: VS Verlag für Sozialwissenschaften, pp. 37–49.

Sáenz, Rogelio, and Karen Manges Douglas. 2015. A Call for the Racialization of Immigration Studies: On the Transition of Ethnic Immigrants to Racialized Immigrants. *Sociology of Race and Ethnicity* 1: 166–80. [CrossRef]

Silva, Andrea. 2016. Neoliberalism Confronts Latinos: Paradigmatic Shifts in Immigration Practices. *Latino Studies* 14: 59–79. [CrossRef]

Smart, Noelle, Adam Garcia, and Nina Siulc. 2021. One Year Later, We Still Don't Know How Many People in ICE Detention Have Been Exposed to COVID-19. *Vera Institute of Justice*. Available online: https://www.vera.org/blog/one-year-later-we-still-dont-know-how-many-people-in-ice-detention-have-been-exposed-to-covid-19 (accessed on 3 September 2021).

Sullivan, Laura. 2010. Prison economics help drive Ariz. immigration law. *National Public Radio*. Available online: http://www.npr.org/2010/10/28/130833741/prison-economics-help-drive-ariz-immigration-law (accessed on 1 November 2016).

TRAC Immigration. 2019. Immigration and Customs Enforcement Detention: ICE Data Snapshots. Transactional Records Access Clearinghouse (TRAC) at Syracuse University. Available online: https://trac.syr.edu/phptools/immigration/detention/ (accessed on 11 September 2021).

UCLA Law. n.d. COVID Behind Bars Data Project. *UCLA*. Available online: https://uclacovidbehindbars.org/ (accessed on 12 June 2021).

Wang, Emily, Bruce Western, and Donald Berwick. 2020. COVID-19, Decarceration, and the Role of Clinicians, Health Systems, and Payers: A Report from the National Academy of Sciences, Engineering, and Medicine. *JAMA* 324: 2257–58. [CrossRef]

Ward, Julie, Kalind Parish, Grace DiLaura, Sharon Dolovich, and Brendan Saloner. 2021. COVID-19 Cases Among Employees of U.S. Federal and State Prisons. *American Journal of Preventative Medicine* 60: 840–44. [CrossRef] [PubMed]

Watkins Liu, Callie. 2018. The anti-oppressive value of critical race theory and intersectionality in social movement study. *Sociology of Race and Ethnicity* 4: 306–21. [CrossRef]

Weaver, Vesla. 2007. Frontlash: Race and the Development of Punitive Crime Policy. *Studies in American Political Development* 21: 230–65. [CrossRef]

WHO. 2021. March 30. WHO-Convened Global Study of Origins of SARS-CoV-2: China Part. Available online: https://www.who.int/publications/i/item/who-convened-global-study-of-origins-of-sars-cov-2-china-part (accessed on 12 June 2021).

Zarrugh, Amina. 2020. The development of US regimes of disappearance: The war on terror, mass incarceration, and immigration deportation. *Critical Sociology* 46: 257–71. [CrossRef]

MDPI
St. Alban-Anlage 66
4052 Basel
Switzerland
Tel. +41 61 683 77 34
Fax +41 61 302 89 18
www.mdpi.com

Social Sciences Editorial Office
E-mail: socsci@mdpi.com
www.mdpi.com/journal/socsci

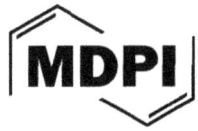

www.ingramcontent.com/pod-product-compliance
Lightning Source LLC
LaVergne TN
LVHW070046120526
838202LV00101B/829